FACTS AND VALUES

AN INTRODUCTION TO CRITICAL THINKING FOR NURSES

FACTS AND VALUES

AN INTRODUCTION TO CRITICAL THINKING FOR NURSES

Stan van Hooft
MA, PhD, DipEd,
Associate Professor of Philosophy,
Faculty of Arts, Deakin University

Lynn Gillam
BA (Hons), BA (Oxon),
Research Assistant,
Monash University Centre for Human Bioethics

Margot Byrnes
RN, B.Hlth Sc, MA,
Lecturer, Faculty of Nursing,
The University of Sydney

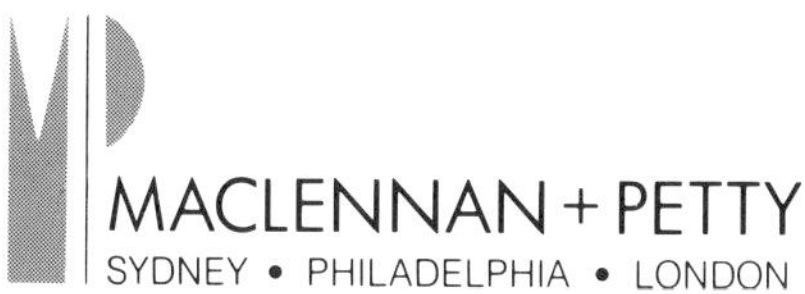

MACLENNAN + PETTY
SYDNEY • PHILADELPHIA • LONDON

First published 1995

MacLennan & Petty Pty Limited
80 Reserve Road, Artarmon, Sydney NSW 2064 Australia

National Library of Australia
Cataloguing-in-Publication data:

van Hooft, Stan
Facts and Values:
An introduction to critical thinking for nurses

Bibliography
Includes index

ISBN 0 86433 107 X

1. Critical thinking. 2. Logic. 3. Reasoning
4. Nursing – Decision making.
I. Gillam, Lynn. II. Byrnes, Margot. III. Title.
160

Printed and bound in Australia

CONTENTS

PREFACE

This book has been developed out of the experience of its authors in teaching critical thinking to nurses in a number of universities in Australia. While there are many fine text books on critical thinking and informal logic on the market (see the listings under 'Suggested Reading' at the end of each part of the book), we have found that no one book quite meets the requirements of a nursing program. Not only are many of these books too detailed in matters of logic, but also their scope is often limited to the purely cognitive aspects of thinking. What is often missing is a discussion of the practical contexts and outcomes of thinking, and of the place of ethical values and principles in the deliberations of critical thinkers. As well, many of these books fail to cover the areas of science which are central to the professional lives of nurses. Accordingly, we have sought to provide a text which has the scope and depth required for courses in critical thinking for both undergraduate and postgraduate nursing students. Our book covers formal and informal logic to a depth that is useful for health professionals, gives a description of scientific method and explanatory thinking of the kinds used in clinical settings, and constitutes a primer in the concepts and arguments used in ethics as it pertains to health care.

A survey of nursing faculties and schools throughout Australia has found that teachers of critical thinking are looking for a text with the following features:

- introductory level
- easy to read
- good presentation and explanation
- practical
- issues-related
- locally relevant examples
- examples from nursing and related disciplines like psychology and bio-medical sciences
- use of scenarios and case studies
- contemporary nursing context
- discussion questions and exercises
- discussion of the methodology of science
- statement of aims and objectives
- nursing research focus
- critical thinking applied to ethics
- discussion of fallacious argument

- models of clinical decision making
- awareness of feminist 'ways of knowing'
- role of reflective thinking
- up-to-date bibliography
- teachers' resources.

We believe we have met each of these demands.

As well, we have sought to provide a text which can be used in a variety of ways. We have given a large number of exercises for students to do and have written a *Teachers' Manual* to accompany the text so that instructors have the assistance of suggested solutions to the exercises. Some institutions may want students to use both books so as to give them self-instructional material for use in the context of learning contracts or distance education. Such students can use the *Teachers' Manual* to monitor their own progress.

The *Teachers' Manual* also contains suggestions as to how the material might be used in the classroom context.

A number of points should be noted. Firstly, we have not sought to adjudicate the current debate about whether it is better to refer to consumers of health services as 'patients' or as 'clients'. By and large we have used the word 'patient', but without prejudging the issue.

Secondly, we have sought to avoid sexist language by using plural pronouns wherever possible. Where this has not been possible we have used 'he' or 'she' indiscriminately rather than the cumbersome 'he or she' or even 'she/he'.

Lastly, we are aware that some of the exercises admit of solutions other than the ones we have given. Please feel free to explore other options and if you think that ours are inadequate, we would be happy to receive suggestions for improvements in future editions of this book.

Aims of the Book

The aim of this book is to assist students and practitioners in the field of nursing and related fields to acquire and develop the critical thinking skills required for ethical, scientifically based nursing practice. The book aims to help students and health professionals develop the ability to think clearly, argue cogently, give reasons for actions and decisions, and make rational choices and evaluations, both in a diagnostic context and in ethically sensitive situations.

Having worked through this book, students and practitioners should be able to:

1. understand and explain the structure of simple arguments, and differentiate between premises and conclusions;
2. evaluate simple arguments in terms of the extent to which the evidence/reasons actually support the conclusions drawn from them, and recognise unsound arguments;

3. construct, present and refute simple arguments on various aspects of nursing;
4. understand the logic of scientific discovery in areas of bioscience and medical science;
5. distinguish sound scientific thinking from pseudo-scientific thinking;
6. understand the basic lines of reasoning employed in diagnosis and problem solving;
7. be aware of the place of values in their professional lives;
8. be able to distinguish between the forms of ethical thinking and the substantive values involved;
9. be able to make, and argue for, ethically sensitive decisions in the nursing setting;
10. develop strategies for ensuring that their working conditions do not jeopardise their ability to think critically.

With the development of critical thinking skills, nurses should be able to:

1. respond flexibly to new situations;
2. be effective advocates for patients and for policies within institutions;
3. deal with and resolve conflict;
4. contribute effectively as an equal participant in health care teams;
5. function as a professional in health care and in the community;
6. question current practice and improve it;
7. perceive health care situations sensitively and accurately;
8. increase their personal independence, self-confidence and self-awareness.

This set of abilities adds up to the empowerment of the individual nurse as a professional, able to make caring and responsible decisions and able to play a full part in the health care of patients and clients.

ACKNOWLEDGMENTS

The authors wish to acknowledge the help that their students have given them over the years at Deakin University, Monash University, the University of Sydney and the Victoria University of Technology. Without the enthusiasm and questioning attitude of these students, the ideas in this book would never have evolved to the point where they could be presented in book form.

Some of our colleagues have also been particularly helpful and encouraging in developing the ideas and curriculum concepts in this book. We thank Jo Boney, Milly Ching, Terry Godfrey, Lois Gorman, Tui Muir and Emil Neven in particular.

Thanks must also go to various publications for permission to reproduce materials: David Syme and Co, editors of *The Age* newspaper in Melbourne and two journalists, Gareth Boreham and Caroline Milburn, for permission to reproduce news items; the following writers of letters to *The Age* which have been used or adapted in this text—Professor Max Charlesworth, Peter Coghlan, Philomena Horsley, Julienne Lauer, Les Tate, Dr David Wignall, Elisabeth Williams, and Stephen Yolland; *The Independent Monthly* for permission to use an item and an illustration as Figure 3.1; the editors of *Nursing Times* for permission to use portion of an article.

The authors and publisher have made every effort to contact copyright owners concerning material used in this book. If, however, we have erred, we welcome advice, and undertake to make appropriate acknowledgment at the earliest opportunity.

PART ONE: INFORMAL LOGIC

Chapter 1

Introduction: The Role of Critical Thinking in Nursing

This chapter uses the concept of professional autonomy in order to argue for the necessity of critical thinking skills in nurses.

In recent times, the nursing profession has undergone profound change. In the past, the image of what a nurse should be drew upon a variety of streams of thought, including the idea of an ideal woman as care-giver and helper, the notion of a helpmate to the medical practitioner, and the military ideals of obedience, sacrifice and service. In contrast, nursing is now seen as a profession, with all the ideals of autonomy and responsibility which that entails.

A professional such as a nurse is someone who has a set of abilities based upon knowledge and skills not available to the general public and requiring a high degree of sophistication. Of course there are many fields of endeavour that could fit this description. A carpenter has knowledge and skills that most people do not have. Yet most people have some understanding and ability in this area and the number of people who engage in do-it-yourself carpentry is very large. In contrast, not many people engage in do-it-yourself by-pass surgery, or do-it-yourself litigation. The knowledge and skills required in these fields is of such sophistication that they are not available to the lay person.

Because they have knowledge which their client groups do not have, professionals have considerable autonomy. Clients are dependent upon them and, in the main, must accept their services without question. Because of the complexity and depth of the knowledge that professionals have, their client groups do not find it easy to scrutinise or evaluate their performance. This is well illustrated in the case of the law, where it is exceedingly difficult for a lay person to criticise, let alone understand, the complex practices which lawyers engage in on their clients' behalf. Because of this, accountability for the professions is largely secured by the professions themselves through their own organisations and systems of peer review (although governments have involved themselves in these matters in recent times).

It follows from this situation that professionals have a responsibility to be clear and ethical about their own practices. Professionals are not only people who have acquired knowledge and skills which they place at the service of the community. They must also reflect, individually and collectively, on their practice, understand their goals, be aware of the expectations of their peers and of their clients, and make informed and responsible decisions. Simple training in knowledge and skills does not make a professional. A professional must also be able to think clearly, creatively, ethically and responsibly. In the absence of effective systems of accountability from outside the professions, the onus is on the professionals themselves to develop a level of thinking which accompanies, informs and scrutinises their operational thinking. This level of thinking we call critical thinking.

Another feature of the life of professionals is that their work is not routine. As opposed to the process worker who performs a small and simple task as part of a larger productive process, and as opposed to the employee who works under the close direction of supervisors, a professional works in a highly self-directed manner. Given the depth of understanding of the task that they have, professionals do not need constant direction and can take responsibility for what they do. But along with this responsibility comes the need for decision making which is informed by clear thought, and for deep sensitivity to the values inherent in the situations that confront the professional. Once again, there is a need for critical thinking.

A third relevant feature of the life of a professional is that the knowledge base of the profession is not taken for granted. A professional will not only have the knowledge needed for professional practice but will also know how that knowledge was developed, and will be able to contribute to further developments of that knowledge. Professionals continue to study the fields of knowledge with which they are concerned and keep up with the latest developments in their field. Moreover, they continue to contribute to the knowledge base of their profession with their own research and with reports of successful practice. This, too, is a part of critical thinking.

What is Critical Thinking?

Because the word 'critical' is connected to the word 'critique', the first thought that this phrase might suggest to you is that critical thinking is thinking designed to criticise. So you might suppose that a film critic in the newspaper thinks critically when he or she offers us their assessment of the worth of a movie. But this is not the sense in which we are using the term. Again, it might be thought that the term is being used in the way that it often is in political contexts. Here one is said to be thinking critically when one questions policy and points out harms that it might lead to, with a view to having that policy changed. This kind of thinking can take place in institutions at all levels and sizes ranging from the state down to business enterprises, public enterprises like hospitals, or even families. Again, this is not the way we are using the term, though this usage is relevant to our concerns.

The first important element in our notion of critical thinking is rational thought. Bandman and Bandman[1] define critical thinking as 'rational examination of ideas, inferences, assumptions, principles, arguments, conclusions, issues, statements, beliefs and actions'. This definition presents a list of contents of thought which we will be explicating in due course. What it says of these contents is that they are to be examined rationally. This is a crucial element in the definition and it points to the distinctive role of reasoning within critical thinking.

For its own part, the word 'reasoning' covers a variety of intellectual activities including:

1. analysing the use of language;
2. formulating problems adequately;
3. clarifying and explicating assumptions;
4. weighing evidence;
5. evaluating conclusions;
6. discriminating between valid and invalid arguments;
7. perceiving a situation correctly and sensitively;
8. discerning any practical implications of conclusions reached.

Of these, 4, 5, and 6 explain the connection with the word 'critique'. Central to critical thinking is evaluating the points of view of others.

Of course, one should not offer a critique of something without making the effort to understand it thoroughly first. Seeking to comprehend what others say and do is an important part of critical thinking. Perceiving a situation correctly and sensitively is also crucial. One health worker might see a patient as a person who is suffering, another as simply a case to be dealt with. Our view of critical thinking would suggest that only the first of these represents critical thinking at its best. Critical thinking does not consist only of rational cleverness. It includes empathy and sensitive perception. It is the contention of the authors that the intellectual skills we have listed can be taught and it will be our aim, especially in the first section of this book, to teach them. But they are not all there is to critical thinking.

Robert Ennis, head of the Illinois Critical Thinking Project at the University of Illinois, provides the following definition of critical thinking: 'Critical Thinking is reasonable reflective thinking that is focused on deciding what to believe or do.'[2] One virtue of this definition is that it stresses the practical aspect of critical thinking. Amongst other things, it is thinking focused on deciding what to do, and such deciding involves making a practical commitment of some degree of importance to the thinker. The thinker is not just engaged in an intellectual or theoretical exercise, but in a professional life in which decisions have to be made and where they should be made rationally.

Further, this definition not only uses the word 'reasonable', but also 'reflective'. Critical thinking is thinking that is aware of its own presuppositions and points of view. Critical thinkers reflect upon their knowledge, ideas, decisions and commitments in order to improve them and make them consistent with the knowledge and expectations of others where that is appropriate. Critical thinkers are also aware of the attitudes, points of view or value commitments that they themselves bring to bear on issues. In this way critical thinkers are very self-aware.

But what Ennis' definition does not highlight sufficiently is the willingness to step outside one's own frame of reference in order to fully appreciate the point of view with which one is in disagreement. The issues that face us on a day-to-day basis are seldom matters of fact. More often they encapsulate attitudes and values. While it sometimes happens that people debate and decide upon issues of fact in the way that scientists might be thought to do when they seek to find out the truth about certain matters, this is not typical. Most often (and this is true of scientists also) people are passionate rather than impartial about the points of view they hold. They debate issues because they feel strongly about them, have strong preferences for one outcome rather than another and deep commitments to the values and points of view which these entail. There are at least two components to any point of view on an issue. There is the knowledge that one has of the matters at hand, and there are the interests, value commitments or attitudes that one brings to bear on that issue. The self-awareness, which we have already suggested should be a part of critical thinking, is an awareness of the way our interests and values colour and intensify our points of view on a range of issues.

But there is a further form of awareness that should be a part of critical thinking. The other party to a debate also has interests and value commitments, and we must be aware of them. It is one thing to be able to think and argue rationally about matters of fact with awareness of one's own value commitments or attitudes, but it is another thing to be able to think and debate about issues with real empathy for the point of view of the other party. Most often when we disagree with somebody else, we also shut ourselves off from their point of view. We might be very clever in the way we use logic and rational thought to argue our case and attack that of others, but in doing so we may lack a sympathetic understanding of our opponent's point of view. Critical thinking includes such understanding. It does not call for compromising one's own commitments, but it does require a sensitivity to the point of view of the other.

This last point implies that critical thinking has an ethical dimension. A critical thinker is not only aware of the views of others but is fairminded and willing to be swayed by stronger argument. A critical thinker is not a fanatic or a bigot. Although critical thinkers are committed to their values and points of view, they are not closed minded and will give new facts or points of view due consideration. Critical thinkers are good listeners as well as good debaters. They seek to understand the point of view of others. In this sense, genuine dialogue is central to critical thinking.

In summary then, critical thinking is:

1. rational
2. practical as well as theoretical
3. committed
4. self-aware

5. sympathetic to the commitments of others
6. conducive to dialogue.

Exercise 1.1

Identify the attitudes inherent in the following news items and letters. Do you share the attitudes? Can you understand them and see the value of those attitudes even if you disagree with them?

The following is an excerpt from a newspaper article.[3]

1. The Health Minister, Mrs Tehan, yesterday signalled that the in vitro fertilisation program would not be widened to accept de facto and homosexual couples. Mrs Tehan, who appears to have hardened her stance on IVF availability, said children were best raised in a 'stable, married, heterosexual couple arrangement'.

   Speaking on 3LO, Mrs Tehan said she had not been persuaded that the program should be expanded, even though de facto couples could be considered married and eligible under equal opportunity laws. 'This is very expensive technology. It is very demanding, not only on the scientists, but particularly demanding on the couples themselves,' she said. 'I am not persuaded that there is any great advantage in advancing or increasing that group beyond what it currently is, which is the technology available for married couples.'

   Mrs Tehan said her opposition to the widening of the program was a personal view and the advice of the State Government's IVF standing review and advisory committee would be considered.

The following are two letters to the editor of the newspaper, in response to the above item.[4]

2. The recent statement by the Health Minister, Mrs Tehan, that only married couples should have access to IVF programs raises serious questions about the rights of infertile couples. Fertile people may have children almost in any way they please: they may be married or in a de facto relationship, or even in a homosexual relationship, or they may be in stable union or in a single parent situation or in reconstituted families after the divorce of one or both parties. No one argues that the 'best interests of the child' or the considerable expense (of providing health care, divorce and family court procedures etc) involved in fertile people having children, gives the State the right to interfere in and to restrict the reproductive choices of fertile couples. Indeed, most people abhor the policies of countries which do have such restrictions.

   When, however, infertile couples enter IVF programs they are restricted in all kinds of ways that the fertile would never tolerate and they are, in effect, treated as second-class citizens.

   The Victorian Standing Review and Advisory Committee on Infertility, of which I was a member when amendments of the present legislation were formulated, made a small step in recommending that de facto couples be allowed access to IVF programs. It would be a pity if even this were to be denied and the rights of infertile people continued to be flouted.

3. It is some relief that Health Minister Tehan's views on eligibility for IVF treatment represent only her personal views. But it is disturbing that planned legislative amendments seem unlikely to broaden the scope of access under Victoria's 1984 Infertility (Medical Practices) Act.

   Rsearch for the past 30 years has consistently disproved the myth that single mothers provide inadequate parenting. At the same time it appears that the 'stable married, heterosexual couple arrangement' Mrs Tehan favours is the source of much of the sexual abuse and domestic violence involving children in Australia today. Where is the logic in her argument?

   Even more interesting is actual research conducted with children of lesbian and gay parents that indicated that there is no evidence to suggest that the development of these children is compromised in any way comparative to the children of heterosexuals. Indeed, there is evidence that there are distinct advantages.

   For instance one study found that children of lesbian parents were seen by parents and teachers to be more affectionate, responsive and more protective of younger children than children of heterosexual parents, and another shows that they spend more time with their fathers and other males than children of heterosexual women.

   Pople are, of course, entitled to their personal views on 'non-traditional' parenting. But when government decisions are taken that involve access to health services funded by all taxpayers we are entitled to question their logic. To deny certain individuals access to parenting on the basis of marital status or sexuality is blatant discrimination.

Critical Thinking and Nursing

We have indicated in general terms why professionals need to be critical thinkers, but we should now focus on the more specific question of what role critical thinking might play in the professional lives of nurses.

To do this it will be suggestive to point to yet another meaning of the word 'critical'. Health workers use this word in such contexts as 'critical care', or being in a 'critical condition'. In this context the word is related to the notion of 'crisis' rather than 'critique'. The professional lives of nurses frequently involve dealing with crises of various kinds and there is very little room for mistakes of judgment in this context. It is vitally important, therefore, that nurses think clearly and well. And this is true not just in relation to factual or diagnostic judgements that nurses have to make, but also in relation to value judgements and policy decisions. In the professional life of nurses, thinking is always critical in this new sense. For this reason it is imperative that it be critical in our earlier sense as well.

There are at least three major areas in which critical thinking skills are important for nurses. Firstly, there is the task of acquiring and keeping abreast of the knowledge base of nursing practice. This knowledge base will include various aspects of the life sciences, psychology, sociology, ethics, management and even accounting, to name a few. Nurses have to be literate and critical in a wide range of sciences and disciplines; literate in order to be able to keep up with the literature, and critical in that, in an area where 'miracle cures' are frequently sought and sometimes announced, it is necessary to distinguish sound scientific thinking from quackery.

A second sphere of critical thinking for nurses is in making up their own mind on an issue. Examples of this are not hard to find. One is making up one's own mind when one is reasoning about an issue where one has to make a decision but is in doubt about what to do. In such circumstances we might engage in a silent conversation with ourselves, in which we weigh up considerations for and against a particular course of action. We might be wondering about how to interact with a client; for example, how to talk to them about their not taking their medication, or whether to tell them about the risks of the procedure which they are about to undergo. Or we might be wondering whether the rise in temperature of a patient with quadraplegia is due to an underlying infection or whether it is simply due to the patient's environment. In each case we go through steps of reasoning to which there is a rational pattern and which can be engaged in more skillfully or less so. We might call this kind of thinking 'problem solving'.

Thirdly, nurses frequently have to engage in critical thinking when they seek to persuade others. They might be urging a policy to be followed in the future or they might be seeking to justify a decision made in the past. The matter at hand may concern values and attitudes or it may be a discussion about some factual matter such as an explanation for something that has happened. Parties to such discussions might include:

1. patients or clients and their families, as when nurses advise people about treatment regimens or self-care procedures;
2. other nurses, as when there are discussions about nursing diagnosis and care, allocation of tasks and sharing the work load, and so forth;
3. other health care professionals such as doctors and physiotherapists, as when patient management is discussed;
4. administrators, as when there are discussions about resources and amenities, staffing issues, rosters and so forth;
5. government agencies and bureaucrats, as when there are discussions about funding needs, the setting of standards, etc;
6. multi-disciplinary committees within institutions, such as ethics committees, planning and policy groups, etc;
7. industrial groupings such as unions in which there are debates about seeking improvements to conditions of employment, etc;
8. the general public, to whom it might be necessary to make representations through political action or publicity efforts on issues relating to

government policy on health funding, health insurance, hospital conditions and provision of resources.

Such a list could go on indefinitely, but what is clear is that in these sorts of cases there is a need for clear and rational communication as well as sensitivity to the points of view of others.

The caring with which one enters into these discussions and debates and opens oneself to the input of others cannot be systematically taught, although much can be done in educational settings to enhance it.[5] What we attempt to do in the chapters that follow is help nurses develop the intellectual skills required for clear and rational communication, scientific literacy, problem solving and ethical decision making. The features of critical thinking described above should always be present when these intellectual skills are exercised.

One last feature of critical thinking needs to be mentioned. A critical thinker is rational, creative, sensitive and independent. But what if the institution in which this critical thinker is working does not encourage such qualities? What if unquestioning obedience is demanded? What if there is an institutional ethos in which hierarchy and tradition are stressed rather than independence and innovation? We have no easy answer to these questions. We recognise that the professional lives of health workers will include struggles for power within institutions and other associations. At their best these struggles will be engaged in ethically and rationally. But whether they are or not, it is clear that critical thinking involves risk. It involves the risk of being out of step with others. It involves the risk of putting oneself on the line, of committing oneself to a position that one may have to defend. It involves the risk of committing oneself ethically, possibly against the prevailing norms. It involves the risk of accepting responsibility when matters do not turn out as one had intended. In short, it involves the risk of having to exercise responsible and sensitive judgement.

Exercise 1.2 (Revision and Discussion)

What are the defining features of 'critical thinking' and why are these important to nursing practice?

NOTES

1. Bandman Elsie L., Bandman, Bertram, *Critical Thinking in Nursing*, Norwalk, Connecticut, Appleton & Lange, 1988, p. 5.
2. Ennis, Robert, 'Rational thinking and educational practice' in Soltis, Jonas F. (ed.), *Philosophy and Education* (Eightieth Yearbook of the National Society for the Study of Education, Part 1), Chicago, NSSE, 1981.
3. *The Age*, Melbourne, 9 February 1994.
4. *The Age*, Melbourne, 11 February 1994.
5. van Hooft, Stan, 'Moral education for nursing decisions', *Journal of Advanced Nursing*, 15, 1990, pp. 210–215.

Chapter 2
Elements of Communication

This chapter describes the roles of authors, audiences and contexts in linguistic communication. The importance of interpretation on the part of audiences is stressed. It assists students to discern meaning in language by distinguishing categories of language use, including: informative, narrative, imperative, interrogative, evaluative, expressive, emotive, hortatory and persuasive. Mixed forms of these are also discussed. The use of signposts (such as 'firstly', 'therefore' and 'indeed') to indicate the structure of communication is explained.

It will undoubtedly seem obvious to say that communication occurs in a communicative context. Yet this point has considerable importance because it implies that it is not possible to understand a communication without understanding that context and that it is not possible to communicate to others successfully without giving due regard to the context.

A communicative context includes several elements. Firstly, there is the person who is doing the communicating. This person will be a speaker or a writer depending on whether we are dealing with a spoken or a written text. For the sake of brevity we will refer to this person as the **author**. The author does not always have to be present at the communication. The communication might take the form of a letter, a book, an audio tape or a movie as well as an event of speaking at which both author and audience are present. Once again, for the sake of brevity we will refer to the actual means of communication as a **text,** irrespective of what form it takes. The text is the second element in a communicative context.

Thirdly, there is the **audience**. This is the person or group who receives the communication. The audience may be a single person or a group of people to whom a speaker is speaking, or it may be the readership of a book. Even in the event that the text has not been read by anyone, the writer can still be assumed to have had an audience in mind when he or she wrote it.

A fourth element in the context of communication is the common body of knowledge which every communication presupposes. This body of knowledge is difficult to delineate exactly because it includes everything that parties to the communication can be expected to know and which they would need to know in order to understand the communication. One obvious element in this body of knowledge is a shared language. For a communication in English to be successful, both author and audience must be functionally literate in English. Such literacy consists not only in being familiar with the meanings of words, but also with the grammar of a language and with the logic inherent in its use. Knowing how to send and receive communications includes knowing how some statements imply others and how certain things cannot be logically coherent. It includes knowing that if something is green it must be coloured, and that it makes no sense to say that it could be not green as well. (Logicians call this the law of non-contradiction.)

Of greater interest is the variety of bodies of facts that people who communicate must share. It is difficult to communicate with someone who believes that the earth is flat and that the moon is made of green cheese. It is difficult to give health care advice to someone who thinks that disease is caused by the casting of evil spells. A further illustration of this aspect of shared bodies of knowledge is illustrated by the various professions. When one hears lawyers 'talking shop', one is aware of a body of knowledge that one might not share oneself. Again, when they are discussing their work and formulating strategies for patient care, members of a health care team make use of a body of knowledge which lay people would not normally share. Health practitioners need to be especially aware of this when they communicate with their patients.

Also relevant, but more difficult to specify, are shared attitudes. Parties to successful communication must share attitudes in order to understand one another fully. It sometimes happens that we are puzzled by what someone says to us, not because we cannot understand the words they use or the facts that they allude to, but because they seem to be expressing attitudes which are strange to us. Imagine a hospital worker who asks a patient to fill in some admission forms just as they are being brought in for emergency treatment after a serious accident. Such a bureaucratic attitude can be confusing to those whose primary concern is the welfare of the patient.

The attitudes of author and audience which must be sufficiently similar for communication to take place successfully might include deep beliefs of a spiritual kind. It will be easier for a clergyman to comfort a religious believer whose child has died from an incurable disease than it would be for an atheist. And an atheist will draw little comfort from the sorts of things a religious believer might say in a time of crisis.

A further aspect of what is shared between author and audience may be a practical task. There are many cases in which people communicate with each other while working together on a common project. Nurses in a hospital ward will be an example of this. In the course of their work they will say things to each other that can only be fully understood in the context of their shared tasks. The surgeon in the operating theatre who says 'scalpel' will be understood and the scalpel given to her because, in that setting, that is how that utterance should be responded to. To an outsider not familiar with the routines of the theatre, such an utterance may seem either rude or puzzling.

A fifth element in the context of communication is difficult to describe in abstract terms. It is the ethics of communication. Parties to a communication have certain responsibilities in regard to it. Somebody who tells me something has an obligation to tell the truth. And I have an obligation to pay attention and to take what he tells me seriously. Authors and audiences must have appropriate intentions for a communication to succeed, and these are requirements of an ethical kind. There are values inherent in communication. It is important to notice that these sorts of requirements can make a difference as to whether a communication succeeds. (There are also obligations that relate to etiquette. For example, one should say 'please' when making a request.)

A sixth element in communication is the actual content of the communication. What is the speaker or writer trying to say? We can only regard the communication as successful if the audience has grasped this content and responds to it in the ways intended by the author. However, while this may seem obvious, the fact is that authors sometimes do not say what they intend to say, or say things that are the contrary of what they intend to say. Accordingly, we need to be aware of a further element in communication.

This seventh and final element in communication might be described as levels of meaning. Most of the time we take what people say and write at face value. What the text says is what the author wants to tell us. But at other times the author may be being sarcastic or ironic. On a rainy day, someone might say to us, 'Nice day isn't it', or when a nurse drops a tray of surgical instruments, a colleague might say, 'Well done.' It is clear from examples of this kind that the meaning of the statement must be discerned from the context in which it is made, rather than just drawn from the meanings of the words being uttered. In these cases there is an element of tone in the way the statement is spoken or written which should alert us to the presence of irony or sarcasm.

Another example is one that tricks people more frequently. This is when an author, usually in an extended text, mentions a fact or a point of view with which that author disagrees. The author might then go on to argue against that view or to marshal evidence against that fact. But if the audience has not noticed that the statement is being mentioned rather than being proposed for the audience to agree with, then that audience will be fooled into thinking that the author holds that view. Scholarly and scientific writing frequently makes use of this device. In order to argue for a particular conclusion, an author needs to refute alternative views. And in order to refute them, the author needs to mention them and describe them in full. He may even tell his audience all the reasons why other people take this view seriously. If he does this over a number of pages, the audience might well fail to notice that the author does not support the view being mentioned. There may be no sarcasm or irony in the tone of the text and yet the author is saying something which he does not himself believe. Once again, it is the context of the particular statements in the text which needs to be noticed in order to see what the author's communicative intention really is.

In summary then, the elements of any communication are:

1. author
2. text

3. audience
4. shared body of knowledge, including:
   - language
   - grammar
   - logic
   - shared body of facts and opinions
   - attitudes, values and 'cultural ethos'
   - deep beliefs
5. ethical requirements and etiquette
6. content
7. levels of meaning.

Exercise 2.1

Read each of the following passages (some of which are taken from the references given in the *Lecturer's Manual*) and answer the following questions:

a. Who or what kind of person do you suppose the author might be? (You may not be able to give a precise answer; just describe the author as best you can.)
b. Who is the intended audience?
c. In what sort of context would you expect to find this text? What are your reasons for your answer?
d. Are there any other elements of communication present?(See the above list.)

1. It might be objected here that permitting conscientious objection is not conducive to the efficient running of hospitals and other health services. There is, however, little support for this kind of claim. In the case of military service, for example, it has been found that objectors are rarely amenable to threats, usually make unsatisfactory soldiers if coerced, and that in fact there are generally not enough objectors to frustrate the community's purpose (Benn and Peters 1959, p. 193). I would suggest that something similar is also probably true of objectors in nursing. As some of the examples in this text have shown, nurses have preferred to resign and risk dismissal rather than perform acts which they find morally offensive. Further to this, those nurses who have been coerced have not wholly complied with given orders (for example, I know of nurses who have resuscitated patients in cases of controversial NFR orders, and not resuscitated patients in the case of controversial CPR orders. A more common disobedience, however, involves night nurses who secretly feed defective newborns on whom a medical order has been given to withhold nourishing fluids). It is also unlikely that there are enough objecting nurses to obstruct the efficient running of the hospital system. Lastly, it is likely that conscien-

tious objectors would gain considerable community support if the extent of their personal and professional suffering were made public. I would argue, then, that it would be mutually beneficial to both the State and the nursing profession for formal procedures recognising conscientious objection to be adopted. By doing this, professional nurses can be spared the unnecessary and morally costly dilemma of whether to obey controversial lawful orders; employers, in turn, can optimistically look forward to achieving a morally tolerable and harmonious clinical reality for both their employees and the communities they are serving.

2. The nurses had to cut my clothes from me in casualty. They had been clean when I left home. The dark blue cords and the black sweater were taken away and burned.

   The shoes, smeared with engine muck, were sent home from the hospital in a brown paper bag. Months later, when I was trying to wear shoes again, I found them in my wardrobe. Inside, hiding like two miserable memories, were my socks crusted with dead blood. I lowered them gently into a rubbish bin and shuddered just a bit.

   As they wheeled me into the emergency area, I looked around blankly and felt grateful that none of it had anything to do with me. I didn't have to rush to resuscitate anyone or hurry to insert intravenous lines or tubes.

   Quite quickly a young doctor, whom I had taught as a medical student, took the first necessary step and, using a local anaesthetic after shaving the hair, put the tube into my chest to help expand the collapsed lung. I wasn't certain if it was inexperience or deference which caused him to be hesitant, but he relaxed when I said, 'You are just about to help save my life with that tube. Go for it, I'm glad I got here and it's you and not me that's doing it.'

   He did it easily.

3. Use of Restraint

   The resident's freedom of movement must not be restricted except where the safety of the resident or others is at risk. Restriction of movement should be avoided in all but the most urgent circumstances. Before use, all types of restraint, including chemical restraint, must be carefully considered and authorised by the resident's medical practitioner. Only in an emergency should restraints be used without medical authorisation. This should be obtained as soon as possible after the use of the restraint has been initiated. The type of restraint used should restrict the resident's movement only to the extent required to prevent him/her from injuring himself/herself or others. Total restriction of movement would rarely be necessary.

   Where restraint does occur there should be clear understanding by all concerned, as well as a detailed record, of the reason for restraint, the circumstances when restraint may be used, as well as the type and duration of the restraint. Intellectually competent residents should not be restrained against their will. When residents with diminished intellectual competence are restrained it is particularly important to involve their representative in the decision.

A detailed record of the circumstances, type and duration of the restraint should be kept. The need for restraint should be reviewed frequently.

4. In this International Year of the Family, many issues will doubtless be addressed, including, we hope, the increased burdens born by carers, families (often ageing parents) and people with a wide range of disabilities.

   The issue of supportive accommodation for people with disabilities, in a secure, affordable and appropriate environment is a matter of prime concern for many who sometimes feel relegated to the 'too hard basket'.

   The desire for independence, coupled with the need for varying levels of support, requires response and commitment on the part of the whole community.

   ADPACC (Accommodation for Disabled Persons under the Auspices of the Christian Church) is a task group not claiming a particular fait accompli, but rather a vision and challenge for church and community to continue to explore and develop a co-operative approach to an ever-growing need, especially in the use of property and people resources.

   Let us hope that in this Year of the Family, we may bring a measure of relief and hope to those who depend on us for added support.

5. Why do we continue to keep silent? Why do we stand by and watch as doctors do things we know to be wrong? Why do we avoid the questioning eyes of our patients, trying to find something non-committal to say? Why do we so fearfully avoid the truth? Or worse, why do we lie to cover up their mistakes?

Kinds of Communication

Our next task is to describe various kinds of communication. There are many classifications possible, and examples in real life will often include mixtures of classifications, but we would suggest the following:

1. Informative

As the name suggests, informative texts convey information. A simple informative text is called a statement or a proposition while longer and more complex cases might take the form of lectures, magazine articles or books. In each case the content of a text or proposition is factual information. Such information can be about a range of matters and take a number of different forms. There might be everyday information such as whether it is raining or at what time the train is due to arrive, or there might be technical information such as whether a patient is suffering from one kind of disease or another. There might be information about persons such as their age, occupation and address and there might be information about things such as where they are located or how they work. Some information is concrete in the sense that it is about something which is real and present while other forms of information are abstract in that they are expressed in scientific or mathematical formulae that can apply to a range of cases.

Many more distinctions might be made but the crucial point is that an informative communication is an attempt by an author to convey to an audience information which, it is assumed, that audience does not already have. The communication might be an answer to a question, or it might be an article in a scientific journal, but the communicative intent will be to increase the store of knowledge in the audience.

2. Hypothetical

Hypothetical communications (sometimes referred to by logicians as 'counter-factual' or 'conditional' statements) are a special kind of informative statement in which facts are described which are not actual. We might say, 'what if we did such and such' and go on to consider what would happen. We might ask what would have happened if we had done something other than what we in fact did do. Or we might say that we could have done something which we did not do, or that we would have done if only we had had the chance. These are all hypothetical statements.

Another form of hypothetical statement that frequently occurs is the 'if . . . then' statement. An example might be, 'If we administer penicillin to this patient without checking their medical history, we might cause an allergic reaction.' General scientific facts are frequently expressed in this form, as in, 'If you put a small amount of salt into water and stir, it will dissolve'.

3. Imperative

An imperative communication occurs when the author issues a command or directive for the audience to follow. A charge nurse giving instructions to a more junior nurse would be an example. Instances can range from the barked command of a drill sergeant on a parade ground, to the courteous request hedged with such qualifiers as 'please' and 'if you wouldn't mind'. In all cases along this range, the author is trying to get the audience to do something.

4. Interrogative

An interrogative communication is a request for information or, more simply, a question.

5. Expressive

An expressive communication is one that gives expression to the author's attitudes and feelings. Swear words are good examples, as are cries and groans (although these last are not, strictly speaking, instances of language). Although the grammatical form of such an utterance might be that of an informative statement ('You are a rotten so and so') or of an imperative ('Drop dead!'), the real function of these utterances is to express the anger of the speaker. There are calmer forms of expressive utterance, too. A speaker might say, in dejected tones, that she feels quite sad about something. This not only informs us about her condition, but also expresses it.

This last point is interesting because it indicates the possibility of the expressive meaning of an utterance having nothing to do with its content. I may be telling you that the sun is shining, but in such a glum tone of voice and with such a doleful expression, that you become aware of my sadness. Here the expression is not in the content of the utterance but in its form. However, in such cases it is not typical that the speaker will have intended to express their feelings. When there is an expressive intention, the text will usually be formulated to convey the speaker's feelings directly, as in, 'I am enjoying myself today'.

But expressing one's own emotions or feelings is not the only instance of expressive communication. Many casual conversations are of this kind. When we meet a friend and say 'How are you?', or 'Nice weather today, isn't it?', we are not typically asking a genuine question in the first case, or conveying information in the second. We are engaging in an exchange, one purpose of which is to express our friendship and reinforce our relationship with each other. In this sense, the exchange is an expression of our relationship. A vast number of our conversations are of this kind. Most conversations in the hospital staff room, or with family members, are more concerned with the formation and expression of relationships than with the content of those conversations. Their primary goal is not to be informative or imperative, or any of the several functional forms of communication. Nor is it exactly to be expressive of emotion, although this element may be present. Rather, it is a form of reinforcement of our relationships which is not self-conscious. As such the content of these communications is of secondary importance. What is more important is that the conversations reflect the nature of our relationships. These conversations are expressions of the people who are engaging in them in that they demonstrate, evaluate, and reinforce the relationship that these people have. We are not concerned to give or receive information about the weather when we say 'Nice weather today, isn't it?', but we are concerned to express the relationship that we have with the person to whom we are speaking.

6. Reflective

A reflective communication occurs when authors are primarily concerned with themselves. Indeed, we are stretching usage a little bit to call these communications at all since their primary intention is not to convey something to others, but rather, to reflect upon one's own experience. Reflection may take the form of thoughts in the author's own mind, or it may take the form of a diary. The content of a reflection will be the author's own experience and activity. The intention will be to evaluate it or to consider how it might be improved, or to integrate it into the values and objectives of one's life. Nurses who reflect upon their professional practice with a view to improving their performance, or who think about a decision that they have made with a view to considering whether that decision is consistent with their deepest values are engaging in reflection. In these cases, author and audience are the same.

However, there are other instances of reflective communication where the author and audience are different. People can reflect upon their relationships by talking to one another about them. People who have an intimate relationship will want to talk to one another about that relationship from time to time, while in an institutional setting there will be discussions about how certain staff members should relate to others and how team activities might be engaged in more effectively than they are. These reflective communications will also involve aspects of the expressive mode of communication just described, in that the form of the conversation will be expressive of the nature of the relationship: intimate conversation on the one hand, or formal committee meeting on the other. But the crucial point about them is that they have the relationship itself as part of their content.

7. Emotive

We use the word 'emotive' to describe communication which is designed to arouse emotion in the audience. This contrasts with expressive communication which, although it might indeed arouse sympathetic emotions in the audience, has as its communicative intention the expression of the author's emotion. In contrast, emotive communication has as its communicative intention the creation of emotional states in the audience. The orator who moves his audience to pity and sympathy for the sufferings of others, or the politician who moves his audience to nationalist fervour, or the sports coach who moves his team to greater determination to win, are all instances of emotive communication. Emotive language is the central technique in the creation of propaganda.

The objectives of emotional communication are secured by the use of suitable rhetorical devices which manipulate the feelings of the audience. Authors ranging from lawyers, clergymen and politicians to cheats are adept at using the techniques of rhetoric to create states of excitement and commitment in their audiences. Very often, emotive communication is seen as the enemy of rational discussion, although there may be occasions when its use is justified.

It is interesting to reflect for a moment on the conditions of the audience which makes successful emotive communication possible. The audience needs to be receptive to the seductive language that the author puts forward. This receptiveness may arise from a number of states. Firstly, there is fear. If the audience is afraid of something, it will be easy for an author to channel this fear into hatred of that which is feared and to distract the audience away from careful consideration of the issues at hand. Secondly, there is group pressure. Everyone achieves part of their self-esteem from the groups of which they are members and with which they identify. As a result, rhetoric that appeals to the values, symbols, rituals and beliefs surrounding such groups, be they our nation or our favourite football club, will have an impact on us. Similarly, appeals to the values of the group of which we are a part, whether it be nurses versus doctors, clinicians versus academics or women versus men will elicit our response.

Thirdly, there is guilt. We may have the feeling (individually or as a group) that we are responsible for some wrongdoing (even when we are not directly involved). When this is so, our thoughts and behaviours can be totally directed toward ridding ourselves of this feeling of guilt. The debate about Aboriginal land rights in Australia is frequently marred by this influence.

Lastly, we must not ignore self-interest. Authors can easily manipulate greed by asserting that someone else will get something that we want if we do not act immediately in the way the author suggests. Similarly, scarcity can be manipulated to have an affect upon us. The attractiveness of an object can be increased by making it appear scarce and unavailable, or by erecting barriers that make the object difficult to obtain. Advertisers use these tricks when they call something a 'limited edition', announce a 'closing down sale' or say that an offer is available 'for a limited time only'.

8. Evaluative

An evaluative communication is one where the author conveys an evaluation of something. Examples, include:

a. This is a good watch.
b. That patient causes a lot of problems.
c. It was a great movie.
d. It is important to be efficient in one's work.
e. Government funding for hospitals is inadequate.

Notice that some of these statements are about individual things or people (a,b,c), while others are about things in general (d,e). In many cases, the statement can look like an informative communication (b, e and the others to a lesser extent), and in some cases there can be elements of expressive communication (a and c, which could be paraphrased as 'I like this watch' or 'I really enjoyed the movie'). Evaluative communications are cousins of expressive communications because they convey the attitudes of authors.

However, what these statements all have in common that makes them different from expressive statements (which convey subjective feelings) is that the author is evaluating the matter at hand, or making a claim about its (objective) value. This means that the author is making a judgment. The basis for this evaluation, or value claim, might be subjective, as in 'I like this watch' or 'I really enjoyed the movie', or it might be objective as in,

'Management theorists agree that it is important to be efficient in one's work' or 'The existence of long waiting lists for elective surgery shows that government funding for hospitals is inadequate'. Example b is somewhat ambiguous in this regard in that it may be the expression of a nurse who is annoyed by that patient, or it may be a statement being made at a health care team meeting reviewing the problems that have to be faced in the coming week.

To go back to example a, the way that 'this is a good watch' differs from 'I like this watch' is that only the former statement is being urged upon the audience in order to get the audience to appreciate the watch. The former statement is about the watch and makes an objective claim about it with which the audience is being asked to agree. 'I like this watch' is about the speaker and does not make a claim with which the audience is being asked to agree.

But if an evaluative statement, or value claim, implies a judgment with which the audience is being asked to agree, then a reason for that judgment must be available. If somebody asked you why you thought your watch was a good one and you said, 'I don't know, I just like it, that's all', then your statement would not be a genuine evaluation, but simply an expressive utterance. The reason for an evaluative judgement must be based on the standards of excellence appropriate to the thing being evaluated. If the watch is being described as a good watch, there must be standards of excellence for watches which this watch meets. It is because the audience knows about these standards that it can agree or not with the author's evaluation of this particular watch. It would be odd if the author said, 'This is a good watch because it flies through the air beautifully when you throw it'. Whereas it makes perfectly good sense to say, 'This is a good watch because it keeps accurate time.' And this shows how an expressive statement is different from an evaluative one. To say, 'This is a good watch because I like it', is not to give the kind of reason that is required to ground the judgment or to impress it upon the audience.

While 'good' and 'bad' are the most common words used for evaluation, there are many others that carry the same connotation. Examples above are, 'efficient' 'inadequate', 'important', 'problems'. These words imply a standard of judgment. If funding is deemed inadequate it is because there is an implied standard of adequate funding. If a patient is said to cause problems it is because there is an implied standard of patient behaviour which does not cause unnecessary problems. It will be found that a great many apparently informative words can carry evaluative connotations, and audiences should always be aware of this possibility.

9. Hortatory

Hortatory statements, or exhortations, are statements that say what ought to be done or what a particular person should do in a given situation. The most common word in hortatory communications is the word 'ought'. Examples might include:

a. Nurses should always keep an efficient watch with them as they work.

b. Nurses ought to be efficient workers.

c. The government should provide more funding for health care.

What is common to all these cases is that the audience, or some other party, is being urged to do something by the author, whether this something is a specific course of action currently available, or whether it is a policy that should be adopted for a range of cases. Also, while some exhortations are directed at specific individuals or groups ('you', or 'the government') other such statements are directed in a very general way, as in:

d. They ought to do something about the roads.

That this last statement is very similar in meaning to:

e. The roads are in a bad state of disrepair

shows that exhortations are closely related to evaluative communications. Indeed, if you consider the statement:

f. I hate these rough roads

as another possible equivalent, then you will see that expressive statements are also closely related. However, the more focused one becomes in an exhortation, as in:

g. Nurse Jones should attend to patient Smith immediately

the fewer elements of expression or evaluation will be present. However, this example does show an affinity with imperative communications. Change g to:

h. Nurse Jones, you should attend to patient Smith immediately

and you will have a clear instance of an instruction or a directive. The difference between an exhortation and an imperative is that an imperative is expressed in the second person (it is a 'you' statement), while an exhortation is usually written in the third person (as in examples a, b, and c, above).

Like value statements, exhortations require reasons to support them. If it is claimed that the government should provide more funds for health care, then reasons for this should be offered.

10. Narrative

A narrative communication is when the author tells a story of some kind. The words that help identify a narrative include 'then', 'and then' and 'later'. These words are usually indicators of the time or sequence in which things happened. Examples of narrative communication occur in news broadcasts, in nursing reports which describe a patient's progress, various forms of research (such as studies which show how people change over time under the influence of various factors) and in everyday conversation. In these cases we would describe the narrative as an informative one.

But narratives also occur in novels and in movies. We would call these poetic narratives. A poetic communication is one which has the main objective of creating beauty, entertainment or aesthetic worth. Not only poems, but also narrative prose, songs and other artistic forms are instances of poetic communication. Some art theorists subsume poetic communication under the category of expressive communication, but this would suggest that an artist has to feel the emotion which her work conveys or evokes, and this is an idea which many practising artists deny. Artists are usually well aware that the most important contribution they make to their work is excellence of craft skills rather than emotion. In any case, where the art form involves telling a story, we would call it a poetic narrative.

11. Performative

Performative statements are statements that have an effect in and of themselves. When a marriage celebrant says, 'I pronounce you man and wife', she does not describe a situation, or exhort the couple to create it. Nor does she express her wish that they be man and wife. She actually makes it so by virtue of her pronouncement. This is a performative statement. Another example might be when the chairperson of a committee meeting says, 'I declare this meeting open'. By virtue of this statement, the meeting is opened and any further idle chat becomes an interruption. As the name suggests, performative statements (they are seldom long texts) actually do what they say.

One class of performatives which is of more concern to people who do not have official positions like those in the examples above, is the making of a promise. When you say, 'I promise to come to relieve you in the wards at noon', you are binding yourself to a course of action. If you fail to show up at noon, you will not only have caused inconvenience, but you will have broken your word—the performative word with which you had bound yourself to do what you promised.

One of the key features of a performative utterance is that the intentions of the speaker are not relevant to its efficacy. Even if the marriage celebrant thought that the couple before her were badly suited to each other and would do better not to marry, her words would still have their effect. And even if the chairperson of the meeting secretly wished she were lying on a beach somewhere, her words would still have the effect of opening the meeting. More importantly, even if you thought to yourself, 'But I won't do it' as you spoke your promise, you would still have made the promise and it would still be binding upon you. The reason for this is that saying the words does the job. In the case of the promise, saying the words creates the expectation in others that you will do what you promised and so you have a duty to fulfil those expectations.

12. Persuasive

A persuasive communication is one where the author seeks to convince the audience of something. This something could be an attitude, a point of view, a value, a fact, the wisdom of a course of action or even the appropriateness of an emotional response. The key element in a persuasive communication is that the author has to offer reasons which will lead the audience to adopt the author's point of view.

Persuasive communication most frequently occurs when the audience is not already convinced of the point of view that is at issue, and even actively disagrees with it. There is a resistance within the audience to the point which the author wishes to present, and so the author has to overcome this resistance in order to convince the audience. If the author were to present a policy for action or a fact which the audience readily agreed with, it might be a case of hortatory or informative communication. The overcoming of audience resistance is a defining feature of persuasive communication.

To be convinced of something is not to be caused to believe it or agree with it, but to see that there are reasons for agreeing with it and that these reasons are sound. An author might get an audience to believe something by way of the power of oratory, but this would be emotive communication or perhaps even poetic communication. We only have a genuine case of persuasive communication when the audience is able to make up its own mind and come to agree in the light of the considerations that have been presented (and in the light of the background knowledge and attitudes held by both author and audience). This is why persuasive communication must present reasons for the point of view that is being presented.

It will be the task of the following few chapters to set out the forms and protocols of persuasion in some detail. For the moment it is enough to note that if reasons are added to any of the forms of communication already described, they will become persuasive forms of communication. So we might have

a. persuasive/informative statements where evidence is offered for factual claims;
b. persuasive/imperative statements where reasons are given to the audience by the author to convince them to do what they are being asked to do;
c. persuasive/hortatory statements where reasons are given for why something should be done;
d. persuasive/evaluative statements, where reasons are given for valuing something;
e. persuasive/reflective statements, where the author gives himself reasons for adopting a particular point of view in his private soliloquy.

Note that not all communications can be supported with reasons. Expressive and poetic utterances, in particular, would be compromised if reasons were offered, and it would not make sense to offer reasons for a performative statement.

Exercise 2.2

How would you classify the kinds of communication in the following utterances?

1. Doors can only be closed if the hinges are properly lubricated.
2. Close the door!
3. There are more wards behind that door.
4. I wish he'd close the door.
5. It is estimated that 73% of all internal doors in this building are regularly left open.
6. If the door were closed, it would be a lot quieter in the room.
7. Isn't that a beautiful door?
8. That door is open.
9. I sometimes wonder why I get so annoyed when the door is left open.
10. People who don't close doors are as despicable as those who spit on the floor.
11. Bill came into the room and pointedly left the door open. He sat down, lit a cigarette, and stared angrily at the nurse behind the desk. In his mind, he dared her to make him close the door.
12. I always close the door when I enter a room.
13. Courtesy is one of the finest qualities of a human being and nothing is so annoying as a door to a waiting room left ajar. Accordingly, people should close the door behind them when they enter a waiting room.
14. People should close doors more often.
15. How many doors were left open today?
16. It gives me great pleasure, in opening this door, to declare the new wing of the hospital open.
17. I love you.
18. You ought to be more sensitive with that problem patient.
19. Twenty research subjects were chosen at random to answer the questionnaire. Only seventeen replied, and eleven of those agreed that caring is an important attitude for nurses to have. Later, after the seminars, the number of respondents who agreed with this proposition increased to fifteen.
20. The rate of suicide among males aged 15 to 19 in NSW country towns with populations between 4000 and 25,000 rocketed from 7.2 per 100,000 in 1964 to 41.9 per 100,000 in 1991.

Exercise 2.3

Go back to Exercise 2.1. How would you classify the kinds of communication in those five texts?

Form and Content in Communication

In any communication it is possible to distinguish form from content. The content, as we have already explained, is what the author is trying to say. The form, in contrast, is the way the author is saying it. Obviously, in order to convey anything to us, the author has to use some form for doing so. The most general such form is the language itself, with its vocabulary and its grammar. But it is possible to focus upon the form of a communication more explicitly and to learn a lot from it. There are many forms of communication ranging from books and magazine articles, to lectures, conversations, poems and so forth. The list is almost endless. While it is not our purpose to describe these forms in detail, it will be useful to point out particular formal features which can help the audience to understand the communicative intentions of the author.

The features that we will now describe for you are called **signposts**. Signposts are words or phrases that tell us how the contents of a text are organised. There are many kinds of signposts, having a variety of functions.

1. In informative texts, signposts may be used for listing points or for showing the order of priority in a series of points, for example:

firstly	fourthly
in the first place	finally
the next point to note is	moreover

2. They may show that the author is about to offer an illustration of an idea or an example of it:

for example	for instance
let's take	suppose
an instance/example of this was	

3. When the text has a narrative content, signposts may be used to indicate a time relationship:

then	while
when	after that
later	next

4. An important class of signposts is one which shows that the author is about to sum up what she is trying to say, or a part of it:

if I could just sum up	in other words
to summarise	it amounts to this
what I have been saying is that	

5. Signposts may be used to re-phrase what has already been said, to introduce a definition or to clarify:

let me put it this way	that is to say
to put it another way	in other words

6. Signposts may be used to emphasise or draw attention to important points in the text:

it is worth noting
let me emphasise that
particularly
most importantly
especially

7. Or they may be used to indicate that a point is not a crucial part of the exposition:
   as an aside, we should note that
   in parenthesis, it is worth noting that
   (in written texts, the use of parentheses or brackets)
8. Signposts can indicate hypothetical or conditional statements:
   if . . . then
   unless
   suppose that
   assuming that
   would only happen if
   provided that
9. They can indicate a relationship of implication between one idea and another (such relationships will be described more fully in the next chapter):
   because
   thus
   so
   therefore
   since
   it follows that
10. Signposts can introduce an idea which is contrary to what has just been said:
    nevertheless
    but
    and yet
    on the other hand
    although
    however
11. They can introduce an idea that the author wishes to mention but does not agree with:
    some people claim that . . . but
    it has been argued that . . . on the other hand
    in his important book, Smith (1994) says . . . but
12. Signposts can also indicate attitudes:
    unfortunately
    it is regrettable that
    luckily
13. Some signposts are logical connectives which indicate inclusion or exclusion, or possible alternatives:
    and
    neither . . . nor
    only
    or
    either . . . or
    nothing but
14. Signposts that indicate exhortation include:
    ought
    should
15. Along with the many words that can be used in evaluative communication, clear signposts of evaluations are:
    good / better / best
    bad / worse / worst
    effective / efficient / successful
16. Some signposts are used to qualify the strength with which a statement is being made:

might — probably
it is likely that — may

17. While others serve to place a stress on a statement (especially when the audience might be expected not to have known it before):
    indeed — in fact
18. Some signposts indicate causal relationships or that an explanation is about to be given:
    by — because
19. Some signposts indicate that the author is appealing to the audience to agree with a statement because that statement is one that everyone might be expected to agree with:
    it goes without saying that
    of course
20. A group of signposts that is often taken for granted is the group which indicates negation:
    not — never
    none — nothing

Our list of signposts could be even longer, but the key point to note about them is that if you fail to notice them and their role in a text, you will almost certainly fail to understand the content of that text. It is also important to note that many authors do not use as many signposts as they could or should. In this case, a careful audience has to implicitly provide signposts in order to understand the text correctly.

Lastly, it is important for you as authors to become accustomed to using signposts. It is our experience as teachers that many students write essays which are little more than lists of points, without any indication of how those points connect together. This makes it very difficult for the audience to understand the train of thought that lies behind the text. Writers of research papers, reports, journal articles and memos can fail in similar ways. It can be a useful exercise to go over a text that you have written and to deliberately add as many signposts as you can. Gradually you will get used to the idea and put the signposts in as you write. This will also result in your own thinking being clearer than it was before.

Exercise 2.4

Identify the signposts in the following text[1] and specify (by referring to the list above) what job the signpost is doing (for example, 'emphasis', 'listing points' or 'negation').

> It has been argued that sugar paste is a useful wound care product because it is easily available and comparatively cheap. However, it does need to be changed at least twice a day to be effective. Not many nurses realise that the simple measure of a once- or twice-daily bath

or soaking is much more beneficial, particularly for chronic wounds (which are inevitably colonised with bacteria). As an aside we might note that a 'clean' procedure is probably all that is necessary for chronic wounds provided the usual precautions to prevent cross-infection of other patients' wound are taken. In fact, a pair of non-sterile gloves may be used and discarded after each patient rather than sterile forceps.

Some dramatic changes have occurred in the search for the ideal dressing. For example, there is now a move away from dry dressings towards occlusive dressings. What is exciting about these newer products is that they create an optimum healing environment by controlling crucial factors such as humidity, temperature and gaseous concentration. Moreover, they protect the wound from infection and secondary trauma.

Perhaps even more importantly, the hydrocolloid and hydrogel types of 'wet' dressings have the added advantage of relieving pain and discomfort in the wound. This is because dry dressings and some of the so-called non-adherent and tulle-type dressings cannot avoid damaging newly formed epithelial cells on removal, sometimes making it necessary to administer drugs or even a general anaesthetic in order to perform the task.

These occlusive dressings greatly reduce the need for routine wound cleansing, which can in itself hinder the healing process rather than encourage it, by allowing the wound surface temperature to drop. There is no excuse for the hospital practice of leaving a wound uncovered for long periods to await the consultant's ward round, since this allows the temperature to drop and the surface to become dry. On the other hand, allowing the consultant to 'peek' under the corner of a dressing is dangerous, as he may be tempted to do the same thing on the next patient without washing his hands first.

The ideal dressing has been defined as a material which, when applied to the surface of the wound, provides and maintains an environment in which healing can take place at the maximum rate. Such a dressing should firstly provide a moist environment; secondly, it should be comfortable for the patient; thirdly, it should remove any necrotic material; fourthly, it should promote the production of granulation tissue; fifthly, it should stimulate re-epithelialisation; and last but not least, it should be cost-effective.

The selection of the right dressing for the treatment of wounds at different stages of healing is extremely difficult. No two patients are the same and no two wounds heal in the same manner or at the same rate, so that observation and experience are essential. Unfortunately, some consultants are reluctant to move away from what they feel is safe, reliable and cheap. They argue that new dressings are expensive, ignoring the fact that they need changing far less frequently and that they reduce the healing time considerably. So nurses must take the lead in advising on wound management and recommending wound care products.

Exercise 2.5

Re-read the five texts in Exercise 2.1 and:

a. Highlight the signposts that you find there.

b. Explain, in your own words, what function they are serving.

NOTE

1. Adapted from the first section of an essay by Glenys Griffiths entitled, 'Choosing a dressing', in *Nursing Times*, 87, 36, 4 September 1991, pp. 84–90

Chapter 3

Form and Content in Communication

In this chapter, the notion of a topical outline (or précis) is introduced as a means of summarising content. The usefulness of this for the development of study skills will also be stressed. We then look at persuasive uses of language and argument. Argument is defined as the offering of reasons for conclusions, where such reasons might include evidence or premises. (Evidence will be discussed in Part Two.) We then explain how an argument is displayed in its outline. The strategy of outlining arguments is the key to this part of the book. Outlines display the premises, points of contention, and conclusions of arguments. They show nested conclusions and assumptions and identify the premises from which the conclusions are drawn. Premises within arguments can be factual claims, exhortations, or they can affirm values. (The discussion of values is resumed in Part Three.)

Having described in the previous chapter how to recognise some of the formal mechanisms whereby texts are organised, we now turn to the matter of understanding the content of texts. The way that we describe the content of a text is to develop a summary of that text. Taking lecture notes or reading notes is an example of this. We call such a summary an **outline.**

Topical Outlines

There are at least two kinds of outline of a text, corresponding to two of the kinds of communication which we discussed in Chapter 2. When the text you are dealing with is purely informative in nature, as might be a chapter in a bioscience text book or the report of a new scientific discovery, you might want to write a summary of the main points in your journal to allow you to retrieve the information at a later time. Similarly, as you are reading paragraphs of books or journal articles (but not newspapers, since paragraphs in newspapers are often very short), you should be able to pause and state what the main point of that paragraph was. To achieve these aims you would write a **topical outline**. Such an outline would consist of a listing of the main points. A topical outline condenses the information into a brief and manageable form. It is a précis of the original text concentrating on the major points. It omits the minor points, leaves out the examples, and ignores the details of the exposition.

Of course, in order to select the main points and distinguish them from the incidental ones, you need some familiarity with the area of knowledge you are dealing with and you need to have some interest in the area yourself, in the light of which you will select what is of most interest to you. If you are reading a text about neurosurgery without a basic knowledge of that area, you will not know which points are important and which are not. Similarly, if you are reading about something that you are not interested in, you will not be struck by the importance of one point as opposed to another.

It can be helpful when writing topical outlines to use categories and headings to organise the information. However, it is important not to be too brief, since you will want to go back over what you have written at some future time and you must then be able to understand it. If you have written only headings, or single words, you may not be able to fill in the missing information at a later date. For this reason it is useful to write whole sentences rather than mere points or notes. Sum up the information you have read in your own words and write it out in full grammatical sentences.

It is also useful to split the contents of the text into separate parts. To do this you must become aware of the structure of the text you are reading. Some points will be subsidiary to others. Some facts will be offered as examples or illustrations, while others are asides which merely set up the context in which the information is being conveyed. (For example, descriptions of research methodology, previous research or information about the researchers). You should be particularly careful to notice points that are being mentioned only to be refuted or questioned later. Some articles will explain alternative views quite fully before going on to show that they were wrong. A topical outline that lists such a point without further comment could be quite misleading. If you have time, it is useful to read the whole text through first in order to understand what is important in it. It should be clear that in order to make these kinds of discriminations, you need to be very attentive to signposts.

Example 3.1

The following is an item from a newspaper.[1] (We reproduce it without its heading, since headings tend to lead the reader to interpret texts in a particular way.)

> Marriage for men is a source of happiness but for women there are more important things in life, according to a book on wealth in Australia, released yesterday.
>
> When asked what makes them happy and gives them a sense of achievement, men rate matrimony as important on both counts.
>
> But for women, marriage just doesn't rate. Instead, good friends, good health and family support are ranked by women as the most important sources of happiness.

The findings are contained in a new book, *Living Decently, Material Wellbeing in Australia,* which examines poverty and wealth during the '80s.

Dr Peter Travers, co-author of the book, said that married men seemed more content with their lot than older, single men.

'Marriage for men was a strong predictor of whether they were happy or not, but it was not a significant predictor of happiness for women,' he said.

'This seems to suggest that women who are alone can cope much better than men who are alone.'

The research found rich people were only slightly more likely to be happy than poor people.

Men and women associated being in a higher socio-economic class with doing well but did not associate it with happiness.

Money and possessions were not very important to most of the 1697 Australians who were asked to describe what made them feel content.

As long as there was enough money to get by on, people cited non-material things.

Good friends, health, social standing, marriage and not being worse off than previously were all important factors.

In no case did education levels, being unemployed or having recently experienced unemployment or a high debt ratio affect people's feeling of doing well or being happy. The research covered 1987–89, a period largely unscathed by the recession.

And in a hint about who shoulders most of the domestic work, paying the bills was cited as another difference between men and women in the happiness stakes. Men did not report a link between feeling stressed when paying bills and feeling unhappy, but women did.

He said the research showed Australians adjusted to their financial circumstances and overseas studies revealed a similar pattern among rich and poor citizens.

'On the one hand material things certainly matter and on average richer people are somewhat happier than poorer people, but the main reason is that people adjust to their level of material wellbeing,' he said.

'If people are thinking that increased money brings increased happiness, they are deluded.'

Dr Travers is a senior lecturer in public administration at Flinders University. Dr Sue Richardson, who co-wrote the book, is a reader in economics at Adelaide University.

Their research also uncovered pockets of misery.

People with incomes in the bottom 20 per cent were far more likely than the richest 20 per cent of Australians to have multiple problems. The richest group had very little likelihood of having more than one problem in the areas of happiness, health and social participation.

Those surveyed for the study were aged between 20 and 74.

A topical outline of this piece might read as follows:

1. Marriage is a source of happiness for men.

2. Women find good friends, good health, and family support more important as a source of happiness.
3. Source: *Living Decently, Material Wellbeing in Australia,* by Peter Travers and Sue Richardson.
4. Rich people are only slightly more likely to be happy than poor people.
5. People (including the unemployed) adjust to their level of material wellbeing.
6. People in the poorest categories are less happy.

Points 1 and 2 are interesting in that they indicate some of the elements that make people in Australia happy. We have included point 3 even though it is not strictly something that the article is about, because we may want to find out more or we may want to cite these findings in the course of writing an essay later. In these cases we will want to know where to find more details and we will want to be able to offer a citation for the information. Notice that we have used a heading, namely 'Source', when writing this point. This will tell us later that what we have written is the source of this information. Point 4 describes a relationship between wealth and happiness which some may find surprising, and so we have included point 5 which offers an explanation for this point. Point 6 qualifies point 4 somewhat and should be included for that reason.

Notice that in numbering our points we have largely followed the order of exposition in the article itself. You may want to note points in a different sequence. (For example, point 3 might appear last.) Notice also that a person with different interests might have highlighted different points. Nurses, having a special interest in health, might be expected to notice the point that many people in the study found health to be more important to their happiness than money. Lastly, notice that there is an example in this piece of a point which is mentioned but refuted, namely 'increased money brings increased happiness'. Of course, in this instance, the fact that the authors do not agree with this is clearly signposted.

As you become more aware of the structure of informative texts you will notice that such texts frequently include arguments. Facts will be cited, but the evidence for them, or the reasoning that led to their discovery, will be described also. In this way, informative texts can contain, not just the information, but the reasons which persuaded people of the truth of that information. A topical outline typically does not include those arguments. Topical outlines are used to record the facts in summary form and therefore do not need to recount the evidence or arguments in support of them. It is important to note this, since the evidence for facts will also be factual in nature. As a result, there will be a temptation to list these facts as well without noticing that they are of a subsidiary nature. If you are listing all the facts in a text, then your list will include them without showing the logical relation between the facts. This could lead to confusion. In a topical outline, it is only the conclusions that have been established which you need to note down, not the facts which support those conclusions. If you do note down both kinds of facts, then you should also show how the supporting facts lead to the conclusions and when you do this you are writing a **logical outline**. This is a second kind of outline and we will describe it in the next sections.

Exercise 3.1

Write a topical outline of the following item which appeared in *The Independent Monthly* in November 1993.

Medicos Shocked By Miracle Cure

POST-TRAUMATIC Stress Disorder is a recent name for shell-shock, the condition suffered by many people after traumatic experiences ranging from armed hold-ups to the Vietnam War. The number of people diagnosed with the condition has increased rapidly since the name was coined in the 1970s, and the condition is now being used as a basis for claims of compensation in the courts.

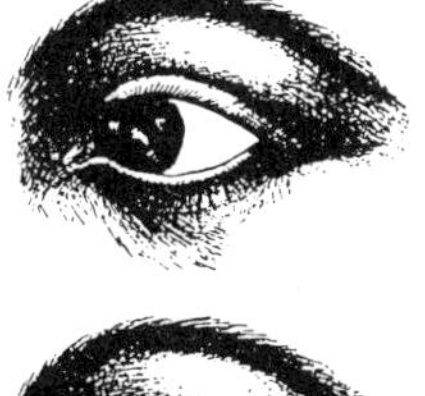

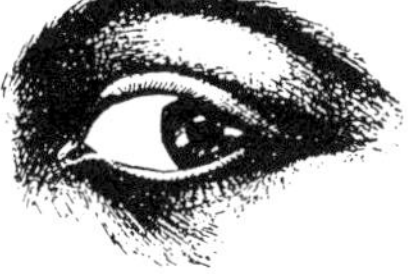

An unlikely cure has just emerged. In 1987 Francine Shapiro, a Californian clinical psychologist, was walking in the park and noticed that disturbing thoughts were no longer depressing when she moved her eyes from side to side. She went on to develop a therapy called EMDR—eye movement desensitisation and reprocessing. The patient recalls the traumatic episode and the therapist moves an index finger rhythmically from side to side about 40 cm from the patient's face. The patient follows the movement with his or her eyes and the distress associated with the memory is gradually reduced.

The reaction of Gary Fulcher, who runs the psychology department at Sydney's Concord Hospital, was perhaps typical. "I wondered if it was just a wank," he recalls. The procedure seemed too simple to be plausible. But then he tried it out. "I had been seeing one particular patient for two years," he says. "She had multiple problems, she had been sexually abused by a doctor and a priest. She's been put in a psychiatric hospital and was abused there too . . . She threw herself off a carpark roof and broke her back. Anyway, we had worked together for two years and she had progressed, but not very far. I suggested we try EMDR. Twenty minutes—maybe the session was 20 minutes long. It changed her life. She goes out almost every day now, she looks me in the face. She laughs—she's able to take charge." Other therapists have achieved similarly good results. "What makes them optimistic," says Jac Brown, secretary of the Sydney branch of the Australian Psychological Society, "is when they've been working on a lot of emotional stuff for a long time and it hasn't shifted, and then they do a few sessions with EMDR and it's gone."

About 1,000 Australian psychologists have now been trained in the technique, which seems to be successful with a range of conditions apart from PTSD. Some observers are critical: one suggestion is that th. subjects think they are better but in fact are not. One problem is that no one knows why the technique should work, although there has been speculation that there may be a link with the rapid eye movement that occurs during sleep, which is thought to be associated with the brain's processing of information. But, as Sydney University psychologist Bob Boakes says: "No one knew how aspirin worked for 50 years or so, but it cured quite a few headaches along the way."

Figure 3.1

What Is an Argument?

We said in Chapter 2 that persuasive communication involves offering reasons for points of view, for believing certain statements, or for adopting policies of action. In Chapter 2 we explained the role of signposts, including those that show that one proposition 'follows' from another. In this section we will develop a deeper analysis of these points.

Let us focus on the form of persuasive communication. The most common term used to describe an instance of persuasive communication is the word 'argument'. However, you should not be tricked by this word into thinking that every case of persuasive communication is a dispute or a quarrel. The form of a quarrel is:

The sky is blue
No it isn't
Yes it is
No it isn't

and so forth. The central feature of this quarrel is that it consists of statement and counter-statement without reasons being offered. In a dispute like this the person with the loudest voice or most stamina wins.

Another feature of quarrels or disputes is that they are competitive in the sense that participants in them have an emotional stake in winning. Sometimes it hardly matters what the quarrel is about. It only matters to the disputants that they win a victory over their opponent. In contrast to this, the audience in a genuine persuasive communication must not prejudge the issue and must be willing to be convinced if the arguments are sound. They must also be willing to offer genuine reasons for their own position in an attempt to refute the claims of the author. There must be a shared desire to end up with the truth or with the best policy. It must not be a competition motivated by the desire to win at all costs.

In fact, the word **argument** is used by logicians not to describe a conversation or an exchange, but to describe what an author says to an audience when what that author says is supported by reasons. A text that supports a point of view with reasons will be said to contain an argument.

What then, is the nature and structure of an argument? We define an argument as a linked set of statements designed to lead to a conclusion. The first of the crucial terms here is **linked**. An argument is not just a list of statements in the way that the newspaper article in Example 3.1 was. The statements that make up an argument must be connected in such a way that they add up to a set of considerations or reasons. Any statement that is not linked in this way is said to be irrelevant to the argument. The statements that make up an argument can also be referred to as **propositions,** but the best and most technical way of describing them is to use the word **premise**. A premise is any statement or proposition which the author is offering as a reason for supporting the conclusion.

Of course, it will be for the audience to judge whether the premise actually does support the conclusion or not. For its part, the **conclusion** is the fact, theory, policy or course of action that the premises lead the audience to accept. When arguments have been effectively mounted, the conclusion will also be what the author wishes to convince the audience of. The key word in the above definition is 'lead'. The premises must lead to the conclusion. They must induce the audience to believe or support t he conclusion in cases where they did not do so prior to having heard the premises. This relationship of leading to the conclusion is called an

inference. From the premises we should be able to infer the conclusion.

So, with this terminology in place, we can now describe the structure of an argument as follows:

Premises $\Rightarrow$ Conclusion

where the arrow designates the inference or the process of being led by the premises to the conclusion.

Premises need not always be propositions or statements. We might see a situation and immediately draw a conclusion from it. For example, a nurse might see a damp area in the middle of a patient's abdominal dressing and conclude that the dressing needed changing. Or we might have information on the basis of a report and draw a conclusion from that. So, a nurse looking at a patient's chart might conclude that the patient needs further medication. Again, evidence might be given for a particular conclusion by way of reports of scientific experiments or observations. But whatever form it takes, anything that leads one towards a particular conclusion can be called a premise.

Similarly, a conclusion need not always be a statement or a proposition. We have already indicated that people can argue for points of view, for facts, for scientific theories or for policies of action. But a person who hears an argument in favour of a particular action might respond to it by simply doing that action. One nurse might say to another, 'That patient's dressing is wet; the charge nurse should be told about it,' and the other might respond by simply going to tell the charge nurse. In this instance, the action itself is the conclusion of the argument. More usually however, the conclusion of an argument is something that the audience agrees to, and most often this will be expressed as a proposition or statement. We will see in Part Two of this book that another form of conclusion is an explanation. Explaining why something happened involves giving reasons for expecting it to happen.

We have already mentioned some signposts which indicate arguments. We can now be more specific. Signposts that identify premises include:

since	because	for
for the reason that		due to

while signposts that identify conclusions include:

therefore	then	this shows that
so	it follows that	this means that

Exercise 3.2 (Revision)

In your own words, describe what an argument is. What is the structure of an argument and how would you define the terms used to describe that structure?

Logical Outlines

In order to display the structure of an argument we write what we call a **logical outline** of that argument. A logical outline contrasts with a topical outline. Whereas the latter merely gives us a summary listing of points, a logical outline displays the premises, points of contention and conclusions of an argument. It shows nested arguments and identifies which premises the conclusions are drawn from. (We will define these terms below.) A logical outline reconstructs the line of thought or argument in a text. It emphasises the connection between the parts of a text and displays which of the premises support the conclusions.

Logical outlines are not only useful in understanding persuasive communications. It is also possible to write a logical outline of an informative text where that text also supplies information about how a particular conclusion was reached. Most scientific writing should take this form. Reports in scientific books and journals not only tell us about facts or theories that have been arrived at, but also about the reasoning used in arriving at them and about the evidence that was gathered to support them. We will return to this matter in Part Two.

But the most important context for writing logical outlines is the context of persuasive language, where a particular point of view, factual conclusion, value or policy for action is being urged upon an audience by argument and persuasion.

There are a number of steps that one should take when writing a logical outline of a text.

1. Identify the Point of Contention

The point of contention is the single most important element in any argument. It is what the speaker or writer of the text is trying to persuade us of. It is what they are trying to say, or what they are trying to persuade us to do. Sometimes it is called 'the issue' in an argument. In a well prepared speech, essay, research paper or scientific report, the point of contention will be stated near the beginning of the argument as part of the introduction to it and may even be restated at the end as part of the summary.

A point of contention should always be a single proposition. There should be no signposts such as 'and', 'or', 'because' or 'since'. Signposts would indicate subordinate clauses which, if they are relevant at all, should be part of the argument and therefore identified separately as premises. However, it is possible for a point of contention to take the form of a question. There may be arguments where the issue is what I should do to solve a problem. Henceforth we will refer to the point of contention as the **POC**. Let us take a very simple example.

Example 3.2

'It's very stuffy in the ward today; let's open the windows.'

The POC here is that the windows should be opened.

This may seem a very simple matter, but the unfortunate fact is that in everyday communications speakers and writers are often clumsy in making clear what it is that they are trying to say. Sometimes they do not state it at all, at other times they say it unclearly or ambiguously. In a well-formed argument, the POC will be the same as the conclusion, but sometimes people state a conclusion to their argument which is not what they actually wanted to say (we will explain how to identify conclusions presently).

In order to identify or formulate the POC, it is important to read the whole text, or at least all of the relevant section of the text, first. When you are listening to an argument, rather than reading it, this will be more difficult because you will not have the luxury of being able to read it all and then go back over it to look at it in closer detail. However, you can glean a lot from the context in which the statement is made, from the tone of voice and from the identity of the speaker (for example, are they an authority or a person in charge?).

Example 3.3

'It's very stuffy in the ward today.'

If we take it that the context in which this statement is made is similar to that of Example 3.2, and that the speaker is someone in charge, then we can conclude that the POC, once again, is that the windows should be opened. Only this time it was not stated explicitly.

Exercise 3.3

Write down the POC in each of these arguments.

1. Since the bacteria count on urban beaches increases greatly after heavy rain, we can conclude that it is safer not to swim at these beaches after a storm.
2. The dangerous effects of smoking are now well known in our community. Therefore, people who smoke are very likely to be aware of the risks that they are taking.
3. I wonder if I should take Friday off. I've been tired and short tempered lately. I think I will.
4. A mothercraft nurse is talking to her assistant (who has turned the TV on in the créche play room) in disapproving tones. She says: 'Watching violence on TV makes young children behave violently.'
5. Scientific studies have shown that green plants remove toxins from the air, so it would be sensible to put indoor plants in hospital wards.

2. Identify Premises

A premise is a proposition that supports the conclusion or POC of an argument. To identify the premises in a text, you need to identify those statements from among the points made which lead to the conclusion. You can do this as you read the text so that what you write down are just the premises. Alternatively, you can write out a topical outline of the text and then note which points lead to the conclusion and which do not. If you have listed all the points made in the text, you will need to decide which of them are premises. This sounds simple, but it involves a complicated judgment on your part. You have to decide which point leads you towards the conclusion. Which point or points make the POC persuasive or conclusive?

Example 3.4

'It's very stuffy in the ward today; let's open the windows.'

The premise here is that the ward is stuffy.

3. Number and Label the Premises

The standard form of a logical outline is a numbered list of propositions with a label attached to each of them in brackets. In a moment we will illustrate how this should be set out.

There are different kinds of premises and it is important to understand these if you are to understand arguments. Most books on logic say that premises fall into two broad categories, namely, factual claims and value claims (hence the title of our book). If we were to use our terminology from the previous chapter, we would describe premises as informative, hortatory or evaluative. However, to make the kinds of distinctions we need, these categories won't quite do either. Accordingly, the labels that we use to classify premises in logical outlines are as follows:

- fact
- assertion
- value
- exhortation
- side comment
- assumption.

Let us discuss each of these in turn.

Facts

Any informative proposition in an argument that you can agree with you should label as a **fact**. (There may be other informative propositions in the text which you consider contentious and you will label them differently.) The clearest examples of premises which are to be labelled as facts are informative propositions with which you can expect anyone (including yourself) to agree. By labeling a premise as a fact you are signalling that you agree with it or acknowledge it is an item of general knowledge which you accept. A premise labelled 'fact' will not be contentious and if you should want to offer a critique or refutation of the argument, you will not be inclined to challenge the facts in it.

Example 3.5

> 'It's very stuffy in the ward today; let's open the windows.'

Let us take it that everyone is walking around in the ward perspiring and the patients are showing signs of discomfort and heat stress. In that context, the premise that it is stuffy in the ward can be taken to be a fact. (Of course, the POC that the windows should be opened might not be established as the conclusion of the argument, because it might be hotter outside or there might be better ways of cooling the ward down such as switching on the airconditioning.)

Another instance of a premise that should be labelled as a fact is when the author offers credible support for it. One way in which this is frequently done is by citing research or other sources. The point in question might have a footnote or a citation attached to it which gives you the source from which it was drawn. This gives you the opportunity to look up the book or article in question should you want to. Even if you do not look it up, you can be confident that the point has appropriate backing in research and scholarship and you should accept it as a fact. It does not do to be excessively sceptical when reading texts, otherwise you would never learn anything new. On the other hand, if the whole argument rests upon a point which is drawn from other sources in this way, the author would do well to support that point by telling you how it was arrived at in the first place.

Example 3.6

> 'It's very stuffy in the ward today, and recent research done by Professor Sweaty has shown that hospital airconditioning units can carry dangerous bacteria; let's open the windows.'

The point about the dangers of the airconditioning is a premise because it leads to the conclusion that the windows should be opened and it can be deemed a fact because the research which established it is cited (albeit without full bibliographical details).

Assertions

In contrast to a fact, an **assertion** is an informative proposition which the author of the text has put forward without argument, but which might be contentious. Typically, it will be contentious because the author has not provided enough evidence for it, or because there are reputable sources of information which affirm different and incompatible informative propositions. In short, you, as reader of the text, are not fully convinced of the informative proposition in question. You label this premise an assertion and should you want to criticise the argument you will suggest that more support is needed for this proposition. Sometimes we respond to an assertion by saying or thinking that the author is merely assuming that proposition to be true. And this way of speaking might lead us to label such a premise as an assumption. However, that is not the way we use the word 'assumption'. As we will explain presently, an assumption is a premise that is not stated at all. When an informative premise is offered without adequate evidence we call it an assertion.

Whether you label a premise as a fact or as an assertion will depend on your own knowledge of the field in question and on your perception of what could be expected to be commonly accepted background information. (This is why shared background knowledge is an important element in communication.) It might also depend upon your confidence in the authorities cited in support of the proposition, or on your knowledge of the speaker. This is a matter for subtle judgment.

Example 3.7

> 'It's very stuffy in the ward today, and it's dangerous to use the airconditioning; let's open the windows.'

In this version of our example, let us take it that the speaker is an older person who is known to be very suspicious of modern technology; 'new fangled gadgets' she calls them. Notice that the speaker has offered no reason or authority for the view that the airconditioning is dangerous. In this case, while the proposition that the airconditioning is dangerous is a premise in that it is intended to convince you of the POC, you should label it as an assertion.

Values

You should label as a **value** any proposition on the part of the author which expresses what the author finds important, or valuable, or regrettable or deplorable. In short, any proposition which expresses the author's attitude, or a generally held attitude, to the matter at hand should be labelled as a value statement.

Example 3.8

> 'It's very stuffy in the ward today, and it is important that patients don't suffer heat stress; let's open the windows.'

In this version of our example, there is a new premise, namely that it is important that patients do not suffer heat stress. On account of its wording (note the signpost; 'it is important that'), this premise expresses a value and should be labelled as such. Value premises can be very complex or subtle.

Any expressive proposition which conveys the author's attitude or feelings about the matter at hand should be labelled as a value statement.

Example 3.9

'Gosh, I hate this heat in the ward today; let's open the windows.'

In this further variation on our example, the speaker has expressed her or his dislike for the heat. This is the reason for the POC and so it is a premise. It should be labelled as a value.

To identify a value premise can require subtle judgment. Values are frequently hidden in propositions that look informative. For example, to say of an incident that it is a case of murder might look like an informative description . But, even if it is, it also conveys the author's attitude to the incident in question because most people disapprove of murder. (A premise can also be a definition and we will discuss this kind of premise in Part Three of this book.)

Exhortations

One should label as an **exhortation** any proposition in which the author says what should or should not be done. An exhortation urges people to act. Accordingly, we should also include under this classification the imperative or directive communications which we discussed in the previous chapter.

Example 3.10

'Windows should be opened when the ward is stuffy. It's very stuffy in the ward today; let's open the windows.'

Yet another argument for our POC. This time there is a premise which expresses a general policy as to what should be done in particular circumstances. This premise is an exhortation.

Policies can be expressed with the use of such words as 'should' or 'ought' and are therefore clearly identifiable as exhortations. However, we can also express an exhortation by saying such things as, 'It is a good idea to open the windows when the ward is stuffy'. Notice the word 'good' which makes such premises sound like value statements. However, they are clearly hortatory in nature because they urge us to do certain things.

Exhortations do not frequently occur as premises in scientific texts, but they do occur very often in texts which are concerned with public policy issues or with advocating a particular course of action to solve problems. Such texts will also make frequent reference to the values in pursuit of which certain things should be done, or to the attitudes of the author. In short, value premises are common in hortatory texts. For this reason value premises and hortatory premises can be hard to distinguish from each other and many logic text books do not distinguish them. We will discuss these distinctions more fully in Chapter 12.

Just as value statements can look like informative ones, so too can exhortations. One can think of cases where an exhortation might be accepted as a fact. If we say that it is the responsibility of the government to provide adequate health care for all, we are saying, in general terms, what the government ought to do. As such it may seem like a hortatory statement. However, it is now so widely accepted in our kind of society that this is indeed a responsibility of government, that it can be taken to be a fact that the government has that task. Just how the government ought to exercise that responsibility—what policies it should put into effect—is more contentious, and the various proposals put forward will depend upon the value positions of their proponents. Such proposals will be exhortations.

Example 3.11

> 'State enrolled nurses are useful assistants in the hospital system.
> They should always follow instructions from registered nurses.'

In this new example, the POC is that State enrolled nurses should always follow instructions from registered nurses. This is an exhortation. The premise certainly looks grammatically like a factual or informative statement (the word 'are' appears), but it is an example of a definition which specifies what State enrolled nurses should do. As such it implies an exhortation. (Again, we will return to definitions that have hortatory effects in Chapter 12.)

Exercise 3.4

The following propositions could form premises in an argument. Label each of them: fact, assertion, value or exhortation.

1. It is vital that drips be monitored carefully.
2. Epilepsy does not interfere greatly with the daily life of most sufferers.
3. Peppermint tea cures bed sores.
4. Hospital funding should be increased.
5. People with dementia have poor short-term memory.
6. Nursing students ought to have longer clinical placements.
7. Back pain really gets me down.
8. Abortion is murder.

Side Comments

In a well written text, any point which is relevant to the POC should be a premise. Any point which does not lead you to be convinced of the POC is irrelevant. The special name we give to such points is **side comment**. Strictly speaking a side comment need not appear in your logical outline, since it is not part of the argument. But since most people write their logical outlines by first writing a topical outline, the irrelevant points also get listed. This is acceptable provided that such points are then identified as being side comments.

Many texts begin with a section which sets the stage, as it were, for the argument which follows. The author might recount the incident which set him or her off on the train of thought which follows. Or they might give a summary of previous research in the area in question together with a description of some problems which that research has left unresolved. Letters to newspapers frequently refer to items in that newspaper to which the letter writer is responding. Such matters are important for understanding the text, but they are not part of the argument. As such, they can be left out or, if listed, labelled as side comment.

Example 3.12

'I had a very hot and uncomfortable trip into the hospital today. Gosh, isn't it stuffy in the ward; let's open the windows.'

This further version of our now somewhat overworked example is more complex than it looks. The POC is still that the windows should be opened. One way of reading this text is to see it as offering two reasons for the POC: that the ward is stuffy, and that the speaker is hot and uncomfortable. In this case, both these propositions would be premises, with the latter being a fact (if we can all see that the speaker is in heat-related discomfort). But we envisage that the speaker has mentioned her trip to work merely to make conversation. In this case it is side comment. (Yet the comment is not completely unrelated to the POC because it refers to the heat of the day. If she had told us that she had gone to the movies the night before, her comment would be totally irrelevant.)

Like facts, assertions, values and exhortations, side comments should be identified by putting that label in brackets at the end of the numbered premise in your logical outline. We will illustrate this in a moment.

Assumptions

An **assumption** is a proposition which is not openly stated, but which the author of the text takes for granted. It can be an assumption about some matter of fact, about a value or about what the author thinks should be done. It is difficult to use this term without confusion in critical thinking because it is used in many different ways in modern English. Moreover, different books on informal logic and critical thinking define this and other terms differently. Some say that an assumption is something which is stated, but without support. Others define an assumption as a proposition, explicit or otherwise, that refers to background knowledge which can be taken for granted. We would argue that in the latter case we should label the explicit proposition as a fact, while in the former case we should label the unsupported proposition which is contentious as an assertion.

In everyday speech, many people use the notion of an assumption to describe a proposition that they disagree with or which they think has no support. They will say that an author is just assuming that something is the case without having enough evidence or warrant for saying it. In the present context this usage of the term is misleading. Lastly, some authors use the word assumption to identify an axiom or a supposition which the author wants the audience to accept for the sake of the argument. They might say, 'Let us assume that . . .', and then go on to draw conclusions from that axiom. In our usage, such a statement should be labelled as an assertion.[2] These differences in terminology and meaning can be confusing and annoying to the beginning critical thinker. But don't give up. The important thing is to choose a set of terms, say what they mean, and then stick to them consistently. This is what we do here.

The defining characteristics of an assumption in our terminology are that it is not stated and that it is crucial to the argument. As such, an assumption is a hidden premise. Usually, the author makes assumptions because he or she thinks that the audience shares the point of view in question so it does not need to be stated. If an author were to state such a point of view, it would be signposted with some such phrase as, 'of course . . .' or 'it goes without saying that . . .'. (But these signposts do not appear in the text in order to identify assumptions because, by definition, assumptions are not stated.)

Assumptions are usually harmless. As we explained in Chapter 2, every communication depends upon a body of shared knowledge which does not need to be stated. Take this example:

Example 3.13

> A patient says to a nurse finishing her shift: 'There are clouds coming up, so you had better take your umbrella.'

Now, the POC is that the nurse should take her umbrella and the premise is that there are clouds coming up. But if you look more carefully at this argument, you will see that there are also a number of unstated or hidden premises. These include:

- Clouds indicate that rain is likely.
- Rain will cause you to get wet.
- It is undesirable to get wet.
- Umbrellas protect you from rain.

It would be time consuming and boring to state all of these premises every time we wanted to advise someone to take their umbrella. They are part of the background knowledge and attitudes we all share. There is no reason to state them.

The problem arises when an assumption turns out to be false, controversial or not shared by the audience, even though it seems completely obvious to the author of the argument. In Example 3.13, it is possible to imagine this arising with both the value assumption and the informative assumptions. Let's take the value assumption first. The patient has assumed that it is preferable not to get wet. But the nurse may not share this attitude. Perhaps it is a very hot sultry summer day, and she would be happy to get wet—it would cool her down a bit after working in the un-airconditioned ward. Or take the last of the informative assumptions. It may be that the nurse's umbrella was blown inside-out in a storm the day before and is now totally useless. Here again, what the patient thought was obvious turns out not to be. It often happens that the source of disagreements between people is hard to find because, while they agree on the premises that have been stated, they disagree on the hidden assumptions. (We will return to this matter in the next chapter.)

But there is an important point to be made here. A logical outline must occasionally supply premises which are not actually present in the text, but which are necessary for the argument to be complete. Once again, the audience of the text has to exercise subtle judgments here. A principle of generosity should apply. We should not refuse to supply premises which it is reasonable to attribute to the author, simply because the author has not stated them. We must assume that the author is intelligent, and we must acknowledge the shared background knowledge that we all have with the author, which makes it unnecessary to supply all the information needed in the argument. On the other hand, one should not supply hidden premises to an argument which it would be unreasonable to expect the author to agree with. This would be too generous.

Example 3.14

'It's very stuffy in the ward today; let's open the windows.'

If the suggestion to open the windows makes any sense to its audience, it must be assumed that there is a relatively cool breeze outside. If everyone knows this, it will be taken for granted. But if you, as the audience for this utterance, do not know it, then you might wonder whether it is so. You will certainly take it that the speaker assumes it to be so. In this instance, your outline should include that proposition as a premise and you would label it as an assumption.

In order to leave room for such labels as fact, assertion, value or exhortation, assumptions should be identified by placing them in brackets in your logical outline.

Exercise 3.5

In each of the following arguments write down the important assumptions that the author is making. State whether the assumption is a fact, assertion, value or exhortation.

1. There has been a car accident on the freeway. Therefore we need more staff in the emergency department.
2. A recent study by the Australian Institute of Family Studies showed that 40% of mothers work outside the home. To correct this problem, the government must increase family allowances.
3. Many of the patients in this hospital were born overseas, so we need to recruit more nurses who speak languages other than English.
4. This child does not want to have an injection, so it would be wrong for the nurse to give it to him.

4. Identify the Conclusion

The **conclusion** is the point that the premises lead you towards. In a well formed argument, it will be the same as the POC. You identify it by putting in brackets after it, not the word 'conclusion', but the numbers of the premises from which it follows.

With our terminology in place we can now offer a simple example of a logical outline.

Example 3.15

'It's very stuffy in the ward today; let's open the windows.'

The logical outline of this simple argument would be:

POC: The windows should be opened.
1. It's very stuffy in the ward today. (fact)
(2. There are no other ways of cooling the ward.) (fact)
3. The windows should be opened. (1,2)

One matter which complicates things considerably is that many arguments reach subsidiary conclusions before they draw the final conclusion. Various premises will lead to conclusions which are needed as premises in their turn before the final conclusion can be reached. You should note these conclusions in your outline. You may even have to formulate them yourself, if they are not drawn explicitly by the author, just as you did with hidden premises or assumptions. The number that you have assigned to such a **nested conclusion** should then appear as one of the premises from which the final conclusion is drawn.

Perhaps it is time we illustrated all of this with some examples. Take the following argument:

Example 3.16

Regular colonoscopies can reduce the risk of colon cancer, because they can detect and remove pre-cancerous growths called polyps. But very few people are aware of the advantages of colonoscopy. Therefore the government should introduce an advertising campaign to educate the public.

For this argument we would suggest the following outline:

POC: The government should introduce an advertising campaign to educate the public.
1. Regular colonoscopies can detect and remove pre-cancerous growths. (fact)
2. Colonoscopies can reduce the risk of colon cancer. (1)
3. Few people are aware of the advantages. (side comment)
(4. More people should be aware.) (exhortation)

5. The government should introduce an advertising campaign to educate the public (2,4, exhortation)

We call premise 1 a fact because we take this to be well known or at least something that the audience would be inclined to agree with. Premise 2 is a nested conclusion drawn from 1. In the argument, this is signposted with the word 'because'. We might have drawn the conclusion directly from premises 2 and 3, but we thought that there was an assumption being made, namely that more people should know about this procedure. We think that premise 4 is an assumption without which 3 would not be relevant. Indeed, with the assumption spelt out, premise 3 becomes a side comment. It is the assumption that leads to the conclusion. The relevant point is that more people should know about colonoscopies.

We could have expressed premise 4 as a value (as in, 'It would be good if more people knew about it') rather than as an exhortation (as in the form we have given it). But, as we will explain more fully in Chapter 12, we needed an exhortation among the premises if the conclusion was going to be an exhortation.

Now here is a more extended example. This is a text of the kind that often appears as a letter to a newspaper.

Example 3.17

> The practice of multiple organ donation should stop, at least until there has been full and frank public discussion of the matter. The public in general does not know what really happens in organ donation, and it is not acceptable to go on pretending that there is public support for something which the public has no knowledge of.
>
> The retrieval of organs is not a dignified process, even though the families of organ donors are assured that the body of their loved one is treated with respect. In fact, it is treated more like a supermarket, with retrieval teams racing in, cutting out a liver or a kidney, then racing out again. Often, more than six organs are removed, by six different teams.
>
> How would the family feel if they could hear all this talk about 'harvesting the organs'? On many occasions, the family does not even have a chance to say a proper goodbye to their loved one, since the hospital is more interested in retrieving as many organs as possible than in assisting the family's grieving.
>
> Nurses find the practice disturbing, especially those who are responsible for monitoring the 'beating heart cadaver'. There should be more study of the effects on those who are involved in the practice of organ donation before it is allowed to continue.

Now, let us write a logical outline of this text together. The first question to answer is, what is the point of contention (POC)? We would suggest that the POC is:

> The practice of multiple organ donation should stop until there has been a full debate on it.

The premises that lead to this conclusion are:

1. The general public doesn't know what happens. (assertion)
2. There is no public support for multiple organ donation (1)
3. The cadaver is treated like a supermarket. (value)
4. Families often do not have a chance to say goodbye to the deceased when there is multiple organ donation. (fact)
5. Multiple organ donation is not a dignified process. (3,4, value)
6. Multiple organ donation disturbs nurses. (fact)
(7. There has not been enough study of the effect on those who are involved.) (assertion)

And the conclusion is:

8. The practice of multiple organ donation should stop until such a study is done. (2,5,6,7, exhortation)

Notice firstly, that this conclusion is not exactly the same as the POC. It is sufficiently similar for there not to be a problem, but it would appear that the author has gone off the point slightly. Perhaps the author is a nurse who, having mentioned the reaction of nurses to the practice, then focuses upon it to the detriment of the main thrust of the argument. What he or she should be advocating is a full public debate, not just a study of the effects on those involved, particularly nurses.

We call premise 1 an assertion rather than a fact, because the author has not presented evidence for it. Are there surveys of public knowledge and attitudes? On the other hand, the audience might feel that this point is not contentious, in which case it would be accepted as a fact. We think premise 2 is a nested conclusion drawn from premise 1. Premises 3 and 4 are put forward by someone who knows. If one assumes that the author is a nurse who has seen what happens, then we can accept that what is being said is true. On the other hand, if we thought the author was a lay person who is merely surmising that what goes on is as undignified as this, then we should label those premises assertions and we would be justified in asking for evidence. (Notice the importance of having some idea of who the author is.) Premise 5 is a nested conclusion drawn from these premises even though there is no signpost in the text which would indicate this.

We call premise 6 a fact because, once again, we assume the author is a nurse who is in a position to know this. We would call it an assertion if we doubted the ability of the author to be sure that this was true.

Premise 7 is not formulated in this form in the text. The statement in the text is an exhortation that more study should be done. In this form it would be an irrelevant side comment. If it is to add to the argument as the author clearly intends (he or she says it should be done 'before [the practice] is allowed to continue'), then it must be rendered in the form that we have given it.

We call premise 7 an assertion because no evidence has been presented for it. In fact, it is very hard to present evidence for negative statements like this. The author would have had to scour a vast body of scientific and sociological literature to know how many studies had been done and then he or she would have had to decide that this was not enough. But how do we decide how much is enough? There is a vagueness here which vitiates the argument somewhat. It would have been better if the author had been able to say that the studies which had been done showed that the effect on nurses was harmful. This would have strengthened the conclusion considerably.

With these examples before us, we can now summarise how to write logical outlines.

Hints for Writing Logical Outlines

1. Look for 'signposts'.
2. If these are absent you may need to supply them yourself (though be sure that you do not change the meaning if you do).
3. Supply any unstated premises. (Such premises should be necessary to the argument and put in brackets as assumptions.)
4. Notice any 'nested' arguments (where a premise is the conclusion of a previous argument).
5. Do not assume that the POC will be stated or will be the same as the conclusion.

Exercise 3.6

Write a logical outline of the following argument, numbering and labelling the premises and indicating any assumptions or nested conclusions.

> This institution is about to suffer a major funding cut. Clinical staff numbers are already critically low, so no further cuts can be made in that area. So we suggest that administrative staff have dry biscuits for morning tea, instead of their current Danish pastries.

Exercise 3.7

Write a logical outline of the following imaginary letter to a newspaper.

> It is appalling that there is a waiting list for elective surgery of almost two years at some public hospitals. The Government is clearly not providing adequate funds.
>
> Every citizen has a right to adequate health care. Whether you are a victim of a road accident, or an elderly person needing a hip replacement, this right is not lessened simply because the surgery is 'elective' in only the second case. Needless suffering is being caused by the failure of governments to address this issue.

Exercise 3.8

Write a logical outline of the following item which is based on a letter to a newspaper at about the time of the Los Angeles riots.

> Brian Harris claims that the ever-increasing preponderance of young over old in Australia will be corrected if the Federal Government ceases to fund 'more than 60,000 abortions a year'. Yet the writer of the leading letter in the same paper, Bill Walker, warns that Australia's 'swelling masses of unemployed' could explode into the sort of violence and bloodshed we have witnessed in Los Angeles.
>
> With jobs both scarce and precarious when held, how will the extra 60,000 children Brian Harris wants born annually be supported? Perhaps Mr Harris envisages that unemployed parents will offer their babies for adoption? But adoptive parents can become unemployed, just as they can become widowed or divorced. And women I know who have experienced both adoption and abortion say that they find the former the more traumatic.

Exercise 3.9

Write a logical outline of the following item which is based on another letter to a newspaper at about the time of the Los Angeles riots.[3]

> While watching the news from Los Angeles last week, a friend commented to me that 'it could only happen in America'. I was stunned. How obviously wrong he is. It is so easy for me to imagine the same riots here after similar injustice is passed by our legal system.
>
> How close to America we are. How similar our bloody history, how well-disguised our racial tensions behind a veneer of egalitarianism. How horribly unequal is our equal society. And how little our governments are interested in changing that. I sit in my safe, white middle-class suburb, but I can hear the wind blowing, and I feel it is merely a matter of time.

Exercise 3.10

Write a logical outline of the following item which is based on a letter to a newspaper.

> I am appalled that the debate on medical provision in Australia has now reached the level of 'What patients shall we let die because their treatment is too expensive?'
>
> I am certain that if the vast mass of Australians realised that the debate had moved to this point, there would be an outcry. Sadly, I suspect the debate will be the preserve of the well-educated, the better-off, the bureaucrats and the politicians, and those who read 'quality' newspapers.
>
> How shameful that one possible area of cuts is neo-natal intensive care. Tiny babies can't argue with cold financial experts. Middle-aged smokers needing coronary bypasses can. Guess who will lose out.

I have a better suggestion. Double the tax on cigarettes to pay for illnesses caused by passive smoking. And make those with smoking-related illness who smoke themselves pay for their own treatment, if they can. If they cannot, tough. They cannot say they have not been warned.

My daughter was in a neo-natal intensive care unit for five days before she died. The wonderful, saintly staff, and the unbelievably brilliant technology, gave her a chance to survive.

Anyone who thinks she should not have had that chance can come around to our place any time and debate it with my wife.

Exercise 3.11

Write a logical outline of the following text:

> Discussing their impending death with patients is never easy, but nurses must nevertheless not shy away from this vital task. Some nurses may believe that such discussions are always best left to the experts—the social worker or the chaplain—but this is not so. In many ways, the nurse is the best placed to talk about these matters. The social worker and the chaplain, while in some senses better trained to deal with discussions of death, are simply not always there when the patient wants to talk. And more importantly, the patient may not *want* to talk to them: many a chaplain has experienced the suspicious silence or false cheeriness of a dying patient, only to learn from the nursing staff later that the same patient has spent hours talking to one of the nurses, or even a nursing student. The reason is not hard to find, of course: the chaplain is a stranger, and perhaps represents an institution which the patient has rejected, whereas the nurse is familiar, more like a friend, and non-threatening. So if nurses shy away from talking with a patient about death, they may be leaving that patient with no-one to talk to: and surely this is something none of us would want to have happen.

Exercise 3.12

Go back to Exercise 2.1 and write a logical outline of the first of the five texts listed there.

NOTES

1. *The Age*, Melbourne, 2 November 1993.
2. This label does not fit very comfortably since the proposition is not being offered for the audience to believe. There would be no harm in expanding our terminology to fit this and other cases that seem to fall outside of our categories. In this instance, you might want to label the premise as a 'supposition'. But in either case the effect on the audience is the same. As with an assertion, the audience will seek assurance that it is true before it accepts any conclusions drawn from it.
3. Letter to *The Age*, Melbourne, May 1993.

Chapter 4

Debate: Mounting and Evaluating Arguments

This chapter describes strategies for developing your own arguments and for offering critiques of others' arguments. Some premises in an argument will be crucial, and it is suggested how these are identified. Other strategies include asking questions, exploring implications and proposing better alternatives.

In the previous chapter, we described how to write logical outlines of arguments to demonstrate the structural elements in an argument and how the conclusion of the argument has been reached. One purpose of this exercise is to ensure that you have understood the argument correctly. But another possible purpose is to enable you to dispute the argument effectively. There will be many occasions in which you find yourself disagreeing with what someone has said to you or with something that you have read. If you are to do more than merely state your disagreement or counter with a different point of contention of your own—a response which would turn the communication into a quarrel or dispute on the model of, 'yes, it is', 'no, it isn't'—then you must identify what you think is wrong with the argument that has been presented to you and mount a critique. You may also want to offer your own point of view supported by reasons. If all this takes place you would be engaging in a **debate**.

We define a debate as a juxtaposition of two (or more) arguments with opposite or inconsistent points of contention. Usually these two arguments will have different authors, although people can debate with themselves, as it were, such as when they deliberate over a difficult matter and present themselves with different reasons for doing different things. Debates can take place in face-to-face situations or through written texts such as books or newspaper articles. Most often, a debate has the purpose of reaching an agreement. There are debates which are engaged in as formal competitions in which the verbal skills and wit of one team are pitted against those of another. We will not be primarily concerned with this notion of a formal debate, although much of what we say will be applicable to this sort of contest. Our primary focus will be upon discussions where debaters are genuinely concerned to convince one another about a point of view, an explanation, a policy or a particular course of action, and where only one resolution is being sought. In this context, there will be winners and losers only in the sense that one point of contention ends up being agreed to by all parties to the debate.

Of course such debates should be marked by genuine dialogue so that everyone is listening sympathetically to the point of view of others. As a result a decision can be reached which represents a compromise between the different positions initially urged by the various participants.

As we noted in Chapter 1, debates are not the only contexts in which nurses use critical thinking skills. As a nurse, you might write a memo to your supervisors, a letter to the newspaper, or a prepared speech. There are many occasions in the professional life of a nurse where it is necessary to prepare and develop cogent arguments to convince others of your point of view, including those which involve the many responsibilities that a nurse has in relation to health education. Another significant professional area in which the skill of formulating an argument will be relevant is that of writing nursing reports. All too often nursing reports consist of jottings about everything that has happened to a patient, everything that a patient has done and everything that the nurse has thought about this. There should, however, be some discrimination and judgement on the part of the nurse as to what is important and relevant to such a report.

And, of course, if you are a student, you should be developing your debating skills in every student essay that you write. You should always imagine that you are trying to convince an audience of people like yourself (rather than imagine that you are trying to impress your teachers). With an imaginary audience in mind you can anticipate what that audience needs to know and how they might possibly object to what you are trying to say. As a result, you will support your contentious points and develop clear lines of argument.

Whatever form a debate takes, there are at least two possible approaches to debating the point of contention that someone else is proposing. Sometimes one approach is used, sometimes another, and very often a debater will use both. There is a negative approach in which the debater seeks to question or undermine the conclusions of the other, and there is a positive approach in which the debater seeks to establish their own point of contention with sufficient force to convince the other party of it. We will begin by describing this positive approach first.

How to Develop Your Own Arguments

The part of a debate which involves offering reasons in support of your point of view is easy to understand. It is a mirror image, as it were, of writing a logical outline of an argument. You start with the outline and develop the argument from that. In conversational contexts, you would do this spontaneously and without too much deliberation, but when you are able to prepare an argument ahead of time you should take the steps that correspond to those of a logical outline.

1. Identify the Assumptions of the Audience

Before we go on to describe the steps involved in outlining your own arguments, it is important to ask yourself a question: What do I actually need to argue for in this debate or presentation? The import of this question is that you should have some idea of who your audience is and what views they already have on the matters at hand. If you are a nurse engaged in a health awareness campaign and you want to convince your audience that it is important to wash their hands before eating, it will make a difference whether your audience is a group of primary school children or a group of homeless people. You would expect that the basic attitudes to personal cleanliness, and the receptiveness to messages about cleanliness, will differ for these two groups. So you have to make an educated guess about what assumptions your audience will bring to the discussion, and you should begin your presentation on the basis of these assumptions. You can take it that the primary school children will assume that cleanliness is important, or at least that anything the visiting community nurse tells them is important, and so all you really need to tell them is how to do it. With the homeless group, on the other hand, you will need to reach further back, as it were, and you will need to establish in their minds the importance of cleanliness. And you could only do this by appealing to attitudes which you can assume them to have, such as positive attitudes to survival. You might argue that they will only maintain the strength to survive on the streets and do the things they want to do if they maintain their health, and this requires a degree of cleanliness.

The only basis from which you can convince somebody of anything is the basis of the attitudes, beliefs and values that they already have. If you do not build your argument on this basis, but begin with different assumptions, then you will not be convincing. So the first step in developing your argument is to be aware of what your audience already believes and what they take to be important.

2. Identify Your Point of Contention

It goes without saying that you should be clear in your own mind what it is that you want to argue for. In an essay, it is always a good strategy to tell your reader right at the beginning what the essay is about and what point it will be trying to establish. Similarly, in a spoken discourse, it helps both you and the audience to focus on the issues at hand if you announce what your point of contention is.

You should plan you argument or your essay carefully. Public speakers often use little cards or other forms of written notes, and writers also use notes jotted down to indicate the outline of what they want to write. In some cases such notes might take the form of topical outlines, but where the text contains an argument and is being put together in order to convince the audience of a point of view (student essays can be of either type), the planning of that text should take the form of a logical outline. You should know ahead of time exactly how you are going to draw your conclusion and what the premises are that you are going to draw it from. Your plan, like an outline, will consist of a series of numbered statements which are labelled so as to identify their logical status (fact, value, etc.)

and it will show the nested and final conclusions of your argument by identifying the premises that lead to them.

3. Use Signposts

As you develop your argument, is it helpful both to yourself and to your audience if you make clear how your points relate to the point of contention. The best way to do this is to use lots of signposts, especially ones that demonstrate logical relationships such as, 'because', 'therefore' and 'so'. You could even make your reasoning very explicit by using such phrases as, 'In support of my claim, I offer the following considerations, firstly, . . .' and so forth.

We have found in our experience as teachers over the years that students very often write essays which have next to no signposts in them. These essays read like a series of points, and it takes considerable effort for the reader to detect how the points are linked and what is the structure of thought that lies behind them. Such essays do not do well, and their authors are not likely to be critical thinkers. The same problem is shared by some writers of journal articles, research papers, nursing reports and so forth. You must make the structure of your argument just as obvious as its content. Your audience must find it easy to identify which of your statements are premises, which are side comments and which are conclusions. Nested conclusions should be identified with such signposts as 'It follows from the conclusion we have just drawn that . . .', and so forth. You should also identify assumptions in your own thinking and, if you think that your audience may not share them, you should state them clearly and support them if you can. In this way, they will no longer be assumptions in our sense of that term, but factual or value claims for which you are prepared to argue.

4. Anticipate Possible Objections

This is a logical strategy which we have not discussed before but which is used by many debaters and writers of essays and articles. In the course of arguing for your own position you might imagine, or know from past experience, what your opponents are going to say. You might know how they usually argue for the position that you disagree with because you have read their books and articles, or you might know what attitudes they have and how they differ from yours. And so you are in a position to steal their thunder, as it were, and anticipate their objections. To do this you will have to mention their point of view and, in order to avoid possible confusion, you should signpost this clearly. You do not want your audience to think that you are espousing the view that you are going to mention. Suitable signposts are:

It may be objected that . . .
My opponent will say that . . .

And you might follow the statement of your opponent's view with:

Against this, I argue that . . .
The objection assumes that . . .

and you then mount an argument against the assumption or objection so as to rob that objection of any force.

You should not begin your speech or begin writing your article or essay until you have written out a thorough plan on the model of a logical outline.

Summary of Features of a Good Essay or Article

1. States the POC clearly at the beginning.
2. Offers arguments in favour of the POC.
3. Uses evidence to support these arguments.
4. Raises possible counter-arguments or objections.
5. Deals with these counter-arguments.
6. Uses plenty of signposts to make the structure clear.
7. Uses plain, clear English, and avoids unnecessary jargon.
8. Does not contradict itself: argues consistently for the same POC throughout.

Exercise 4.1

Write out the plan/logical outline of arguments which you might present for or against the following propositions.

1. Nurses should be protected by law if they assist a patient to die when that patient is terminally and painfully ill, requests assistance to die and is competent to make such a request. (Imagine that you are addressing an audience of nurses.)
2. Condom vending machines should be placed in all secondary schools. (Imagine you are a health worker addressing a meeting of school principals.)
3. In general, wealthy people tend to be healthier than poor people. (Imagine you are a student writing an essay.)
4. Nursing students and medical students should study together for the first two years of their courses. (Imagine that you are a nurse educator writing a submission to a government inquiry.)
5. Alcohol should be made illegal. (Imagine you are engaged in a conversation with your uncle, who is a publican.)

Evaluation of Arguments

We turn now to the negative part of the craft of the debater, that of evaluating and attacking the arguments of one's opponents. From the very start, remember that you are engaged in a dialogue. It can sometimes happen that, after spending more time trying to understand an argument you disagree with, you come to see its value and change your own position. For this reason, we do not describe the negative approach to debating as 'critique', as this seems to assume that you will find the author to be in error just because you have disagreed with them. Rather, we will describe the process as evaluating an argument, which leaves it open whether you will criticise it or agree with it. It is important to be openminded, even when you evaluate an argument that you disagree with.

However, the process does usually start from disagreement. You might be listening to a speaker, or reading an article or book, and you are struck by a feeling of disagreement with the author. If you are going to express this disagreement but do more than engage in a mere quarrel, then you will have to be able to show exactly why you disagree. You might not share the fundamental values and attitudes of the author, and in this case there is probably not much room for debate. The best you can do is point out the values which you and the author do not share. But in many cases you may very well agree with the fundamental values of the author, but not with the conclusions that he or she draws from them and from other premises. In this case, you should be able to say at what point in the author's argument you think there has been an error leading to the view that you disagree with. If you disagree with the conclusion and the argument is sound, then you cannot agree with all of the premises. Either there must be at least one premise with which you disagree, or there must be an error in the structure of the argument. In either case, if you are going to argue against the author's position effectively, you must be able to identify the point at which your disagreement begins.

We can sum this up by saying that there are two basic questions you should ask about any argument:

1. Are the premises true?
2. Does the conclusion follow logically from the premises?

However, you will not be able to deal with these questions effectively unless you complete the following steps:

1. Write a Logical Outline

It will be obvious that the first step in developing an evaluation of an author's argument is to write a logical outline of that argument. In this way the structure of the argument will be apparent, as will be the pared-down content of the premises. This content will be subject to our first question above, as we will explain in a moment. The structure of the argument will be subject to our second question above. To answer this question will require familiarity with the rules of logic. We will be explaining these in the next chapters.

2. Identify Assumptions

The most important part of getting the argument clear is ensuring that you have all of it in front of you. To do this you must see whether the author is making any assumptions which are important links in the argument. Such assumptions should be articulated and written down as part of the logical outline. Some sensitivity to the audience is required in order to do this effectively. It is all too easy to take it for granted that the author shares the same attitudes as yourself, especially on matters of value or exhortation. You may need to attend to the text very carefully to see whether this is so. If you find, when you identify their assumptions, that the author has differing attitudes from yourself, then you will have identified an important point upon which to base your evaluation. And you will also have identified a major obstacle to being able to convince this other person of your own point of view.

We have already indicated that, when you develop your own counter-argument, you should begin from the attitudes of your audience. It is at this point that the negative and positive approaches in a debate converge. The negative phase can have as its aim, not just the undermining of the credibility of your opponent's argument, but also the stripping back of their argument to the fundamental attitudes that are inherent in it. Once you have identified the assumptions that an author has made on the basis of their attitudes and discovered attitudes that you can agree with yourself, you can build up your own argument on the basis of those shared attitudes. It would be very rare for parties to a debate to share no attitudes at all. Both advocates and opponents of abortion agree that human life is important. Progress towards agreement can be made when shared beliefs and values are found. A premise that both you and your opponents agree with is the only possible starting point of an argument if you are to reach a conclusion that you can both agree with.

3. Identify Crucial Premises

We turn now to our first question: Are the premises true? Note that it may be a waste of time to ask this question of every premise. Some premises are more important than others. Even though they are premises from which the conclusion has been drawn, some premises could be deleted from the argument without leaving the conclusion unsupported. Such premises are not crucial. For example, take the following simple argument (set out as an outline).

Example 4.1

POC: Should I take my umbrella?

1.	The weather forecast has predicted rain.	(fact)
2.	There are dark clouds gathering.	(fact)
3.	I should take my umbrella.	(1,2)

In this argument, the conclusion could be drawn from either premise by itself. Each of the premises could be deleted while retaining the other and the conclusion could still be drawn. This means that neither premise is crucial.

On the other hand, if there is a premise which, if it were removed, would leave the point of contention without strong support, then that premise is crucial. Take this case:

Example 4.2

POC: Does the patient have breast cancer?

1.	Tests have shown that the lump on this patient's breast is malignant.	(fact)
2.	The patient's family has a history of breast cancer.	(fact)
3.	The patient has breast cancer.	(1,2)

In this case, premise 1 is crucial to the conclusion. If we only had premise 2 (and the patient had presented with a lump on her breast) we would be right to suspect cancer, but the premise would not be conclusive by itself. Premise 2 contributes to the conclusion but is not crucial to it.

It will be clear that if you are intent upon attacking an author's argument, then you should seek out the crucial premises. It is these crucial premises that you must question.

4. Identify Controversial Premises

The next step is to see if any of the premises, especially the crucial ones, are controversial. By this we do not mean that they might be matters of wide public dispute. We simply mean that they are premises which you can, or would be willing to, contest. These are the premises that raise the question, 'Is this premise actually true?' in your mind. By definition, the premises that you have labelled as facts in your logical outline are not controversial. In labeling them as facts, you have accepted them as being beyond dispute. It is the premises which you have labelled as assertions or assumptions that you should now scrutinise. Are there any which are neither supported nor widely believed? Do you have evidence which would counter those assertions or assumptions? Can you argue that they are not plausible? If they are value assertions, can you argue that different values are more tenable or more widely adhered to? In short, you are looking for the weak link in the argument and trying to snap it.

If you are going to dispute informative assertions, you will need to do research to find out the truth of the matter so as to be able to show that the assertions are false. On the other hand, if the premises that you wish to question are value claims or exhortations, then you will need to argue against them somewhat differently: for example, by showing them to be incoherent, out of touch with widespread opinion, or faulty in some other way. The chapters on ethical reasoning in Part Three of this book discuss how to evaluate arguments involving ethical values and exhortations in detail. Alternatively, you could propose an alternative value or exhortation and support it with arguments of your own.

5. Ask Questions

Asking whether the premises are true is not the only strategy for dealing with the content of your opponent's argument. You can also ask your opponent questions. This strategy is not readily available if you are dealing with a written text, but in the context of a face-to-face debate, it is always a good idea to ask questions. Very often, you might be genuinely seeking more information or clarification of the arguments that are being presented. But questions can also help to undermine the argument. A famous example in the history of philosophy is that of Socrates, an ancient Greek thinker who used the method of asking people questions about their beliefs to bring them to the point where they could see that what they believed was actually quite absurd.

A very useful question which can sometimes have this effect is the simple, 'What do you mean?'. This question asks the author to put his point in different terms and this may have the effect of exposing his argument's weaknesses in a way that the original formulation did not. It sometimes even happens that an author does not know quite what he meant. Asking an author to 'unpack' an argument can be helpful too. To 'unpack' an argument is to elaborate on it. It is to articulate the assumptions that might have been implicit in the first and shorter formulation, and to use more signposts in order to demonstrate the structure of the reasoning. Having been asked to do this, an author might well come to see that their argument was not sound.

In relation to written texts where the author is not present to answer questions, a critic can still use questions to score points. In your written response or in your discussion with others about the text, you might ask rhetorical questions, such as 'What do you suppose the author really means by that?', or 'Are the facts really as the author says they are?' You might not expect an answer, but you are at least pointing to possible weaknesses in the argument. While the strongest attack on the author's assertions would be to show that they are false, when this is not possible because relevant information is hard to obtain quickly, it is a useful debating strategy to raise questions about the assertions. Of course, there have to be reasons why these questions are appropriate. The author's assertions have to be unclear to some extent before it is valid to ask for clarification, and they have to be contentious to some extent before it is valid to ask for evidence to back them up.

Questions can also be useful in the positive approach to debating. If you think you have identified the assumptions that an author is making, you could ask her whether they are indeed assumptions that she holds. If she answers in the affirmative, you could ask her what implications she might draw from her assumptions. It may turn out that not only her point of contention, but also your point of contention, would be supported by her assumptions.

Of course, the asking of questions is a technique that is not only used in the context of debate. There are many occasions when the asking of questions can be part of a cooperative effort of research, decision making or deliberation over policies. It is frequently important to ask questions at committee meetings, for example. Indeed, it is a very helpful thing, both for yourself and for others in a discussion, to be able to ask effective questions. All too often a discussion over policy takes the form of one person saying what they think should be done, followed by another person saying, 'Yes, but I think we should . . .', and then another person chimes in and says, 'No, what I think should happen is . . .' and so on. None of these people is actually listening to what the other is saying. They are so intent upon putting forward their own proposals that they are not taking the time to explore the proposals that others are making. What they should be doing is asking one another questions. The second person should respond to the first proposal by asking 'Why do you think that is a good idea?', or 'What exactly do you mean?', or 'Have you considered this possible outcome if we do that?', and so forth. By a mutual exploring of possibilities the best policy will be arrived at. If the discussion just takes the form of proposal followed by counter proposals it will quickly turn into a dispute in which the decision goes to the most powerful. Such a decision would not benefit from the contributions that all parties to the discussion could make. Making your contribution in the form of a question is a more cooperative strategy than making it by way of a counter proposal.

6. Explore Implications

Another useful strategy in debates, and also in discussions such as those that take place in committees, is to explore the implications of what is said. In this case you might say, 'Suppose we accept your point of contention, what would follow from this?' If you can plausibly suggest that what would follow would be unwelcome, then you will have argued against the POC. In the logic text books, this strategy is called 'reductio ad absurdum' which is Latin for 'reduction to absurdity'. Logicians speak of absurdity because, in its strongest form, the strategy consists in showing that the conclusion of your opponent's argument has incoherent or absurd consequences. However, it is usually quite enough if you can show that the consequences are unwelcome or implausible. Notice that in this form of argument, you do not attack the premises or structure of your opponent's argument.

Example 4.3

> Nurse A: Because it would make it easier to organise our meal breaks at a suitable time, I propose that we arrange our shifts as per this diagram.
>
> Nurse B: It may make meal breaks easier, but if we did that, then those nurses who have university study leave would have to leave work too late to attend lectures.

It is interesting to notice that a reductio argument can work as a positive or as a negative debating strategy. As a negative debating strategy, the argument works by showing that the author's proposal has unwelcome or illogical consequences and therefore should be rejected. But suppose that only two proposals are possible. For example, suppose that there are only two possible shift rosters because of the various time commitments of nursing staff. In this case, showing that nurse A's proposal is unsatisfactory will have the effect of promoting the other alternative. If there are only two options and one of them is shown to have unwelcome implications, then the other option must be taken. In this way, the negative argument against nurse A's proposal becomes a positive argument for the other option.

In a similar way, one can argue for a particular conclusion by excluding alternatives when there are more than two possibilities. Suppose that a detective has three suspects for a murder; Jones, Smith and Jackson. If Jones and Smith both have an alibi, then the finger of suspicion will point to Jackson. This argument is called the Method of Remainders and we will explore it more thoroughly in Chapter 6.

7. Propose a Better Alternative

A debating strategy closely related to the previous one is to propose a better alternative to the proposal of your opponent. This would be an instance of a positive approach to the debate, rather than a negative one. Like the previous strategy, this strategy also accepts the premises and forms of the opponent's argument, at least for the sake of the discussion. When you use this strategy you seek to better your opponent's proposal rather than attack their argument. In the above example, Nurse B might have a better roster ready which solves both the meal break problem and the university study leave problem. Of course, Nurse B would have had to possess a fair bit of foresight to have worked all this out ahead of time. A more likely scenario is that, once the problems with Nurse A's proposal are pointed out, Nurse B will propose that the group work on a new roster which avoids all the known problems. This is not such a strong proposal but it is a better proposal than one which is known to produce problems of its own.

The strategy of proposing a better alternative occurs frequently in science. Theories in science are often maintained even when there are lots of problems with them. Newton's laws of gravitation were subscribed to right up to modern times, even though there were known to be phenomena inconsistent with those laws. It was not until Einstein came up with a better alternative that physicists felt able to relinquish the older orthodoxy in favour of the new theory of relativity. Finding fault with established theories seems to be less effective in making scientists abandon them than the proposing of new and better theories.

8. Attack the Author

This strategy may sound a bit aggressive. It may also sound like what many logicians condemn as the fallacy of arguing 'ad hominem' (which is Latin for 'to the man' or 'at the person'). What this means is that the attack is against the person rather than against the argument, and this is deemed to be improper. However, we would suggest that it is not always improper to attack the author of an argument. If the argument concerned a complex medical diagnosis, we would have the right to expect that the author of the argument had the relevant expertise. If we could show that the author did not have that expertise we would effectively and appropriately undermine their argument.

In a similar way, it would be relevant to the debate if the author of an argument had a conflict of interests. Suppose we were reading a discussion of the relationship between smoking tobacco and lung cancer. We might be struck by the forceful evidence that is being presented which seems to suggest that the danger is not as great as we had been led to believe. Then we look at the notes about the author at the end of the article and we find that she is a spokesperson for a tobacco growers' and cigarette manufacturers' lobby group. Would this make us sceptical? This is a difficult issue because we have to be as fairminded as possible. We should not assume without evidence that the author is lying. Yet we might be aware of the subtle pressures to adopt a particular point of view when one's salary depended upon taking that point of view. It follows that, in a debating context, you would score points against the author of an argument if you could convince your audience that the author had an interest in advancing that view. However, the best way of ensuring that you were being fair in using this strategy would be to enquire into the form and content of that author's arguments to see if there were any errors that you could point to. It would be wrong to jump to the conclusion that the author's argument was unsound simply because of the possible conflict of interests.

9. Find Any Formal Fallacies

The second of our key questions above was, 'Does the conclusion follow logically from the premises?' This is a question about the logic of the argument. Logical or formal fallacies are mistakes in the process of reasoning. We will not be able to explain what we mean by this until we have explained the formally correct structures of reasoning in Chapters 6 and 7. For the moment, suffice it to say that the strongest attack you can mount against an argument is to demonstrate that it has committed a formal logical fallacy: that is, that it has made a mistake in the process of inference or reasoning from premises to conclusion. Such a mistake can be made through flouting the formal rules of logical inference, or through misunderstanding the correct meanings and implications of the key words in the premises. (The latter kind of mistake, when made in the context of ethical reasoning, will be discussed more fully in Part Three of this book.) It will be helpful at this point to say that the best way of detecting formal fallacies is to write out the logical outline of an argument. Such an outline, because it displays the structure of an argument, will help you detect any fallacies in it.

10. Find Any Errors in Informal Logic

There are a great many errors of reasoning or ways of introducing irrelevant premises which are described by logicians as fallacies. A 'fallacy' is not just an instance of reasoning which is incorrect on formal logical grounds. As well as formal logical fallacies, authors can commit errors of judgement, they can argue in ways that are not fairminded, or they can introduce propositions that are irrelevant to the point of contention. We call these 'informal fallacies' and we will illustrate these sorts of error in the next chapter. For the moment it is enough to say that if you can pin such an error of reasoning on your opponent, you will have scored an important point in the debate or found an important flaw in the argument which you are evaluating.

We can sum up how to evaluate arguments and how to combine such evaluation with the task of developing your own arguments by suggesting that there are now three basic questions you should ask about any argument:

1. Are the premises true?
2. Does the conclusion follow logically from the premises?
3. Are there better alternatives to the POC?

Exercise 4.2

Imagine that you disagree with the following item which is based on a letter to a newspaper.[1] Write out your plan of attack. In such a plan you will include a logical outline, identify any crucial premises, identify the premises that you will question, indicate questions you would ask if you could, suggest any alternative facts, values or proposals, and so forth.

> Your report on fast food restaurants continues a myth about sugar that really should be laid to rest. An unnamed official of the State food and nutrition program is quoted as saying that 'fat, sugar and salt are linked with certain diseases that are responsible for a lot of deaths and disability in our society, such as heart disease, diabetes and certain types of cancer'.
>
> The role of sugar in human disease has been comprehensively examined by international scientific review committees, independent scientists and professional associations, which have concluded that sugar does not contribute to any chronic disease other than its involvement in dental caries.
>
> More than ever today, the emphasis is on decreasing the total dietary fat intake, especially saturated fat and sodium. There is no scientific basis for including sugar in the same sentence. Current levels of sugar consumption are moderate and are compatible with good health.
>
> [by a nutritionist working for the sugar industry]

Exercise 4.3

Imagine that you disagree with the following item which is based on a letter to a newspaper. Write out your plan of attack. In such a plan you will include a logical outline, identify any crucial premises, identify the premises that you will attack, indicate questions you would ask if you could, suggest any alternative facts, values or proposals, and so forth.

> Two Brisbane psychiatrists are reported as warning of 'significant adverse consequences for the sick person' who is referred to by their doctor as a 'client'.
>
> In modern times, a person attending a medical practitioner is less inclined to be satisfied with an authoritarian, 'one up, one down' approach to medical information and treatment—being in general better informed and having a greater desire to contribute to the decision-making process. Such a person seeks more of a partnership in which both parties play important but different roles.
>
> In respect of this trend, I refer to people attending my practice as 'clients'. The use of this term bypasses, in my opinion, a lot of traditional implications of the label 'patient': a person who is somehow less empowered to determine what treatment he or she may undergo.
>
> Referring to a person as a 'client' rather than as a 'patient' does not change the responsibilities of a medical practitioner in terms of ensuring confidentiality, of providing medical certificates, or of instituting appropriate care with compassion.
>
> Drs Raphael and Emmerson are reported to suggest that the label 'client' 'denotes that the person has a choice in his or her treatment'. What, then, I would ask, is the implication of the label 'patient' as used by these doctors?

Exercise 4.4

Imagine that the following notice has appeared on the notice board at the hospital where you are working. On seeing it, you immediately convene a meeting of the local branch of your union and you and your colleagues decide to prepare a response. Prepare, in outline form, a possible response.

> NOTICE TO ALL STAFF
>
> Due to a recent cut-back in government funding, the management of this institution has no option but to reduce the number of nursing staff. Since funding cannot be obtained from non-government bodies, and regulations prohibit us from increasing the charges for residents, we are forced to cut staff numbers. Cost-cutting measures have been instituted in non-nursing areas, but this will not be sufficient to cover the

anticipated shortfall. Information about a redundancy program will be provided in the near future.

NOTE

1. Letter to *The Age*, Melbourne, February 1991.

Chapter 5
Informal Fallacies

In this chapter, students will be shown how to identify errors in informal logic, such as *ad hominem* arguments, use of emotive language or threats, begging the question, and many others.

Faulty arguments can be persuasive. Indeed, one might sometimes think that they are the more persuasive, the more fallacies they commit. For this reason it is important to develop a keen awareness of faulty argument so that one will not be seduced into accepting conclusions which have not been established correctly. Also, as we suggested in the previous chapter, evaluating arguments requires us to become aware of errors in argument.

As we mentioned at the end of Chapter 4, fallacies are errors in argument which can be grouped into formal fallacies and informal fallacies. Formal fallacies arise when an author makes a mistake in the form of an argument. We will be describing such reasoning in the next chapters. Informal fallacies, on the other hand, are mistakes which can arise in a wide variety of ways, not only in the process of reasoning. There is almost no limit to the varieties of informal fallacy that are possible and books on informal logic make various listings. We will describe those which we consider to be the most common. We will arrange our listing under two broad headings:

- Errors of Reasoning
- Dirty Tricks

even though this division is not a tight one. An error of reasoning is usually the result of incompetence or carelessness, but if it were engaged in deliberately to deceive an audience, then it would become a dirty trick. On the other hand, an author might engage in a dirty trick fallacy through ignorance of correct reasoning processes.

Errors of Reasoning

1. Composition and Division

The informal fallacies of composition and division consist in confusing parts for a whole. They involve attributing properties of a part to a whole (composition) or of a whole to a part (division). Let us explain what we mean. To take composition first:

Example 5.1

Suppose a patient observed that Nurse Jones was doing a very good job on the wards. She was efficient and caring in all that she did and looked after this patient very well. In conversation with friends later the patient says that the hospital is a very good hospital.

Now the problem with this line of thinking is that the patient has taken his appropriate and positive attitude to Nurse Jones and extrapolated from it to the whole hospital. He has attributed a property of a part of the institution—Nurse Jones—to the whole institution. It may indeed be a good hospital and it may be that there is an actual link between its being a good hospital and Nurse Jones' being a good nurse, but the patient has not cited any reasons for his general judgement and so his argument is unsound. It is a case of the fallacy of composition.

The opposite fallacy, that of division, is illustrated as follows:

Example 5.2

An occupational health and safety nurse has an appointment for an interview with an employee called Mrs Tran. The nurse thinks, 'Tran is a Vietnamese name. I'd better arrange for an interpreter.' But Mrs Tran turns out to be a Caucasian married to a Vietnamese.

This nurse commits the fallacy of division in that she takes a general view about a group and applies it without appropriate evidence to a particular member of that group. The fallacy does not consist in having the wrong general view. The general view may be quite true. Likewise, somebody who says that Guido can't be Italian because he does not have black hair is committing the fallacy of division because he is applying the true statement that most Italians have black hair to a particular case.

The way to avoid this fallacy is to make the appropriate inquiries into the particular case. The OHS nurse should not jump to conclusions. The person interested in Guido's nationality should ask Guido or inspect his passport. Relying on general knowledge can often mislead.

The fallacy of division is often present in cases where people have a prejudice against particular races or groups of people.

Example 5.3

A worker of Mediterranean background comes to see the nurse attached to the first aid clinic of a large factory. He complains of a sore back and says that he cannot return to work. The nurse thinks, 'These Mediterranean men are all the same, they try to shirk hard work by complaining of bad backs'. She performs a cursory inspection, gives him a light analgesic, and refuses to write a certificate authorising sick leave.

In this case the fallacy still consists in applying an alleged property of a whole to a part, but it is made worse because the alleged property is based on a value judgement which has been applied to the whole group. In this case the general view is a prejudice about that group. This nurse should not only avoid the fallacy of division and make a thorough investigation of the worker's back, so as to make her judgement on the merits of the individual case, but she should also question her possibly unfounded generalisation.

We need not always judge that the conclusion of an argument which commits the fallacy of composition or division is wrong. The problem is simply that the argument is weak if it is based on this fallacy alone. That Nurse Jones is a good nurse is some sort of evidence for saying that the hospital where she works is a good hospital. But it is not enough. The patient needs more evidence to justify the judgement. And if it were true that most workers of Mediterranean extraction were malingerers, then the factory nurse might be justified in being suspicious about this particular worker. But she still owes it to him and to critical reasoning to inspect his back carefully and to make a judgement independent of this general view. Something more is needed than dependence on the generalisation.

2. Improper Analogy

The fallacy of improper analogy is committed when a property that applies to one category of things is applied without proper justification to a second category of things on the grounds that those two categories are similar in some way or other. A classic example is when, in the past, it was said of nurses that they should obey all instructions of medical staff because they were the 'doctors' handmaidens'. In this case an analogy is being drawn between nurses and servants and the claim is that whatever applies to one category should apply to the other. Because servants are supposed to have the property of being obedient, so too should nurses. The question that this raises, of course, is whether two things that are similar in some respects, are similar in every respect. There may be some similarity between nurses and servants: for example, both groups work for wages, but this similarity does not justify the conclusion that they should be similar in this further respect also. Are nurses really like servants in every respect? What is the scope of the analogy?

Along with the question of the scope of the similarity, there is a further question of whether the analogy is appropriate at all. Nowadays it would be regarded as extremely offensive to think of nurses as servants or 'handmaidens'.

Analogy is an argument strategy which is not always a fallacy. Argument by analogy is frequently used in medical research. When pharmaceuticals are tested on laboratory rats to see if they are safe for humans, the researchers are using this strategy. They are assuming that rats are similar to humans in the relevant ways, so that what applies to the rats will also apply to humans. The reason why this is most often not a fallacy is that there is an argument available to justify the analogy, and the conclusions are drawn on the basis of a limited set of properties shared by rats and humans. Many of the physical systems of rats are indeed similar to those of humans and if the drug being tested acts on those organs that are similar in this way, then the analogy holds. Any unwelcome side effects that arise for the rats can be expected to arise for humans also.

Another distinction that should be noted is between the improper use of analogy and the quite proper use of illustrations. If I am trying to explain something to you or to convince you of a proposal and I use an illustration, then I can be enhancing my communication in a proper way. Suppose I said that a convincing argument works on the mind of an audience like a trap. The audience cannot fail to agree if it sees how the premises lead to the conclusion. The use of the analogy of a trap nicely expresses this idea and so helps to explain it. Again, no molecular biologist really thinks that molecules are like coloured balls held together with plastic rods. Yet it is a very useful teaching device to demonstrate the structure of complex molecules by building models with such materials. Our knowledge of how the DNA molecule is responsible for the processes whereby traits are passed on from one generation to another was made possible by drawing the analogy between the structure of this molecule and that of the double helix.

The difference between a proper and improper use of analogy is that the author must be able to explain just why the analogy is appropriate and also what particular feature of the analogy is being used to illustrate the point of contention. It is only the shape of the double helix that is being used to illustrate the features of the molecule—not the colour of the plastic balls used in the model. Likewise, it is the psychological feeling of entrapment that is being used to illustrate the logical force of a good argument—not the pain that a physical trap might cause. And finally, it is only the features of particular organs or physical systems in the rats that are being used as an analogy for the features of human organs, and this is appropriate because the organs in question are similar in rats and humans. In short, the analogy must be justifiable by argument and the scope of the analogy must be defined.

We will have more to say about the use of analogies in the construction of knowledge in Chapter 7.

3. Changing the Question

People who watch interviews with politicians on television will be familiar with this fallacy. It consists of arguing for something which is off the point. An author may offer a very impressive and cogent argument, but insofar as the argument is for a conclusion other than the point of contention, the author has committed the fallacy of changing the question.

Example 5.4

Interviewer addressing the Minister for Health: 'Sir, how do you respond to the damning report into the provision of community health?' Minister: 'I have nothing but admiration for the splendid staff of community health centres who are working in difficult circumstances and doing a wonderful job.'

If we assume that the intent of the interviewer's question was to ask the minister whether he would provide more funding for community health and why he had not done so up to now, then it is clear that the minister's answer is irrelevant.

For another example, we might refer back to Example 3.17. In this example the author argued for a conclusion which was slightly different from the point of contention. The POC was that organ donation should stop until there was a full debate on the issue, whereas the conclusion was that it should stop until there was more study of the effects on people involved. This is only a slight difference (the results of such a study would be used in the debate that is called for), but it nicely illustrates how there can be subtle instances of the fallacy of changing the question.

It also illustrates how a logical outline can uncover such a fallacy. Any argument of which the outline shows a different conclusion from the POC has committed this fallacy.

4. Begging the Question

One commits the fallacy of begging the question when one assumes what one is trying to conclude.

Example 5.5

Two people, one a religious believer and the other an atheist, are debating the existence of God. The believer says, 'The universe must have had a creator: that creator can only have been God, and so there must be a God.'

Given that the Western concept of God includes the notion that He is the creator of the universe, the believer's first premise, that the universe must have had a creator, assumes that there is such a creator and thus that there is a God. Even if that first premise had been couched in the more neutral form of 'the universe must have had a beginning', it could still imply that something must have begun it and hence that there must be a creator-God.

In actual everyday arguments, the fallacy of begging the question can be very hard to detect. It depends on how a point is being expressed. If it is couched in terms different from the conclusion it may look as if it is not the same point as the conclusion. The solution to this problem is, of course, the logical outline and the enunciation of assumptions which such an outline allows for. If the logical outline shows an assumption which is equivalent to the point of contention, you will have a case of the fallacy of begging the question.

Example 5.6

Let us go back to Exercise 3.7. Our suggested outline for this exercise was:

POC: The Government should provide funding to shorten hospital waiting lists for elective surgery.

Premises:

1. Every citizen has a right to adequate health care. (exhortation)
2. The Government is not providing adequate funds. (side comment)
3. Needless suffering is being caused by the failure of governments to address this issue. (side comment)
(4. Governments have a responsibility to provide adequate health care.) (1, exhortation)
5. Candidates for elective surgery have an equal right to adequate health care. (1, exhortation)
6. The Government should provide funding to shorten hospital waiting lists for elective surgery. (4,5, exhortation)

It is possible to suggest that in this argument premise 4 begs the question. Notice that it is a hidden premise which did not appear in the original text and so we might be being a bit unfair on the author in accusing her of a fallacy based on a premise that she has not articulated. However, that premise is needed if the argument is to work, so it is certainly appropriate to attribute it to the author. The point is that it is a generalised form of the conclusion and POC. It does suggest that the question (that is, the POC) has been begged (meaning that it has been assumed).

Another form of the fallacy of begging the question is where an author places a condition on the point of contention but does not say whether that condition has been or will be fulfilled.

Example 5.7

A hospital administrator: It is possible that the government will provide more money for community health next year. I think we should set up a working party to see how we can make use of such increased funding in order to improve our services.

The plans that this hospital administrator is making are premised upon the condition that the government will provide more money for community health next year. He seems to be going ahead with those plans without making sure that this condition will be fulfilled. In this he is begging the question as to whether those funds will be provided.

5. Argument from Ignorance

An argument from ignorance occurs when the only support someone offers for a point of contention is the absence of any evidence or considerations against it.

Example 5.8

A proponent of an alternative method of treatment for cancer says that his treatment works because there are no tests which have shown that it does not work.

In this instance what is needed is a positive test which shows that the treatment does work. To say that there are no tests which show that it does not work does not support the point of contention. The author cannot conclude that his treatment works unless there are tests which positively support this conclusion.

It is important to distinguish this error from another form of argument which is similar to it, but which is not necessarily fallacious. This is the argument which offers evidence for something and adds that there is no evidence against it. Take the case for the addition of fluoride to water supplies.

Example 5.9

POC:	Fluoride should be added to domestic water supplies.	
1.	There is epidemiological evidence showing that fewer tooth cavities occur when there is fluoride in the water.	(fact)
2.	There is no epidemiological evidence linking fluoride with any other health problems.	(fact)
(3.	Health measures that are beneficial and have no adverse side effects should be adopted.)	(exhortation)
4.	Fluoride should be added to domestic water supplies.	(1,2,3, exhortation)

In this argument, premise 2 sounds like an 'argument from ignorance' and, if it were the only premise offered, it would be. But, in conjunction with premise 1, it adds to the conclusion in a valid way.

A further point to note is that statements of ignorance are frequently assertions because there is no way for the audience to check them. However, in this instance, we call it a fact because the epidemiological studies are on the public record and can be checked by anyone. Computer data bases make it possible, even with the proliferation of research world-wide, to be thorough in one's research into these matters. What the author is saying is that there are no known adverse side effects to offset the known benefits. However, that this premise is not a strong one by itself becomes clear when we note the persistence of the anti-fluoridisation lobby in some parts of the world. Scaremongers need only point to one case where fluoride might have caused some harm to bring this premise into question. The supporters of fluoride will then have to show that the alleged harm was not caused by the fluoride after all. A claim that there is no evidence for something is easily challenged by producing putative evidence and putting the onus of proof onto the original author to show that the case offered does not constitute evidence against his position. But while opponents might counter this negative premise in this way they have greater difficulty in countering the positive premises. The evidence that fluoride produces benefits is very strong. In this way, premise 1 in example 5.9 is a crucial premise and provides much stronger support for the conclusion.

What this example shows is that an argument from ignorance is, at best, a weak argument. It depends on the knowledge base of the author, and the knowledge of any one person or group is limited. It is very difficult to know for certain that there is no evidence for something and hence very precarious to depend on the absence of evidence in an argument. Allegations were recently made in a newspaper that human subjects had been injected with radioactive isotopes without their knowledge, to test the effects on various parts of the body. The government denied the allegations by saying that there were no records of such tests having been carried out. The very next day, a newspaper published details of medical journal articles of the day in which those tests were described. Clearly, the fact that the government did not know of these tests was no evidence for the claim that they did not occur.

6. Argument from Authority (Connected or Disconnected)

An argument from authority is to be distinguished from an argument by coercion, which we will be describing presently. The latter is a dirty trick which depends on the power able to be exercised over an opponent by the author. An argument from authority, in contrast, depends on irrelevant premises that refer to the prestige, charisma or teaching authority of the author. In this context, the word 'authority' does not mean power, as when we say that the nurse in charge has the authority to issue instructions for others to follow. Rather, it means ability to teach or elicit the agreement of others on the basis of knowledge, experience, prestige or age. The fallacy occurs when this authority is the only basis offered for accepting the point of contention.

Example 5.10

> Suppose an Olympic gold medal winner endorses a new headache powder. She appears on your television screen saying that this new wonder drug will relieve pain quickly and harmlessly. Sales of the new product increase dramatically.

What the designers of this advertisement intend is that the affection or admiration you feel for this person as a winner of an Olympic gold medal will transfer across to the product which they are promoting. An endorsement by this sporting hero is an endorsement that will be taken seriously. Clearly, this is not a sound argument in favour of the product. The fact that the powder is used or endorsed by a gold medallist tells us nothing about the efficacy or safety of the analgesic. That this person endorses it is irrelevant to the point of contention. This is called an argument from authority because the authority of this person (acquired by winning a gold medal) is being used to persuade the audience.

Example 5.11

An outline of the argument might be:

POC: Everyone should buy product X.

1.	This gold medallist buys product X.	(fact)
2.	Everyone should do what this gold medallist does.	(exhortation)
3.	Everyone should buy product X.	(1,2)

Setting out the argument in this way makes it clear that while there is no formal fallacy in it, it depends on a crucial premise—premise 2—which is highly contentious. We would regard this premise as irrelevant, not because the conclusion does not follow from it (in which case we would have labelled it as a side comment), but because it posits a highly contentious point which is not relevant to an intelligent judgement about whether the headache powder is effective and harmless.

A further point to note is that this is also an example of 'disconnected' authority. What this means is that there is no connection between being good at sport and knowing anything about analgesics. It is merely the prowess of the sporting hero which is being used to support premise 2.

This can be contrasted with 'connected' authority, where the nature of the authority of the person does have a connection to the product being endorsed. Take, for example, an advertisement in which a dentist endorses a newly designed toothbrush. In this instance the authority of the endorser is relevant to the product. However, it is still an informal fallacy because the fact that one person (even one whose authority derives from relevant expertise) uses the product is not a very strong argument for concluding that the product does everything that is claimed for it. There are better ways of judging the merits of a toothbrush than relying on the testimony of others. The least we should do is ask why the dentist thinks this toothbrush is better than others. The advertisers should provide us with reasons. These reasons may have extra authority if they are offered by a dentist, but we should not accept them just and only because they are offered by an authority, albeit a connected one. We should be able to make up our own minds.

However, there is room for subtle judgment in cases like this. If there is doubt about a patient's diagnosis and a specialist is brought in to offer advice, then it would be quite appropriate to accept that advice purely on the basis that the person offering it is the appropriate expert. In this case, because the non-specialists are not able to decide the issue, there is no other source of information available and credence should be given to the person with authority.

Even in a case like this, however, we should not believe what is said just and only because the person who says it has authority. Either we should seek independent evidence, or that person should also offer reasons for the point of contention, and we should be able to see that these reasons are sound.

Dirty Tricks

7. Argument against the Author (Argumentum ad Hominem)

We have already mentioned this form of argument, though without calling it an informal fallacy. The argument consists in calling the credentials or credibility of the author into question. It is a frequently used debating strategy but, by itself, it is seldom fair. It is a case of introducing considerations which are, in most cases, irrelevant to the conclusion.

Example 5.12

> Suppose a report has been written about the state of community nursing which finds that government funding is inadequate and inefficiently used. The government minister for health responds by pointing out that the author of the report had worked as a research officer for the nurses' union some years earlier. He means to imply that the report was biased because of this. But he offers no evidence from the content of the report to suggest that the report is flawed.

This would be a case of the informal fallacy of ad hominem argument if it were all that the minister said. But if he went on to point out some genuine flaws in the report, he would be arguing against it in a valid way. In either case, his casting aspersions on the author is irrelevant to his point of contention. At best, it is a useful debating trick; at worst, it is an unethical strategy.

8. Argument by Coercion

This fallacy is committed when someone tries to force another to adopt a particular point of view or policy by using the authority or power that they have over that person.

Example 5.13

> Let us suppose that the author of the critical report into the community health service worked for the ministry of health. Let us suppose further that a draft copy of the report had gone up the minister. The minister sends back a memo to the author asking that the author change his conclusions so as to reflect more favourably on the government and on the minister, and reminding the author that, as an employee of the ministry, it is in his interest to create favourable publicity for the government. Promotion seldom comes to those who are known to be critical of government performance.

This memo would contain an argument by coercion. Quite apart from the unethical nature of the strategy, the logical error consists in providing a premise which is irrelevant to the point of contention. This can be shown by providing an outline of the minister's argument.

Example 5.14

POC: The report should not be published.

1.	It is not good when reports that harm the government's reputation are published.	(value)
2.	This report harms the government's reputation.	(fact)
3.	You (the author) will not be promoted if you publish the report.	(side comment)
4.	The report should not be published.	(1,2, exhortation)

9. Appeal to Pity

This is an argument which frequently occurs in courts of law during criminal trials. A defence lawyer may urge the jury to find his client not guilty of a murder charge on the grounds that the defendant had a violent upbringing and knows no better way of resolving conflicts than through violence. Now while this argument may be relevant to deciding on a sentence, it is not relevant to whether the defendant is guilty of the crime.

This is also an argument sometimes used by students in talking to their examiners about their results. Students may plead for a higher grade than they actually received by saying that they worked very hard on the assignment. This may be true, but it is not relevant to what grade a student should get. The grade is for the standard that the student has achieved, not for the amount of effort that has been put in. Asking the examiner to take pity on the student, as it were, because they have worked hard is appealing to an irrelevant consideration.

It must not be thought that an appeal to pity is always irrelevant. If a patient is suffering acute pain during the terminal stages of an incurable illness and the proposal is made by the family of the patient, or by the patient herself, that life-sustaining treatment be terminated, the proposal may well be supported by an appeal to pity. The argument may include the premise that the patient is suffering acute pain which cannot be alleviated. This is an appeal to pity. However, it is relevant to the proposal since the very reason why the proposal is being made is that it is the only way in which the suffering can be brought to a halt.

10. Social Identification

This argument is a variation of the argument from authority. It consists in promoting an idea, proposal or product by associating that idea with something that the audience desires or identifies with. This is a rather abstract way of describing what went on in the advertisement for the headache powder in which the Olympic gold medallist endorsed the product. Since we 'identify' with the gold medallist, in the sense that we would like to be like her, we will adopt values and products that the gold medallist adopts. In this way we will feel ourselves to be emulating or identifying with what we admire or desire.

Another common example of this argument used in advertising is to associate a product with a desirable lifestyle or any other desired object. The cigarette advertisement which uses visuals of tropical islands and sailing boats to suggest holidays and relaxation uses this argument, as does the car advertisement that shows a scantily clad model leaning on the bonnet.

In the context of professional practice, a more frequent form of the argument by social identification is signposted by the phrase, 'everybody knows that . . .'. If you are seeking to convince somebody of something, you might simply assert that everybody knows that this is the case, or that this is the way things are always done. This argument will seem to have force if you assume that your audience wants to be like everybody else and does not want to stand out as the one person who has a different view or does things in a different way. We all want to conform to some degree and so we will be inclined to go along with (or to identify with) what the majority say and do.

The fallacy in this argument consists in introducing an irrelevant premise. The fact that a sports star, a beautiful model or the majority of one's colleagues believe something to be true or valuable is not, by itself, a strong argument in its favour.

11. Slippery Slope

The fallacy of appealing to a slippery slope occurs when an author opposes a proposal by alleging, without appropriate evidence, that if the proposal is adopted the consequences would be disastrous. This argument is a form of *reductio ad absurdum* argument but is fallacious because of the lack of evidence needed to support the claim that the unwelcome consequences would inevitably occur.

Slippery slope arguments are very common in the context of debates about abortion and euthanasia. The argument is that if such practices were permitted by law, even with a number of conditions and restraints in place, there would be a reduction in the community's respect for the value of life and hence an inevitable slide into abuse and unjustified killing. The example of Nazi Germany is frequently cited to suggest how inevitable this consequence would be. But one shocking historical example does not prove that these consequences would always occur. Other relevant circumstances are not likely to be similar. So if the author thinks the consequences are inevitable, he or she should offer evidence for this. This form of argument is a fallacy whenever no evidence is given for the claim that the unwelcome consequences of adopting the proposal are inevitable.

12. False Dilemma

The fallacy of false dilemma occurs when an author supports a proposal by alleging that if the proposal is not adopted the consequences will be disastrous. The fallacy consists in suggesting that there is only one alternative to the proposal. One feature of the fallacy is that the author frequently exaggerates the unwelcome consequences of not accepting his proposal. For example, someone might say that the government should ban pornography because otherwise the entire moral fabric of our society will be threatened. In this kind of case, the fallacy consists in suggesting that there is no third alternative or no other way of preventing or ameliorating the unwelcome consequence. Either the proposal is accepted or there will be total disaster.

It can be difficult to distinguish false dilemma arguments from slippery slope arguments. The appeal to a slippery slope also consists in saying that disastrous consequences are inevitable if a proposal is not accepted. But the fallacy here consists in not offering evidence for that claim. In a false dilemma argument the author is saying that the only choices possible are between accepting the proposal or accepting the disastrous consequences of not doing so. But if the author strengthens his case by offering evidence for saying that the disastrous consequences are inevitable if his proposal is not accepted then he is not appealing to a slippery slope, though he is still offering a false dilemma. The fallacy of false dilemma does not consist in not offering evidence for the inevitability of the unwelcome alternative, but in asserting that it is the only alternative to not accepting the proposal. In this fallacy, there is no allowance for other possibilities or other measures (such as legal restrictions on the availability of pornography) to prevent the unwelcome consequences. A policy may be dangerous, but there are often effective ways of controlling the risks.

There is another form of the fallacy of false dilemma which occurs in negotiation situations. In this context the fallacy suggests that there is no room for compromise and no middle ground that might be found by negotiation.

Example 5.15

The nursing union is meeting with the Minister for Health to demand more funding for community health. The union representatives tell the minister that if he does not provide at least an extra ten million dollars, the entire community health service will collapse, staff will go on indefinite strike and the community's confidence in the system will be destroyed forever. The minister feels that there is no point in offering the nine million he had already earmarked for the purpose and closes the meeting.

13. Misuse of Language

This error is not so much a fallacy in reasoning as an instance of incompetence, laziness or even verbal trickery. It consists in not using words clearly or correctly, thus leading to misunderstanding or obfuscation. Misuses of language are a fallacy when used deliberately in an argument to confuse an audience into accepting a conclusion which is actually not supported. If the misuse is inadvertent, then it just represents poor communication skills. There are a number of different kinds of such error:

Use of Ambiguous Terms

There are many words in the language that can have different meanings in different contexts. In differing contexts, the sentence 'There's been an arrest in Ward 3' could mean either that a patient has had a cardiac arrest or that a patient (or nurse) has been taken away by the police.

Use of Vague Terms

This kind of error is more likely to occur than the previous one. There are lots of terms which have meanings that are not very specific and which individuals can understand in a number of different ways. For example, if someone urges you to engage in 'appropriate behaviour', or to be a 'good nurse', it is possible for you to interpret those phrases in ways that reflect your understanding of what appropriate behaviour would be in that context, or of what it is to be a good nurse. And this interpretation might differ from what the author intended.

Use of Slogans

Slogans are words or phrases that have vague meaning but elicit strong positive or negative responses from those who hear them. The most frequent context for the misuse of slogans is politics. Politicians will speak of 'family values', or of preserving 'the way of life of ordinary people'. Naturally, we all respond positively because we like what we hear. But what do these phrases actually mean?

It is worth considering whether words and phrases frequently used in the nursing profession have the characteristics of slogans. What is 'holistic care'? What do we mean by 'the whole person'? And what is 'advocacy' in real and practical terms? The way to avoid allowing these terms to be mere slogans is to think carefully about what they mean and what they imply for professional practice.

Use of Jargon

Jargon is language that is specific to a particular field of knowledge or activity and which outsiders to that field of knowledge or activity do not understand. When mechanics talk to each other about 'camshafts' and 'rocker covers' they are using jargon, and when health workers talk to each other about 'occlusive dressings' and 're-epithelialisation' they are using jargon. Of course, there is nothing wrong with this. It would be longwinded, inefficient and possibly dangerous if mechanics had to constantly use phrases like 'that long thing that goes round and round' or 'the half-bottle shaped thing on top of the engine'. And nurses wouldn't get far if they had to refer constantly to 'dressings that seal the wound' or 'the regrowing of the top layer of skin'. Technical language is clearly necessary in technical and professional fields of activity.

Technical language frequently takes the form of acronyms, where the first letters of a series of words is used to refer to that whole series. In this way nurses might speak of 'IV. TKVO' meaning 'an intravenous line which conveys fluid at a slow rate in order to keep a vein open'.

But because such language is not widely understood by lay people, it can be used to obfuscate or to impress without good reason. When talking to a patient or his family, it may sound impressive to use jargon and your audience may think you are very knowledgeable, but they will not understand what you are saying and your communication will fail. For example, you would not say to a patient with a drainage catheter, 'I'm milking your tube to keep it patent'. Instead, you would say something like, 'I'm manipulating your tube to stop it clogging'.

Professionals who are keen to enhance and preserve the status of their profession frequently use jargon as a means of excluding lay people. Academics in the humanities are common offenders, but even nursing text books use such phrases as 'the epistemological and ontological aspects of caring'. The use of jargon is unhelpful when it is unnecessarily technical or specialist and when it is more likely to obscure information than reveal it. A heading in a popular nursing journal recently announced that, 'Although a promising treatment, embolization followed by single-dose radiotherapy may not obliterate an AVM for two to three years'.[1] Is this an unacceptable use of jargon?

The way to consider whether jargon is being used incorrectly is to consider the audience in a communication. Can the audience be expected to understand the terminology that the author is using? If the answer is yes, then there is no problem. But if the answer is no, then we have a case of obfuscation. In your own communications, whether they be conversations with patients or other health workers, or whether they be written submissions, memos or reports, you should always have your audience in mind and try to imagine how familiar that audience might be with the technical language you use.

Use of Metaphors

The use of metaphors and similes is a frequently used technique in debating. It can sometimes illuminate an issue very well, but it also frequently degenerates into the use of slogans. The main problem with such devices is that they can lead to exaggeration. Metaphors frequently have rhetorical force but not much substance. Common examples in the health field are descriptions of an epidemic as a 'plague', or even a 'curse'. Working to cure those affected by the epidemic and to prevent its spread will be described as fighting a 'battle' against the disease, or even as 'waging war' against it. People who suffer an illness that frequently claims lives will be said to have 'fought courageously' against it (whether or not they survive).[2]

Once again, the use of metaphors and similes will be innocent in most contexts. Indeed, they can be very useful in explaining complex ideas. In this respect they are like analogies. But there will be cases where their use can be a harmful error. For example, the idea that the victim of a disease can 'fight' it, may lead to the thought that the victim will have failed in some blameworthy way if they 'succumb' to that disease. Along with the suffering of the disease itself, there will then be the feeling of failure and loss of self-worth that patients frequently feel when they are ill.

Use of Emotive Language

We defined emotive communication in Chapter 2 as communication designed to arouse the emotions of the audience. Many of the rhetorical strategies that we have just been discussing have this purpose, but there are other ways in which the emotions of the audience can be manipulated. Use of such extreme expressions as 'appalling' or 'disgusting' tends to have this effect, as does a tone of irony or dismissal. Sometimes a definition of something may be offered in such a way as to sway the emotions or shape the attitudes of the audience. For example, euthanasia or abortion might be defined as murder without a justification for such a definition being offered. The problem with emotive language is that it appeals to unquestioned attitudes, and possibly even prejudices, without any use of reason or argument.

Exercise 5.1

Look at the following arguments and identify the kind of fallacy that is being committed (if any) in each one. There may be more than one fallacy in some examples. Moreover, some of the categories of informal fallacy which we have described overlap. Accordingly, there may be more than one correct answer.

1. Sign in a foreign hotel: 'Ladies are requested not to have children in the bar.'
2. Research shows that when certain species of monkeys are crowded together in cages, they become more aggressive towards each other. Perhaps this explains the violence in our inner city slums.
3. Part of being a good nurse is being punctual. Nurse Quick is always punctual and so must be a good nurse.
4. Euthanasia is wrong because it is a case of murder, and murder is always wrong.
5. There is no doubt that the arguments offered for changing the work rosters are sound: patients would receive better care and medical staff

would be able to work more efficiently. However, I don't think the union would accept the changes.

6. The hospital needs to cut nursing staff; either we cut running costs, or we will be forced to close our doors altogether.
7. Who was at the committee meeting today?
   Dr Jones, a neurosurgeon, Nurse Jones and the hospital bursar.
   Were there three or four people present?
8. Chairperson of the Hospital Ethics committee: Before we vote to approve this proposal, I should remind you that the pharmaceutical company funding this research also helps this hospital. It might go badly for us if we refuse their requests.
9. The hospital where I work has a high reputation for caring service. I must be a very caring nurse.
10. Nursing is an art. Yet there are no nursing displays in art galleries.
11. Nursing is a science as well as an art. Nurses should spend more time engaging in research and less time caring for patients.
12. Nursing is a valuable profession because it involves caring for the sick, and caring for the sick is a good thing to do.
13. The way to ensure that this hospital achieves the highest standards of service is to head-hunt the best staff.
14. Nurses who allow terminally ill and suffering patients to die should be charged with wilful neglect, lest the respect for life which holds our whole society together be lessened.
15. This child seems to be suffering so much pain already. Perhaps we should skip this injection.
16. Sister Nguyen thinks *Jaws V* was a terrific movie. I should go and see it.
17. It's no use asking Nurse Bongiorno for an opinion on the new rosters. She's new here and doesn't know the difficulties we have had.
18. It is the responsibility of nurses to care for the whole person of patients.
19. Use the tennis shoes that Steffi Graff uses.
20. The staff at St Oswald's Private Hospital have had a top couturier design their uniforms. We should get new uniforms too.
21. I can think of no good reason to oppose the proposal. Therefore, it must be a good one.
22. The hospital must make every effort to admit more patients even if it means overworking the staff. The people in this region are from poor, unemployed and migrant communities and they are already severely disadvantaged.
23. In response to your argument that we should have a free treatment policy for the poor, I would say that it is a pity that things have got to such a state that such policies are necessary.
24. I'll have to resign from the hospital if you can't allow me time off to pick up my children from school.

25. Use the deodorant that the champions use—Mountain Fresh.
26. Mothers should stay home when their children are young. Everybody knows that professional childcare is harmful to young children.
27. Doctor Theophonous thinks this is the best analgesic available. I will use it exclusively from now on.
28. How could a magistrate, trained in an almost all-male legal profession, be sensitive to women's issues?
29. Human life is sacred.
30. If Nurse Bradford is right about this patient's prognosis, then we had better bring in the emergency support team right away. I'll get straight onto it.
31. Into the actual horizontality of our contemporary urban spaces, Australians have long projected a rich and soaring structure of vertical imaginaries replete with 'tops', 'middles' and 'bottoms'. Into this collective metaphoric imagination, an old discourse and an iconography of 'the underclass' has recently returned.[3]
32. I would argue that, unless we had a free treatment policy for the poor, there would soon be so much social unrest we might have to close our doors altogether.
33. The failure to respect human life is a cancer eating into the very fabric of our society.
34. Nurses should not play God.
35. I don't think we should increase the dosage. You never know what might happen.
36. That suggestion is outrageous.
37. In support of your proposal that we should have a free treatment policy for the poor, I would argue that we should do everything we can to help those who are in need.
38. Physicists have shown that the universe, from the most microscopic levels to the most macroscopic, is marked by a high degree of interconnectivity. Everything connects with everything else. Small wonder then that people feel a deep concern for each other when they are in trouble.
39. In a discussion of the dangers of genetic engineering, Jeremy Rifkin says:'The temptations are great to make more and more radical experiments. Why would we ever say no to any alteration of the genetic code that might enhance the well being of the individual or the species? It would be difficult to imagine society rejecting any genetic modification that promised to improve, in some way, the performance of the human race.'[4]

Exercise 5.2

Write a logical outline of the following letter, and identify any informal fallacies that you find in it.

Few people could fail to be moved by the story of Lore Burmester as recounted by Dr Helga Kuhse. Ms Burmester's condition seems to have been one of those now thankfully rare cases which defy modern palliative care and she showed great courage in coping with it.

But, terrible as they are, we should not let such cases obscure the fact that by legalising voluntary euthanasia we are giving doctors the authority to kill innocent citizens. There are at least two ways in which this may lead to injustice.

The first is the likelihood that people (medical staff, lawyers, JPs, public servants) who regard euthanasia as immoral will be drawn unfairly into the administration of the law.

The second is the problem identified in an editorial in the paper last year: 'It seems almost impossible to devise a law allowing active euthanasia that is not open to abuse.' Once voluntary euthanasia becomes legal, some doctors and relatives will be tempted to pressure vulnerable patients into agreeing to a lethal injection. It is naive to suppose otherwise.

Finally, it should be noted that the moral justification for voluntary euthanasia proposed by Dr Kuhse involves more than respect for personal autonomy. It assumes that the lives of those who are terminally ill and in distress are no longer worth living. Dr Kuhse, I take it, does not propose that we should act on the serious requests for euthanasia of those who face the temporary distress of some curable condition.

But if we can make judgments about the 'quality of life' of competent patients, why can we not do so for those patients who are suffering a terminal illness and cannot decide for themselves—the senile, the demented, the physically and mentally handicapped? Thus, voluntary euthanasia becomes non-voluntary euthanasia. This is not scaremongering; it is the logic of the pro-euthanasia position.

Exercise 5.3

Refer back to Exercise 3.7, imagine yourself to be the government minister for health, and write the outline of a reply that you might make to that letter. Use the various debating strategies discussed so far, including that of accusing the author of informal fallacies.

Exercise 5.4

The following is a conversation actually overheard in a hospital staffroom by one of the authors of this book. Read it carefully and identify any fallacies or other faults of thinking that you think occur in it.

RN: Can I have a word with you? I'm worried about Jane. Since she's been working in this unit she's changed.

Nursing Unit Manager (NUM): Why do you feel that?

RN: She's been late twice this week, then she said she's been losing weight, that's because she doesn't have time for breakfast.

NUM: That doesn't sound like much of a problem to me.

RN: She seems moody, her concentration's poor, she's always tired. I think she made that drug error last week.

NUM: Even though she may have made that drug error, we all take shortcuts with the drug count, we shouldn't really blame her for that.

RN: What about her moodiness and poor concentration?

NUM: Her husband expects a lot of her, she is studying and bringing up the children as well as working.

RN: I've noticed her pupils are pinpoint at times. That combined with her weight loss and poor concentration—I reckon she's on hard drugs.

NUM: Oh no. Maybe it's alcohol. Alcoholics have problems with concentration and weight loss. She's more likely to have that problem.

RN: You can't prove that she's not on drugs, so I think she is. Why not ask Dr Wilson, the Unit Director to see her. He's a good Director and he cares about the staff, he'll be able to sort out what's wrong with her.

NUM: That's a good idea, I'll organise it.

NOTES

1. *Nursing 94*, March 1994, p. 327.
2. A thorough treatment of how metaphors are used to describe illness is given by Susan Sontag in *Illness as Metaphor*, New York, Farrar, Straus & Giroux, 1978, and *AIDS and its Metaphors*, New York, Farrar, Straus & Giroux, 1989.
3. Bessant, Judith, 'Feral policy: the politics of the "underclass" debate', *Arena Magazine*, 10, April–May 1994, pp. 23–24.
4. Rifkin, Jeremy, *Declarations of a Heretic*, Boston, Routledge & Kegan Paul, 1985, p. 66.

Chapter 6
Deduction

This chapter is a little more formal in nature and explicates classic forms of argument used in most reasoning, including practical reasoning, persuasion and scientific thinking. The term 'syllogism' is explained and the formal fallacies resulting from incorrect forms of the syllogism. We also cover deduction by the method of remainders.

Of the several debating strategies which we discussed in Chapter 4, the ninth was that of detecting formal fallacies. It will not be possible to explain what these are until we have described the formal structure of arguments. Only when we know how an argument holds together in formal terms can we describe how authors may depart from that formal structure and make errors of a formal kind.

When we described the forms of argument in Chapter 3 we said that an argument is defined as a linked series of premises that leads to a conclusion. It is time now to talk about those links and how premises *lead* to a conclusion. In a well formed argument, the conclusion follows inevitably from the premises. For the audience there is an experience of being forced to agree with the conclusion if that audience agrees with the premises. Being convinced by an argument is like being caught in a trap. The audience cannot both agree with the premises and not agree with the conclusion. This experience of entrapment is a function of the form of the argument. If the argument adheres to a defined form, then the conclusion will follow with rational inevitability.

There are two major forms of argument: **deduction** and **induction**. We will discuss the first of these in this chapter.

Deduction

In deduction, a conclusion is drawn which is already implicit in the premises. One of the premises in a deduction will be a general statement of some kind and the conclusion will be a spelling out of the information which is already present in that general premise. Here is an example:

Example 6.1

1. All nurses are intelligent. (fact)
2. John is a nurse. (fact)
3. John is intelligent. (1,2)

In this example, the conclusion that John is intelligent is already implicit in the first premise which states that all nurses are intelligent. In this way, this argument does little more than spell out an implication of one of its premises.

Such simple arguments are used in logic textbooks to illustrate what logicians call a **syllogism**. This is the technical term for this simple form of deductive argument and we mention it so that you will recognise the word in other texts. A syllogism is made up of a minimum of two premises and a conclusion. There will be a **major premise** which sets out the general statement from which the conclusion will be drawn. In Example 6.1, this is premise 1. And there will be a **minor premise**, the function of which is to introduce the particular case to which the general statement is going to be applied. In Example 6.1, this is premise 2. It will be clear the **conclusion** follows inevitably.

We have set out the above argument in the form of a logical outline because that is a format with which you are now familiar. In logic textbooks it is more common to see it set out in this form:

Example 6.2

All nurses are intelligent.
John is a nurse.
Therefore, John is intelligent.

where the 'therefore' is sometimes given as a symbol like this: ∴ or the symbol that we will use henceforward, namely ⇒

But it is not only the signpost, 'therefore' which can be rendered with a symbol. Bear in mind that the argument works just by virtue of its form. If we wrote the following argument:

Example 6.3

All fish are blue
John is a fish
⇒John is blue

the conclusion would follow with exactly the same inevitability as before. From premises 1 and 2, the conclusion does follow. It does not matter that the first premise is false and that the second premise is also false (unless my pet goldfish happens to be called John). The argument works whether or not the premises are true because the argument works as a result of the form of the syllogism. It is not the content of the premises that matter, it is the form of the argument. It follows that the argument should be able to be described in terms of its form without any reference to its content.

We describe the form of the argument without reference to its content by using symbols rather than words. Example 6.4 is a description of the argument in both Examples 6.2 and 6.3:

Example 6.4

All x are y
John is x
⇒John is y

In this form of the argument, 'x' can stand for being a nurse or being a fish, or being any other thing, while 'y' can stand for being intelligent, for being blue or for having any other property. In short, 'x' and 'y' can stand for anything. Whatever they stand for, whether the resulting statement is true or even sensible, the argument will still work.

It is possible to display the form of the syllogism in an even more abstract form. We do not need John. All we need is an instance of 'x'. It doesn't matter whether that instance of 'x' be John, or Nurse Ravic or Peter Pan. For any instance of 'x', if all x's are y, then that instance of 'x' will be an instance of 'y'. We write this as follows:

Example 6.5

All x are y
x
⇒ y

And the process of abstraction does not stop here. The statement, 'all x are y' implies that if something is an 'x' then it will be a 'y'. The statement that all nurses are intelligent implies that if something or someone is a nurse, then it will be intelligent. In other words:

'All x are y' is equivalent to
'if x, then y'

Now, there is a formal way of writing the proposition: 'if x, then y', namely 'x ⇒y'. And so the most abstract form of the syllogism that we can write is:

Example 6.6

x ⇒y
x
⇒ y

But this makes very clear just how the argument works. The second and third line of the syllogism, taken together, are exactly the same as the first line. In other words, the whole content of the syllogism is present in the major premise, and the minor premise and conclusion do little more than re-state what is already there. This explains why a deductive argument feels so inevitable. A syllogism is a proof in the strongest sense of that term. If you agree with the premises then you can only disagree with the conclusion at the price of being irrational and seeming silly to others.

Logicians describe this by saying that the conclusion is **necessary** or follows by necessity from the premises. Another way of putting this is to say that a syllogism is a form of **proof**.

Exercise 6.1

Write out the following arguments in abstract form and indicate what the symbols 'x' and 'y' stand for in each case. (Please disregard the fact that many of these arguments are inane.)

1. All nurses wear uniforms. Jones is a nurse. Jones is wearing a uniform.
2. Every person on the train is wearing shoes. Smith is on the train. Smith must be wearing shoes.
3. If you are a nurse you must have a university degree. Ne Win is a nurse. She must have passed her exams.
4. If you give a patient too large a dose of this drug, their heart rate increases. This patient was given a very large dose. We should be prepared to deal with an increased heart rate.

A further benefit of writing the syllogism in an abstract form is that it allows us to detect that form in a number of different contexts. The examples we have used so far have been instances of informative use of language. It has been facts about nurses or about fish that we have been spelling out. This is made clear when we write the sentence, 'All nurses are intelligent'. The verb 'are' indicates that we are describing nurses by attributing the property of being intelligent to them. If the limit of the process of abstraction had been reached when we had written, 'all x are y', then it might have seemed that the syllogism only applied to descriptive statements. But the form of the syllogism can be found in relation to value statements, exhortations and other forms of communication. For example, we might say:

Example 6.7

Every staff member should wear name tags on the wards.
Doctor Lisieux is on the staff.
Therefore, Doctor Lisieux should wear a name tag on the wards.

It will be clear that, once again, the form of this argument is:

$x \Rightarrow y$
x
$\Rightarrow y$

where 'x' stands for being a member of staff, and 'y' stands for having to wear a name tag on the wards. The fact that the major premise contains a 'should' (making it an exhortation) makes no difference. Do notice, however, that when the major premise is an exhortation the conclusion has to be an exhortation also. Whatever logical feature applies to the major or minor premises (whether it be true, false, an exhortation or a value statement), if the argument follows the correct form then that feature will apply to the conclusion. (We will discuss why this is so in Chapter 12.) In Example 6.7, because the major premise is an exhortation, the conclusion must be an exhortation also.

Another more technical way of understanding this point is to see that the 'y' (known as the predicate of the sentence) which is being attributed to the subject 'x' includes the verb. The subject of the major premise in Example 6.2 is 'all nurses' and the predicate is 'are intelligent'. The subject of the major premise in Example 6.7 is 'every staff member', while the predicate is 'should wear name tags on the wards'. So 'y' stands for 'should wear name tags on the wards'. Notice, therefore, that the 'should' is contained in the predicate and will be predicated of the subject in the conclusion also. Hortatory verbs are carried from the premises into the conclusion just as indicative verbs are carried from the premises into the conclusion.

Value statements are carried from the premises into the conclusion in the same say. Suppose we argued:

Example 6.8

All paintings by Manet are beautiful.
This is a painting by Manet.
⇒This painting is beautiful.

(We might imagine an art dealer saying this to a buyer who does not actually see this painting of Manet's as beautiful but is prepared to be convinced that it might be.) In this argument the major premise is a value statement. In consequence, we would expect the conclusion to be a value statement also.

Another feature that is carried from the premises into the conclusion is probability. Consider the following case:

Example 6.9

People who smoke cigarettes have a 60% chance of contracting cancer.
Nurse Smith smokes.
⇒Nurse Smith has a 60% chance of contracting cancer.

It would have been improper to conclude from these premises that Nurse Smith would contract cancer or, indeed, that she would not do so. The measure of probability which is given in the major premise should be carried into the conclusion.

One grammatical feature that need not be carried from the premises into the conclusion is tense. Premises in the present tense can lead to a conclusion in the future tense and premises in the past tense can lead to a conclusion in the present tense, and so forth. It makes no difference to the following example that the major premise is expressed in the present tense and the conclusion in the future:

Example 6.10

All men are destined to die.	(present tense)
John is a man.	(present tense)
⇒John will die.	(future tense)

This point will be important when we go on to discuss predictions and explanations in Part Two.

Exercise 6.2

Write a logical outline of the following arguments and then rewrite your outline as an abstract syllogism explaining what the symbols stand for.

1. All nurses should be punctual. Now that you have embarked on a nursing career, you should develop habits of punctuality.
2. This patient has cancer. You will not be surprised to see how quickly the cancer cells multiply given that such cells multiply at a frightening rate.
3. I'd better keep an eye on Nurse Roussos. Given that he's from a Mediterranean region, he's likely to feign a bad back.
4. The government needs to provide more funds for health care because health is important to the community.
5. Her pupils are dilated and react sluggishly to light, she only responds to painful stimuli, therefore she must be in a coma.

The Practical Syllogism

Deductions which make use of the form of the syllogism also occur in the context of decision making. Several of the exercises in Exercise 6.2 provide examples of this. The conclusions to most of the syllogisms we have been dealing with so far have been statements of fact or of value. But it frequently happens that the conclusion of a deductive argument is a policy or a decision or, even more directly, an action. Take the following example:

Example 6.11

All people who enjoy a high degree of health engage in lots of exercise.
I want to be healthy.
I should get more exercise.

This argument can be seen to be a syllogism of the form:

$x \Rightarrow y$
x
$\Rightarrow y$

where 'x' stands for 'becoming more healthy' and 'y' stands for 'getting plenty of exercise'. The major premise describes a generally true correlation between exercise and health. We can regard this as a factual statement. The minor premise expresses the author's want. We can call this a value statement. The author values improved health. Given these two premises, the author can see what he needs to do. He can express this conclusion in a number of ways:

'I should get more exercise.'	(exhortation)
'I will get more exercise.'	(decision)
'It would be good if I got more exercise.'	(value)
Or he could put on his joggers and go out for a run.	(action)

In each case (but most obviously in the fourth), we have a clear illustration of a practical syllogism.

A further important example of the practical syllogism is thinking that makes use of general principles, including moral or ethical principles. Joe might have the principle or policy that he will always eat a breakfast high in fibre. He finds himself in a foreign hotel in front of a breakfast buffet with foods that are unfamiliar to him. He asks the staff which of these food is high in fibre, is shown a particular cereal product and chooses to eat it. The structure of his thinking here could be represented as:

Example 6.12

Major Premise: Always have a high fibre breakfast.
(or: I should always have a high fibre breakfast.)
Minor Premise: This cereal product is high in fibre.
⇒I should eat this cereal product.
(or: Joe eats the cereal product.)

This can be seen to be a practical syllogism of the form:

$x \Rightarrow y$
x
$\Rightarrow y$

where 'x' stands for 'foods with high fibre content' and 'y' stands for 'should be eaten for breakfast'.

The case of acting from a moral principle would be similar. Let us take the principle, 'It is always wrong to tell a lie'. Helen adheres to this principle but is confronted with a situation in which telling a lie would be to her advantage. She took a day off work without filling in a leave form and the nursing supervisor has asked her where she was yesterday. She is tempted to say that she was at work but at a meeting, meaning that others would not have seen her. She might reason as follows:

Example 6.13

Telling a lie is always wrong.
Saying that I was at work yesterday would be a lie.
⇒Saying that I was at work yesterday would be wrong.

(or: I should not (will not) say that I was at work yesterday.)
(or: She simply tells the truth.)

Once again, we have a form of syllogism in which 'x' stands for 'telling a lie' and 'y' stands for 'being wrong'. The practical reasoning could issue in the judgement that claiming to have been at work would be wrong, or in the decision not to say that, or simply in the action of telling the truth. This and other forms of ethical reasoning will be discussed further in Part Three.

Exercise 6.3

Write out each of the following arguments as an abstract syllogism explaining what the symbols stand for.

1. I had better take my umbrella as I do not want to get wet.
2. It's alright if I steal this small item from this shop. Shoplifting does not cause anyone harm.
3. Nurses should always be prepared to listen to patients so as to provide the caring atmosphere in which patients can achieve healing.
4. Murder is wrong. Therefore active euthanasia should be forbidden.

Various Forms of the Syllogism

So far we have discussed just one form of the syllogism, namely,

$x \Rightarrow y$
x
$\Rightarrow y$

This form is called **affirming the antecedent.** While this sounds like a very fancy phrase which goes perilously close to being a case of the informal fallacy of using jargon, we have found that learning this terminology is helpful in remembering the points that follow and in detecting logical errors. If you look at the phrase: $x \Rightarrow y$, you will notice that the 'x' comes first and the 'y' comes second. For this reason 'x' is called the antecedent and 'y' is called the consequent. It makes even more sense if you remember that '$x \Rightarrow y$' can mean 'if x, then y'. This makes it clear that y is a consequence of x and this also explains why it is called the consequent.

In order to see the other forms of the syllogism, we need to introduce just one more symbol. This symbol is '$-$' and it means 'not', or 'it is not the case that'. In short, it is the symbol for negation. In this way '$-x$' would mean 'it is not the case that x'. If 'x' stood for 'being a nurse', then '$-x$' would stand for 'not being a nurse'.

Now the next form of the syllogism that we would like to discuss is called **denying the consequent**. In schematic form it looks like this:

$x \Rightarrow y$
$-y$
$\Rightarrow -x$

A non-symbolic example would be:

Example 6.14

If you are a nurse, you must have passed your qualifying exams.
(or: All nurses have passed their qualifying exams.)
Jones did not pass his qualifying exams.
⇒Jones is not (or: cannot be) a nurse.

In this example let 'x' stand for 'being a nurse' and 'y' for 'passing the qualifying exams'. It will be seen that this argument exemplifies the form of denying the consequent.

Once you start playing around with the symbols in this way, it will become clear that there are four possible combinations. The two that we have not yet discussed are **denying the antecedent:**

$x \Rightarrow y$
$-x$
$\Rightarrow - y$

and **affirming the consequent**:

$x \Rightarrow y$
y
$\Rightarrow x$

but these two forms of the syllogism are not valid.

Valid is the term logicians use to describe arguments that are logically correct, while arguments which commit formal fallacies are said to be **invalid**. Denying the antecedent and affirming the consequent are invalid forms of argument. Why this is so can be made clear if we use examples in ordinary language. Suppose we said:

Example 6.15

If you are a nurse, you must have passed your qualifying exams.
(or: All nurses have passed their qualifying exams.)
Jones is not a nurse.
⇒Jones did not pass his qualifying exams.

This conclusion would not follow. Jones may indeed have passed his qualifying exams but decided, on completion of the course, to pursue a career in advertising as he felt this was more suited to his talents. One cannot conclude from the fact that someone is not a nurse that he or she failed their qualifying exams, even if it is true that all those who are nurses did pass those exams. So denying the antecedent:

$x \Rightarrow y$
$-x$
$\Rightarrow -y$

is not a valid form of argument.

We could illustrate affirming the consequent as follows:

Example 6.16

If you are a nurse, you must have passed your qualifying exams.
(or: All nurses have passed their qualifying exams.)
Jones did pass his qualifying exams.
⇒Jones is a nurse.

This conclusion would not follow. Jones might have used his university degree to apply for and obtain a non-nursing job. He might not have sought registration as a nurse even though he was qualified to do so. Once again the argument is invalid. It is a case of affirming the consequent and has the form:

$x \Rightarrow y$
y
$\Rightarrow x$

In summary, then, there are four forms of the syllogism:

1. Affirming the antecedent.
2. Denying the consequent.
3. Affirming the consequent.
4. Denying the antecedent.

The first two of these are valid and the second two are invalid. Anyone whose argument can be represented in formal terms using the third form, will have committed the formal fallacy of affirming the consequent, while someone whose argument can be represented in formal terms using the fourth form, will have committed the formal fallacy of denying the antecedent.

Exercise 6.4

In the following arguments,

a. Set out the formal structure of the argument and identify what the x and the y stand for.
b. Identify which form of the syllogism is being used (affirming the antecedent, or whatever).
c. Say whether the argument is valid or invalid.

1. The nurses' strike occurred because people who are denied adequate terms and conditions, and who are treated as servants, will always object.

2. But Joe, you can't be a nurse. Most nurses are women.
3. Marital infidelity is always wrong. Peter (who is married to Pam) should not have gone out with Shirley.
4. Good diet is essential to health. I want to be healthy so I will adopt a good diet.
5. Lung cancer is terminal in most cases. Jones, who smoked a lot, died young. Perhaps he died of lung cancer.
6. All ravens are black. This bird is not a raven so it comes as no surprise that it is not black.
7. Death is the ultimate disaster. Health workers should do whatever they can to prevent it or delay it for as long as possible.
8. Smoking is a health hazard. If you want to be healthy, give up smoking.
9. These symptoms indicate asthma. This patient does not suffer from asthma because he does not have these symptoms.
10. I should check the patients before I finish my shift, since they should be checked regularly.
11. One should not be surprised to see the premier trying to appoint cronies to the judiciary. History shows that when political leaders become so powerful that opposition is ineffective, they will act to entrench that power.
12. We should not permit abortion in any circumstances because abortion is murder.
13. Most doctors have a high income. Mr van Dooren drives a very expensive car. He's probably a doctor.
14. Why should I jeopardise my career to look after my sick mother? I'm not a nurse.
15. If skin cancer is diagnosed early enough, it can usually be treated successfully. It's a pity Guiseppi left it so long to go to the doctor. He is now at great risk.
16. All fat people overeat. No midwives are fat. Therefore midwives do not overeat.
17. I always get a headache and feel irritable when I do night duty. I was on night duty last night, that is why I have a headache and feel irritable now.

The Method of Remainders

There is one further form of deduction which we should mention even though it is not an instance of a syllogism. This is the argument that uses the so-called **Method of Remainders**. When the imaginary detective whom we mentioned in Chapter 4 arrested Jackson for murder, his thinking had been deductive. You will recall that there were only three possible suspects for the crime: Jones, Smith and Jackson. Jones and Smith had alibis and so the culprit must have been Jackson. Given the premise that only these three could have done it (for example, because they were the only ones with access to the victim), and the further premise that Jones and Smith could not have done it (because they were seen elsewhere at the time), there can be no other conclusion than that Jackson is guilty. Of course, the strength of this conclusion depends upon the strength of the premises and in real life situations those premises might not be so conclusive. But so far as the form of the argument is concerned we have the same kind of logical certainty as applies to syllogisms, and hence we call the method of remainders a deduction. The form of this deduction might be given as:

A or B or C or . . . n
−B, −C, . . . −n
⇒ A

where A, B and C stand for alternatives and n stands for any number of further alternatives. These alternatives might be suspects of a crime as in the example we have used, or they might be contending scientific theories to explain a particular phenomenon, or differing diagnoses for a given set of symptoms, or alternative policies to deal with a difficult issue, and so forth. But in each case to argue for one of the alternatives by arguing against the others is, in a broad sense of the term, a form of deduction. It is drawing out implications that are already present in the premises.

Of course, the strength of the conclusion is only as great as the strength of the best alternative. If none of the policies that are being proposed is very good, then the policy that we are left with when we have excluded the worst ones will still not be very good. And if none of the suspects did it, then eliminating two of them will not leave us with the guilty one. There need to be reasons to support all of the alternatives. There must have been reasons to suspect Jackson, Jones and Smith, and for eliminating anyone else. In the case where there are conflicting scientific theories, there must be evidence for each of them. Each of the contending diagnoses must be plausible, and the proposed alternative policies must each have something going for them. The method of remainders is only a valid form of argument when each of the alternatives is strong. To argue for A by arguing against B and C, when B and C are alternatives that no one would take seriously is to commit the fallacy of false dilemma. It is to give A a false degree of plausibility by contrasting it with alternatives that are not plausible at all. These implausible alternatives are like straw men that can easily be knocked over (which is why this version of the fallacy of false dilemma is sometimes called 'The Straw Man Fallacy'). There must be independent reasons for supporting A because it is these reasons that allow us to consider A as an alternative at all. And it is these reasons which ultimately support A, rather than merely the fact that B and C have been ruled out. There must have been reasons for suspecting Jackson in the first place. The fact that Jones and Smith could not have done it is not enough reason by itself to suspect Jackson.

Exercise 6.5

Identify the form of the argument in the following cases and comment on whether the argument is valid. If not, identify the fallacy.

1. As far as I could see, this patient was suffering from either cancer of the bowel or from acute appendicitis. Pathology tests have shown no evidence of cancer, so we had better operate to remove the appendix.
2. It seems to me that in order to solve the staff parking problems in this hospital, we can either charge a parking fee or convert the maternity wing into a car park.
3. Traditional theories in physics require us to account for light either as waves or as particles. However, various experiments have shown that light does not always behave as we would expect if it were made up of waves. Other experiments show that in some conditions light does not behave in the way that particles do. So light must be understood to somehow partake of the properties of both waves and particles.
4. Somebody must have given the patient that wrong dose of medicine. There were only three nurses on duty: Clark, Bussoni, and Larson. Bussoni and Clark are very experienced and have never been known to make such a mistake, so it must have been Larson.

Chapter 7
Induction

In this chapter we discuss induction by complete and incomplete enumeration, as well as errors which can occur in using these methods. Basic forms of statistics are explained and there is a discussion of argument by analogy.

Given that deduction is a process of thinking which draws a particular conclusion from a general premise, we might ask where the general premises come from. How do we arrive at the conclusion that all nurses are intelligent or that if you are a nurse, then you must have passed the qualifying exams? The answer to this is **induction.**

Induction is the form of thinking that leads from particular premises to general conclusions. The basic idea is that we generalise from a relatively small number of instances to a larger number. If we see a number of pigeons in the park which are all a mottled grey colour, we might conclude that all pigeons are mottled grey in colour. Indeed, we might continue to sit on the park bench and notice more and more pigeons, all of which are mottled grey, and feel that our conclusion is warranted. The psychological explanation for this is that, after seeing a certain number of grey pigeons, we get used to their being grey and are not surprised to see more and more grey ones. If we were to see a white one we would be surprised. And of course, we would have to conclude that our generalisation was false. Induction is a form of reasoning that reflects the way our expectations are built up from experience.

However, as a form of reasoning, we must not be content with understanding it at the intuitive level of our expectations. We must understand its structure and be able to evaluate its strength.

The clearest and strongest instance of induction would be that of complete enumeration. If you have a definite number of instances of something and you can study each of them, then it will be easy and safe to draw a generalisation from that data. If the rangers who work in the park had tagged and counted all the pigeons which roost there, it would be an easy matter for them to observe each pigeon, see it is mottled grey and conclude that all the pigeons in the park are mottled grey in colour. Notice that this conclusion refers only to the pigeons in the park and not to other pigeons. The conclusion is based on studying all the pigeons in that group and is therefore a safe conclusion.

The form of this argument may be illustrated in the following way. Let P stand for pigeon and a subscript for a numbered instance of a pigeon. Let g stand for the property of being grey. (Properties are indicated with small case letters and the things which have those properties by capitals.) Assume there are ten pigeons in the park. The form of the ranger's thinking is then:

$P_1g, P_2g, P_3g, P_4g, P_5g, P_6g, P_7g, P_8g, P_9g, P_{10}g \Rightarrow \text{All } Pg$

A 'safe' conclusion in an induction like this is called a strongly **warranted** conclusion. You will recall that in Chapter 6, we described correct arguments as 'valid'. The reason that we use a different term here is that validity is a property of the form of an argument. If the form of a deduction, or the methodological rules followed in an induction, are correct, then the argument is valid. In most cases this is a black or white matter. An argument is either valid or not. Being warranted, in contrast, is a matter of degree. Being warranted is a property of the conclusion of an argument, rather than its form. The conclusion of an argument can be either strongly warranted or weakly warranted depending on the strength of the evidence or the plausibility of the premises. When an argument is valid and the premises are plausible, the conclusion will be strongly warranted. Where an induction is based on a complete enumeration of cases, as with the pigeons in the park, the conclusion will be very strongly warranted while if the evidence is less strong, a conclusion is less strongly warranted.

Warrant is not proof. There is nothing **necessary** about the conclusion of an induction even when the enumeration has been complete, meaning that the conclusion is as strongly warranted as it could be. It is always possible for a white pigeon to take up residence in the park and so render false the conclusion of the argument that all pigeons in the park are mottled grey. We express this idea by saying that the conclusion of an induction is **contingent**, as opposed to necessary. The theoretical reason why this is so is that in an induction, the conclusion usually goes beyond the premises or the evidence to convey more information than is contained in those premises. This contrasts with deduction, where the conclusion does nothing more than illustrate the general point articulated in the major premise.

This point is illustrated by an amusing story told by the philosopher, Bertrand Russell. In the story he refers to an American turkey which had formed the opinion, after some years of careful observation and enumeration, that he would be fed a breakfast of seeds every morning at around sunrise. Given that this had happened every morning without fail for some years, the turkey had thought that it was necessarily true, that he had proven this by way of valid reasoning. However, one Thanksgiving morning, he was cruelly shown to be wrong.

Most cases of inductive reasoning used in everyday life do not depend upon complete enumeration. The usefulness of this form of reasoning depends precisely upon the warrant that it gives for moving from a relatively small number of cases to a general conclusion. We would not have general knowledge if we could not do this. The scientist in a laboratory who notices that pressure builds up in a closed container of gas when it is heated and repeats the experiment a number of times under varying conditions, is quite warranted in concluding that all gases expand when heated. It is simply not possible to test every case of this everywhere in the world, and in the past and future, and it would be quite unnecessary to do so. Research has to extrapolate from the finite number of cases that have been studied to all other expected cases. The form of these more common cases of induction would be:

$P_1g, P_2g, P_3g, P_4g, P_5g, P_6g, P_7g, \ldots P_ng \Rightarrow \text{All } Pg$

where n stands for any appropriate number of cases that have been studied, tested or observed. The finite number of cases that are studied and from which the conclusion is drawn is called a **sample**.

Clearly, the degree of warrant with which a conclusion can be drawn will be a function of the size and nature of the sample. Moreover, if we are to be assured that the conclusion is warranted we must be sure that the sample is representative of the whole class of things that is being studied. Let us see how this might work in practice.

Suppose a sociologist studying the profession of nursing came to a large hospital and observed the nurses at their work. Suppose further that she wanted to interview the nurses about their work but, because of restrictions of time, was only able to interview ten of them. Each of these ten expressed a high degree of satisfaction with their profession in the interview and the sociologist concluded that all nurses are happy in their work. We can illustrate the argument as follows:

$N_1h, N_2h, N_3h, N_4h, N_5h, N_6h, N_7h, \ldots N_nh \Rightarrow \text{All } Nh$

where N stands for nurses and h stands for being happy in their work. In this case, n also stands for the number ten.

Now the issue here is whether it is reasonable to extrapolate from ten cases to all cases. Do ten happy nurses give us enough warrant to conclude that all nurses are happy? It would seem that the sample is much too small. The total population of nurses in this society numbers in the many thousands and a group of ten cannot be regarded as a representative sample.

And there is a second reason why this group cannot be regarded as a representative sample. To be properly representative, a sample has to be varied in the same way that the population of which it is a sample is varied. Nurses work in many different institutions and settings and the nature of their work varies accordingly. To sample nurses in only one institution under one set of working conditions is to ignore the many other kinds of working conditions that might obtain and which will influence professional contentment. To draw the conclusion that all nurses are happy in their work would require that a large sample be drawn from many differing work settings. In this example the group that is being studied—that of professional nurses—is itself large and varied. There are hospital-based nurses, nurses in community health centres, nurses in hospices and geriatric centres, nurses in schools and factories, and so forth. A representative sample would have to be drawn from these various settings.

As an aside, we might mention a further problem which such a study as this one would have. The property that is being studied (being happy in one's work) is rather vague. Does it mean that nurses obtain satisfaction through caring for others, that they enjoy the companionship of other nurses, relish the challenges of a difficult but important profession, appreciate the salary, or what? So long as this remains vague, the answers that the research subjects (that is, the ten interviewed nurses) gave in their interviews relate to the notion of being happy in varying ways. One might say that he hates the patients and the hospital administration but is happy with the salary, while another says that the salary and working conditions are poor but the feelings derived from helping those in need are a great source of contentment. As a result, there might be instances of dissatisfaction which the researcher is able to ignore so as to draw her conclusion that all nurses are happy. The researcher needs to specify exactly what is meant by 'happy' so that the outcome of the research is not ambiguous and vague. So a further lesson to be drawn from this example is that the terms and properties being studied must be carefully defined. But this is true of any research work, whether it follows the form of induction or not.

A further rule of method that is especially important for induction is that a researcher must try to find examples which count against the proposed conclusion. If our imaginary sociologist was wanting to show that all nurses were happy in their work, it would be somewhat self-serving if she interviewed only those nurses who presented themselves as being in high spirits or having a joyful disposition. The researcher ought to look out for nurses who looked glum and dissatisfied and interview them as well. If it turned out that these seemingly unhappy nurses were, as a matter of fact, very happy in their work, then the conclusion would be more strongly warranted. Having looked for disconfirming cases and found none, we can be more confident that the conclusion is correct.

And this is a further reason why a sample should be large and varied if it is to be representative. A large and varied sample is more likely to contain unhappy nurses than a small and select sample. If the conclusion—that all nurses are happy—can be sustained with reference to a large and varied sample, it will be more strongly warranted.

The error of reasoning that our imaginary sociologist has committed has a name. It is the fallacy of **hasty generalisation** and it consists in drawing a general conclusion from a sample that is too small, not varied enough, or in some other way not representative of the population that is being studied.

Another way of ensuring that a sample is representative of the group being studied is to create a random sample. This could be done if our sociologist had a register of all practising nurses and used a computer to select a manageable number randomly, who would then be sent a survey questionnaire. In this way the random sample created would be likely to include nurses who worked in various professional settings. It would contain young nurses who were still optimistic and it would contain older nurses who might be suffering from burn-out. And it would contain nurses who differed from others in terms of other factors that might be relevant to how happy they were in their work. There would be reason to think that such a random sample would be representative of the whole population of nurses, so that whatever conclusions were reached about them could be extrapolated to the rest.

Judging when an inductive conclusion is warranted is a matter for subtle judgement. We suggested in Chapter 2 that any argument or communication is dependent upon the background knowledge of the author and audience. For this reason the audience's judgment as to whether a conclusion is **plausible** will be an important element in deciding whether the conclusion is warranted. Given our everyday knowledge about nursing, we might be sceptical if we read in a sociology journal that all nurses were found to be happy in their work. We might find such a conclusion implausible and it is this reaction that would lead us to ask whether the sample on which the research was based was sufficiently large and varied (and whether the terms used in the research were clearly defined). If, on the other hand, we had read that all nurses wear uniforms on the job, we would not be so surprised and we would not demand that the research be based on a very large sample. If there is some reason for believing the generalisation already, whether that reason is based on previous experience or on some theoretical knowledge about the matters being researched, our demand for evidence will not be so strict. The less reason we have already for believing the conclusion, the larger and more varied should be the sample.

Exercise 7.1

In each of the examples below:

a. Name the kind of inference that is being drawn (eg. deduction, induction, or kind of induction).
b. Comment on whether or how strongly the inference is warranted.
c. Comment on whether any of the relevant methodological or logical rules have been broken.

1. A friend of mine has had irritating eczema for many years. He went to a Chinese herbalist recently, was given some strange herbs to ingest, and found that his skin problems cleared up in a matter of days. Chinese medicine seems to have a lot going for it.
2. I met most of the hospital staff today and found them to be keen and enthusiastic. The morale in this hospital must be quite high.
3. That's the third Mediterranean patient I have had in here today complaining of a bad back. They're all work-shy!
4. There's Judy complaining about the rosters again. She's never happy about anything.
5. I've checked each of the syringes and they're all sterile.
6. A survey done on March 7th showed that every used car salesman in this city was wearing a red tie. This shows that used car salesmen always wear red ties.

7. From a survey of patients in this western suburbs hospital it would appear that not many people take out private health insurance.
8. One hundred people were selected at random out of the phone book and interviewed as to their experience of hospitals. Each person who had a stay in hospital expressed satisfaction with the nursing they had received. It seems that there is complete satisfaction with hospital nursing in this community.
9. People in acute renal failure are anuric. Mrs Smith is anuric. Therefore she is in acute renal failure.
10. The nurses' union has sent a survey to all its members asking them about their terms and conditions. Only 17% of the membership responded but all of these complained that salaries had not kept pace with the cost of living. As a result the union is planning a campaign to gain an increase in salaries.
11. I can't understand why the patient failed to respond to this treatment. The treatment has worked in all other cases where it has been used.
12. Her lips are cyanosed. Her breathing is laboured and shallow. Therefore she has respiratory disease.

Statistics

The arguments that we have illustrated thus far lead from a finite number of cases to a general conclusion of the form 'All S are p' (where S stands for the subject under study and p for the property that is being ascribed to it). But this is not the only form of generalisation which we meet in everyday life, nor even the most frequent. We frequently express generalisations in the form of statistics.

Statistics are not strictly forms of argument. They are ways of presenting information which use numbers. As such they frequently occur in the premises and conclusions of arguments and this is why we should say something about them to clarify how statistics are arrived at and expressed and what concepts are used in articulating them. It will not be our task to explain how to do research that generates statistics or to explain the complex mathematics that is frequently involved in statistical research.

In the general and professional reading that nurses encounter, there occur four main forms of statistics:

1. totals
2. ratios
3. frequencies
4. averages.

1. A **total** is a number that tells you how many items there are of a particular category. It is arrived at by counting. The most frequent example is the population figure of a given region arrived at by government statisticians. The Australian population of about sixteen million as provided by the Australian Bureau of Statistics would be an example of

this. Totals can become more informative if one can compare a number with a different number. So, for example, in the case of population totals, it can be interesting to compare the census figures of one year with those of a previous year or set of years so that one can detect **trends** in the figures. Such comparisons can tell you if the population is increasing or decreasing.

Another example might be figures published by a hospital administration containing such information as that there are 56 nurses employed in that hospital and that when all the beds are occupied there are 218 patients, not counting outpatients. This can be useful information for the hospital administration when ordering supplies and so forth.

2. However, the latter pieces of information can be given in more useful forms for other purposes, such as comparisons with other hospitals. We can compare one hospital with another in terms of how many nursing staff each has or in terms of how many patients each can hold, but this will not tell us much more than relative size. It would be more useful if we could have that information in the form of a **ratio**. In the hospital above the number of patients to every nurse would be 3.9:1. (This is arrived at by dividing the number of beds by the number of nurses. That is 218 divided by 56.) Now suppose there was a much larger hospital in this city which had a nursing staff of 416 and 1955 beds. The ratio of patients to staff in this hospital would be 4.7:1. If these ratios can be accepted as a measure of the excellence of care available to patients, then it is clear that it would be preferable to be a patient or a nurse in the smaller hospital. But this is not because the hospital is smaller, as shown by the total number of nurses and patients, but because of the more favourable ratio of nurses to patients. It is this ratio that is being used as a measure of the quality of care in these hospitals.

3. A **frequency** statement gives the total number of items relative to a larger class of items, while a statement of **relative frequency** gives this same information in the form of a ratio. For example, the statistics issued in the annual report of a hospital might say that of the 108 full-time staff employed by the hospital (not counting medical staff who are not full time), 56 are nurses, 20 are in administration (including managers, receptionists and other general staff) and the remaining 32 are ancillary staff such as cleaners, cooks and launderers. These figures give you a breakdown of the class 'full-time staff of the hospital' in terms of three staff categories and tell you how frequent is the occurrence of each of those categories.

   We could give a different snapshot of the staffing profile of this hospital by devising a statement of the relative frequency with which each staffing category occurred. So, we might say that nurses comprised 51.85% of full-time staff, administration staff accounted for 18.53%, while ancillary staff comprised 29.62% of the total number of staff. These numbers are arrived at by dividing the number in each category by the total number and multiplying by 100.

Once again, the use of ratios here allows us to make comparisons with other similar institutions. Suppose the larger hospital, the one with 416 nurses, had a total staff of 876 of whom 222 are administrative staff and 238 ancillary staff. The percentages at this hospital would be 47.5% nurses, 25.5% administration, and 27% ancillary. This allows us to make comparisons with the other hospital and if we thought that the larger hospital was in need of improvement these figures would suggest a way of making such improvement, namely to increase the proportion of nursing staff.

Information given as frequencies is often displayed in the form of tables, graphs, bar graphs or pie charts.

Frequencies are also often given as **probabilities.** Suppose the statistics showed that of all the deaths that occurred in Australia, a quarter of them were caused by cancer. We could express this finding by saying that each person in Australia had a one in four chance of dying from cancer, or by saying that, for any individual Australian, the probability of dying from cancer was 25%.

4. An **average** is a number which gives a quick snapshot of the significance of a lot of numbers. It can be arrived at in two ways because there are actually different types of averages, depending on what calculation is performed. One common type is the **mean**, and another is the **median**.

The first way of calculating gives us the mean average. Suppose there is a group of nurses whose ages are as follows:

John	19
Nguyen	28
Leslie	24
Joan	22
Guido	25

Now the average age of this group will be the sum of these numbers divided by the number of nurses, namely 23.6. With this average figure we could justify the statement that this was a relatively young group of nurses. This type of average is called the arithmetic mean.

Now let us suppose that one of these nurses was close to retiring age so that the list of their ages looked like this:

John	19
Nguyen	28
Leslie	24
Joan	62
Guido	25

The average age of the group would now be 31.6 and this might give a misleading impression of the maturity and experience of the group as a whole. The one older member of the group has pulled the arithmetic mean upwards.

To avoid this problem we use the median which is the number whose value is in the middle of the other values so that there are an equal number of higher numbers and lower numbers on either side of the median. In the first group the median age will be Leslie's at 24, because she comes in the middle of the five ages when they are listed in order, while in the second group it is Guido's at 25. This second figure gives a more accurate impression of the relative maturity of the group than the mean would.

All these uses of statistics involve induction because they are cases where a general conclusion has been drawn from a number of instances. That the population of a particular city is 24,000 is a conclusion warranted by counting the individuals. That the ratio of nurses to patients is 3.9:1 is information that is not immediately given by counting and so requires an inductive step. The calculation of a frequency is also the drawing of a conclusion warranted by the cases that have been counted. And the snapshot of a group that an average gives us is similarly the product of a piece of inductive reasoning. In each case the conclusion is warranted if the calculation has been performed correctly according to the mathematics required.

A further way in which induction is involved in the formation of statistics is when, as frequently happens, the statistics are based upon a sample of the population being studied rather than a counting of the whole population. A very frequent example of this is the opinion poll in which it might be found that 35% of eligible voters approve of one political leader, 25% approve of another, and the remaining 40% are undecided or do not care. Such polls are usually taken by interviewing a sample of people. The number might only be several hundred. But by choosing a representative sample, the frequency of one opinion or another can be attributed to the whole voting population. Such an extrapolation is a clear example of induction.

There are two warnings that should be sounded about the gathering of statistics and the kinds of error that can be made. Opinion polls provide a good example of one of them. The way that questions are formulated in such a poll can have a bearing on the outcome. If a poll asked voters whether they approved of the Government providing more funds for health care there would almost certainly be a high number of positive responses. But if the poll asked voters if they approved of the Government increasing taxes so as to enable it to increase funding for health care, the number of positive responses is likely to be less. The publication of such polls should be accompanied by a publication of the questions so that we can all assess whether **bias** has been introduced by the formulation of the question.

The second error that can occur in some forms of statistics is when things are being compared which are not exactly alike. Let us go back to our data about the two hospitals to illustrate this point. You will recall that the patient to nurse ratio in the smaller hospital was 3.9:1, while the patient to nurse ratio in the larger one was 4.7:1 and that this made the smaller hospital look better. However, suppose that the totals for the number of nurses in each hospital were arrived at in different ways. In the smaller hospital the count included state enrolled nurses (who are not fully qualified) while such nurses were excluded from the count at the larger hospital. For this reason the smaller hospital unjustifiably seemed to have a better staff to patient ratio than the larger one. So when we are comparing things we must define and classify the things that we compare in a similar way.

Exercise 7.2

Read the following examples and identify the kind of statistics that are being used. Make any comments about how helpful the information is or if any errors in reasoning are involved.

1. According to the Australian Bureau of Statistics, 125 boys and 31 girls in the 15 to 19 age group killed themselves in 1992.[1]
2. In New South Wales alone, the number of boys aged 15 to 19 committing suicide has more than doubled since 1964.[1]
3. The director of the West Australian Research Institute for Child Health was quoted recently as saying that in 1992 in WA there were 43 successful suicides and 1200 attempted suicides by people aged from 10 to 19.[1]
4. See Figure 7.1. The two columns on the left.[2]
5. See Figure 7.1. The two columns on the right.[2]
6. Heart disease kills up to 50,000 Australians every year.
7. The atmospheric concentration of the greenhouse gas methane has more than doubled in the past 200 years, rising over the past 15 years by an average one per cent a year (roughly 17 parts per billion by volume in 1990). But the annual increase rate is slowing down. In 1992, according to measurements just published, the global increase was just 4.7ppbv versus a forecast increase of around 11ppbv.[3]
8. Rates of death from cancer in the United States rose by 7% between 1975 and 1990—a figure adjusted for the changing size and composition of the population. Lung cancer has risen 100% in women; melanoma and prostate cancer are up 80%.[4]
9. One hypothesis as to why women live longer than men is that male testosterone causes a build-up of artery-clogging cholesterol. Not so, according to a German study of the life spans of 50 castrati—male singers relieved of their testicles before puberty to preserve their beautiful voices. They usually lived for around 65.5 years, about the same as the 64.3 years for 'intact' singers of the same period.[5]
10. Figure 7.2.[6]
11. A survey of 741 people between the ages of 14 and 24, commissioned in early April, 1994, asked which occupations were most trustworthy. These are the results:

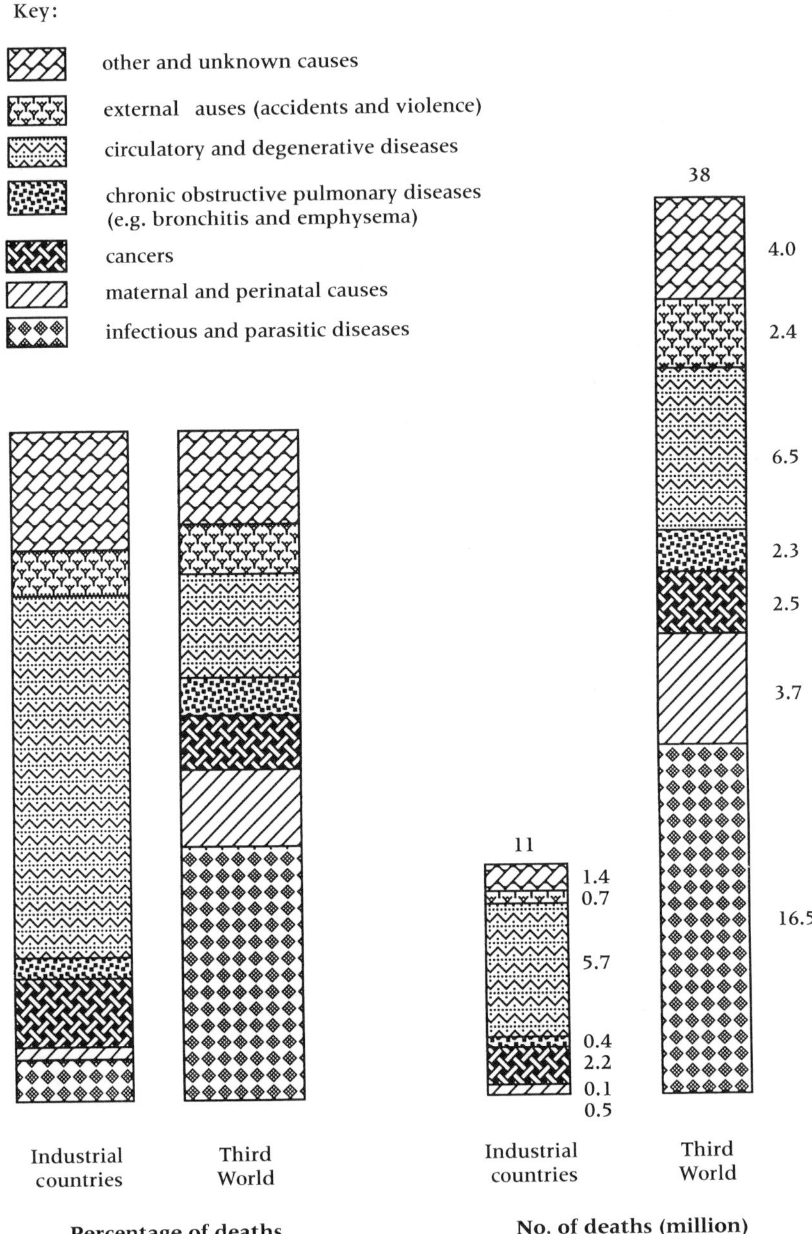

Figure 7.1 Proportional mortality by cause in industrialised countries and the Third World around 1985, together with actual numbers of deaths (in millions).

Occupation	*% Ranking of occupation most trusted*
Doctors	31
Police	20
Teachers	14
Welfare Workers	12
Clergymen	12
Lawyers	4
Musicians	4
Public Servants	1
Journalists	1
Politicians	1

12. Australian Bureau of Statistics figures show that the population density of Australia is two people per square kilometre, which is very low by world standards.

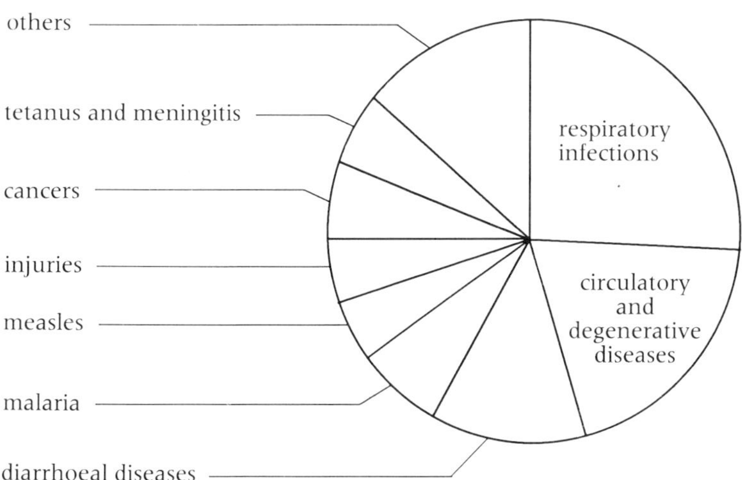

Mortality total: 38.4 million deaths

Figure 7.2 Causes of deaths in the Third World, 1986.

13. Of the seven insurance companies that offer health cover, the premiums of one are only $34 a month for a family. Similar cover from Company A costs $52; from Company B, $49; Company C, also $49; Company D, $54; Company E, $53; and Company F, $51. So it would seem that most people pay about $51 for their monthly family health cover.
14. Nurses in major public hospitals were recently surveyed about their conditions of work. Asked whether they were satisfied with their levels of salary, only 14% answered that they were.

Analogy

Before completing our discussion of induction, we should return briefly to the matter of argument by analogy. We indicated in Chapter 5 that such arguments frequently commit informal fallacies. But they do not always do so and we are now in a position to explain more fully how to distinguish valid from invalid instances.

We are in a position to do this because, although such arguments are often hard to unravel, when we write outlines of them it turns out that they combine deduction and induction. Let us take an example.

Example 7.1

Suppose a medical practitioner was urging you to take an efficient and cost-effective approach to your nursing work and not to 'waste too much time' talking to patients. In the course of her argument she might say that a patient in the clinical setting is a like a car at a garage. The job is simply to fix what is wrong and get it back on the road. This would be an argument by analogy.

If you disagree with it, you need to be able to say why. Without even beginning a formal analysis, we can see at least one apparent problem. That problem is the claim that caring for patients is like fixing cars, which seems to be a case of the informal fallacy of improper analogy which we discussed in Chapter 5. There may be a similarity in some respects, but should we draw the conclusion that they are similar in other respects as well? So even a fairly superficial and non-technical evaluation can reveal one potential flaw in the argument. However, a logical outline and a formal analysis may well reveal more. So let's now proceed to analyse the structure of this argument.

Firstly, here is an outline of the argument:

POC: Caring for a patient can be done without talking to him.

(1.	Fixing a car is a case of fixing something.)	(fact)
2.	Fixing a car can be done without talking to it.	(fact)
3.	All cases of fixing something can be done without talking to it.	(1,2 by induction)

(4. Caring for a patient is a case of fixing something.) (assertion)
5. Caring for a patient can be done without taking to him. (3,4 by deduction)

This outline identifies two assumptions, premises 1 and 4. An argument by analogy says that a property that belongs to one class of things (let us refer to this property as 'q') also belongs to another class of things. But the argument also has to show that the two things being compared belong to the same class or that the things are alike in a relevant respect. The property that makes them alike is called a **middle term** and we will refer to it with the letter 'p'. Let us refer to the two groups of things as A and B respectively. Then the argument has to show that A and B are similar in having the property p even though they are not of the same class. It is usually an acceptable assumption that A has the property—this is what makes the analogy forceful and this is what premise 1 is saying. But the assumption that B is similar in having the same property is more questionable. This is the claim that premise 4 is making. Because it is this premise that asserts that A and B are similar in sharing this middle term, it will be a crucial premise in the argument.

Let us use symbols in the above argument as follows:

A = fixing a car
B = caring for a patient
p = being a case of fixing something
q = involves not talking to what is being fixed.

Then the argument above can be set out in abstract terms as follows:

(1. Ap) (fact)
2. Aq (fact)
3. $p \Rightarrow q$ (1,2 by induction)
(4. Bp) (assertion)
5. Bq (3,4 by deduction, affirming the antecedent)

The argument depends upon an induction and then a deduction, with the connection being a middle term. So the steps in evaluating the argument are: firstly, locate the middle term and evaluate whether that property does indeed belong to both groups of things being discussed, and secondly, evaluate the induction. The latter usually depends on just one case and is therefore weakly warranted. But the crucial premise which asserts that property p applies to B is the one that is usually most open to discussion.

In the case above, this rather abstract analysis can be applied in the following way. The two classes of things are cases of mechanical repair on the one hand and cases of clinical caring on the other. The middle term that is ascribed to both classes is that they are cases of fixing something. This is one point at which the argument is weak and may be challenged. You may object that caring for a patient is **not** a case of 'fixing something' (though you would have to explain why it is not).

The argument has also claimed to show, on the basis of just one class of cases (namely, that of fixing cars) that you do not talk to what you are fixing in all cases where you are fixing something. This is the very weakly warranted induction and so offers another point at which the argument can be challenged. So, converting the argument into an outline and then into a set of symbols has allowed us to see where its weaknesses lie. Premise 3 is a weak induction and premise 4 is a questionable assertion.

Exercise 7.3

Read the following arguments and:

a. Write out the formal structure of the argument (you need only do this once since it will be the same in each case).
b. In each case, identify what the symbols in the formal structure stand for.
c. Identify the middle term which is the basis of the analogy.
d. Evaluate the argument.

1. We should reduce tariffs so that all businesses play on a level playing field.
2. We will have to sedate patient Jones. He's like a pressure cooker about to go off.
3. A hospital is a family. It should have strong central management.
4. Just as a watch must have had a maker, so the universe must have been created by God.

Exercise 7.4 (Revision)

Go back over Exercises 3.6, 3.7, 3.8, 3.9, 3.10, 3.11, 3.12 (which asked you to write logical outlines) and identify whether the conclusions were drawn on the basis of deductive or inductive inference or by the method of remainders or by argument from analogy. Explain your answers.

NOTES

1. Taken from an article on teenage suicide in *Good Weekend: The Age Magazine*, 30 April, 1994.
2. Data from Lopez, A.D., 'Causes of death in the industrialized and the developing countries: estimates for 1985', in Jamison, D.T. and Mosley, H. (eds), *Disease Control Priorities in Developing Countries*, New York, Oxford University Press, 1993.
3. *Nature*, 3 March 1994, p. 19.
4. *Scientific American*, January 1994, p. 118.
5. *Discover*, April 1994, p. 22.
6. Data derived from Walsh, J.A., *Establishing Health Priorities in the Developing World*, New York, United Nations Development Program, 1988.

Suggested Further Reading for Part One

Adams, James C., *Conceptual Blockbusting: A Guide to Better Ideas* (3rd edition), Reading, Mass., Addison-Wesley Publishing Co., 1990.
A zappy guide on how to be creative. Written for the popular market.

Bandman, Elsie L. & Bandman, Bertram, *Critical Thinking in Nursing* (2nd edition), Norwalk, Connecticut, Appleton & Lange, 1995.
We mention this book because of its use of nursing examples, but we do not recommend it unless you want to pursue matters to a much greater depth.

Barry, Vincent E. & Rudinow, Joel, *Invitation to Critical Thinking* (3rd edition), Fort Worth, Holt, Rinehart and Winston, 1994.
Very thorough in its coverage of the same areas covered by Part One of this book.

Boylan, Michael, *The Process of Argument* (2nd edition), Englewood Cliffs, New Jersey, Prentice-Hall, 1993.
Although clumsy in places, this short book was the one used by the authors before they wrote this one. It covers Part One only.

Cederblom, Jerry & Paulsen, David W., *Critical Reasoning* (3rd edition), Belmont, Wadsworth Publishing Co., 1991.
A more thorough coverage of the same areas covered by Part One of this book.

Conway, David A. & Munson, Ronald, *The Elements of Reasoning*, Belmont, Wadsworth Publishing Co., 1990.
A shorter book which covers the topics of Part One.

Fisher, Alec, *The Logic of Real Arguments*, Cambridge, Cambridge University Press, 1988.
More suitable for those interested in philosophical issues.

Fogelin, Robert J., *Understanding Arguments: An Introduction to Informal Logic* (4th edition), San Diego, Harcourt Brace Jovanoch, 1990.
A very thorough treatment more suited to the philosophically minded.

Govier, Trudy, *A Practical Study of Argument* (3rd edition), Belmont, Wadsworth Publishing Co., 1992.
A thorough book with lots of diagrams.

Hairston, Maxine, *A Contemporary Rhetoric*, Boston, Houghton Mifflin Company, 1974.
Rhetoric and logic are traditional enemies, but need not be. This book is especially good in its description of the many ways in which language can be used.

Kelley, David, *The Art of Reasoning* (expanded edition), New York, W.W. Norton and Co., 1990.
Very thorough in its coverage of the same areas covered by Part One of this book.

Missimer, C.A., *Good Arguments: An Introduction to Critical Thinking* (2nd edition), Englewood Cliffs, New Jersey, Prentice-Hall, 1989.

A shorter book with lots of good diagrams and a section on the logic of scientific experiment.

Russell, Alex, *Clear Thinking for All*, Oxford, Pergamon Press, 1967.
A short, clear book written for use in schools. It includes a discussion of science.

Salmon, Wesley C., *Logic* (3rd edition), Englewood Cliffs, New Jersey, Prentice-Hall, 1984.
A classic text on induction and deduction.

Wallace, Michael J., *Study Skills in English*, Cambridge, Cambridge University Press, 1980.
A classic in the field of study skills with chapters on efficient reading, taking notes, essay writing and more.

Waller, Bruce N., *Critical Thinking: Consider the Verdict*, Englewood Cliffs, New Jersey, Prentice-Hall, 1988.
Very thorough in its coverage of the same areas covered by Part One of this book.

Walton, Douglas N., *Informal Logic: A Handbook for Critical Argumentation*, Cambridge, Cambridge University Press, 1989.
A very useful book with lots of examples. Good on fallacies.

PART TWO:
THE LOGIC OF SCIENCE

Chapter 8

The Hypothetico-Deductive Method in Science

This chapter argues that deduction and induction are the keys to understanding how science operates. Reference will be made to examples from the history of medical science, such as Semmelweis's discovery of the causes of childbed fever and Beaumont's study of digestion.

In the first part of this book we explained that the major logical structures inherent in persuasion and argument are those of deduction and induction. It will be the task of the chapters in this part of our book to show how these logical forms are the backbone of scientific thinking. We will do this with reference to some interesting episodes from the history of medical research.

Induction Illustrated

We have already explained that induction consists in the gathering of facts from which a conclusion or generalisation is then drawn. An interesting illustration of how this process works is given by the research of William Beaumont (1785–1853) who was a surgeon in the United States Army between 1812 and 1839.

During this time in the history of medical science little was understood about the digestive processes in the stomach. It had been thought that the process was a kind of cooking relying on heat (until it was pointed out that fish digest their food without generating any heat). Then it was suggested that there was a special 'ferment' in the stomach which was responsible for digesting food. But little was known about the nature of the process. Was it a special 'vital' process belonging to a 'life force' and occurring only in a living body (so as to distinguish it from decay and rotting)? Or was it a process of transformation like other processes that occurred in all parts of nature? In modern terms, was it a **chemical** process to be understood by a science of chemistry which applied to all parts of nature, whether living or not? It was Beaumont who discovered that the process was a chemical one and thereby opened the door to fruitful investigations into the nature of the chemistry involved. Biochemistry could not have developed without this discovery, since the ancient doctrine of 'vitalism' had held that processes in the living body were inherently different from those in the rest of nature. On this view, it could not be assumed that laboratory based knowledge of chemistry would apply to living organisms.

Beaumont's studies consisted of a long series of observations made possible by a gunshot injury suffered by one Alexis St Martin who was an orderly in the army. The wound had opened a hole in St Martin's chest which healed to a point where a sort of valve-like aperture remained just above the stomach. This allowed Beaumont to extract stomach juices from St Martin for use in laboratory experiments. It also allowed him to study the contents of St Martin's stomach without removing them. As a result Beaumont was able to record two sets of observations. One set related to how various foods were digested in St Martin's stomach and the other set related to how St Martin's stomach juices reacted to various foodstuffs in the laboratory.

Beaumont recorded his observations in tables which listed a wide variety of foodstuffs (rice, tripe, liver, lamb and many more), how they were prepared (boiled, roasted, broiled, raw etc.), and the times taken to digest them (that is, to break them down into liquid form). The table showed this information both *in vivo* and *in vitro* (that is, in the stomach and in a laboratory vial). So, for example, it took three and a half hours to digest a hard boiled egg in the stomach, while it took eight hours in a laboratory vial. And baked custard took two hours and forty-five minutes to digest in vivo, while it took six and a half hours in vitro. Beaumont also assembled tables 'showing the temperature of the interior of the stomach in different conditions, taken in different seasons of the year, and at various times of the day'.[1] Beaumont continued his studies, using St Martin, for nine years, making innumerable observations. At the end he was able to conclude that the processes in the stomach and in the laboratory were of the same nature: that is, they were both purely chemical.

In what way does Beaumont's research illustrate induction? The most obvious point is that there were numerous observations and one general conclusion. The more important point is that the general conclusion is supported by the sheer weight in numbers of the observations. A few tests would not have been convincing. Beaumont had a unique opportunity to gather extensive data in that he had a stomach available to him that he could explore virtually at will. As a result, he was able to establish the similarity of the digestive processes in vivo and in vitro, with the only consistent difference being in the time taken.

The logical outline of Beaumont's inductive reasoning would be:

Example 8.1

POC: Digestion is a chemical process.

1. A chemical process can take place in the laboratory (unlike a 'vital' process that can only take place in a living body). (fact)
2. Many observations show that digestion in vivo is similar to digestion in vitro, except that the latter takes longer. (fact)

3. Digestion can take place in the laboratory. (2)
4. Digestion is a chemical process. (1,3)

It is premise 2 which is the inductive step in this argument. Anyone reading Beaumont's book describing his research could not fail to be convinced by the weight of data.

Induction convinces by thoroughness. When there is an overwhelming weight of evidence in favour of a proposition it would be irrational to deny it. Even though it is not proven in the strict sense of that word, there is warrant, or justification, or evidence for asserting it. In such a case, the only justification for denying it would be if one had better evidence for a contrary proposition.

Another Example of Scientific Research

And now another story about early medical research. This story concerns Ignaz Semmelweis (1818–1865) who was a physician at the Vienna General Hospital. Semmelweis noticed that approximately one in ten mothers died in the First Maternity Division of this hospital of an illness known as puerperal fever or childbed fever, while in the Second Maternity Division the death toll from this disease was much lower, about two cases in a hundred. In an attempt to lower the death rate in the First Division, Semmelweis set about trying to find out why there were so many more deaths in that division compared to the Second Division.

Before we describe how he went about this, we should explain the word 'hypothesis'. A hypothesis is a guess, a suggestion or a conjecture as to what might be the nature of a process or what might be causing a problem or puzzling event. In the case of Beaumont's research, his hypothesis would have been that digestion is a chemical process. By itself, a hypothesis is not an explanation. Because it is only a conjecture, a hypothesis should be tested to see if it is correct. This testing might take the form of experiments, or finding further facts in nature which confirm it, or it might take the form of simply thinking through the implications of the hypothesis to see if it could even be true. If the hypothesis is contradicted by the known facts, or is internally incoherent, then it is not even worth testing it by experiment.

For example, there were a number of hypotheses held by hospital staff and by the concerned public to explain the high rates of childbed fever deaths in the First Division. These included the idea that there was an epidemic spreading the fever, that there was overcrowding in the First Division, and that the diet given to mothers in the First Division was to blame. However, thinking about the first of these suggestions, Semmelweis reasoned that if an epidemic had struck Vienna, or even just the areas near the hospital, then the Second Division would be just as affected as the First. Moreover, those mothers who were delivered of their babies as they approached the hospital (a not infrequent occurrence) would also be affected. But it appeared that the death rate amongst these mothers, despite the harshness of the conditions of their birthing, was quite low. Again, on looking into the other suggestions, he found that the Second Division was even more crowded than the First (since mothers who knew of the higher death rates there were keen to avoid the First Division), and that the diet in the two divisions did not differ significantly. It followed logically that these hypotheses could not be true.

The logical outline of the reasoning involved here would be as follows:

Example 8.2

(1. Epidemics affect whole regions indiscriminately.) (fact)
2. An epidemic is causing the deaths in the First Division. (hypothesis)
3. An epidemic would cause equal death rates in both divisions. (1,2)
4. The death rates in the two divisions are not equal. (fact)
5. An epidemic is not causing the deaths in the First Division. (3,4)

Or again:

Example 8.3

1. Overcrowding is causing the deaths in the First Division. (hypothesis)
2. Equal or greater overcrowding would cause equal or greater death rates in the Second Division. (1)
3. The death rate in the Second Division is less. (fact)
4. The Second Division is more crowded. (fact)
5. Overcrowding does not cause death rates to increase. (3,4)
6. Overcrowding is not causing the deaths in the First Division. (5,2)

Exercise 8.1

Write a logical outline of Semmelweis's reasoning regarding the hypothesis that diet was the cause of the higher death rates in the First Division.

It should be clear that these logical outlines display instances of deductive reasoning. We can show this by noting premise 3 in the epidemic argument and premise 2 in the overcrowding argument. These premises can be transformed into general statements as follows.

> If an epidemic were causing the deaths, then the death rates would be the same in both divisions.
>
> If overcrowding were causing the deaths, then the rates of death would be proportional to the rates of crowding.

Notice that these propositions are in the 'If . . . then . . .' form which is characteristic of the general statements from which conclusions can be drawn by deduction (that is, they are major premises). In this instance, the conclusions that are drawn are that the 'if . . .' statements are not true. The arguments are as follows:

Example 8.4

1. If an epidemic were causing the deaths, then the death rates would be the same in both divisions.
2. The death rates are not the same in both divisions.

⇒ An epidemic is not causing the deaths.

Example 8.5

1. If overcrowding were causing the deaths, then the rates of death would be proportional to the rates of crowding.
2. The rates of death are not proportional to the rates of crowding.

⇒ Overcrowding is not causing the deaths.

The form of both these arguments is:

$x \Rightarrow y$
$-y$
$\Rightarrow -x$

where (in the second argument) x = the hypothesis that overcrowding causes the deaths and y = the death rates being proportional to the rates of crowding. (Notice that x and y stand for propositions rather than entities and properties in these cases.) This is a valid form of deduction: a case of denying the consequent. Given that x is the hypothesis, the argument shows conclusively that the hypothesis is false.

What these arguments also show is that, because the death rates in the two divisions are different, it is rational to look for conditions which obtained in one division but not the other (or obtained in both to a difference in degree comparable to the different rates of death). No condition that obtained equally in both divisions could be the cause.

There was a Commission of Inquiry in 1846 which offered a hypothesis that met this condition and was amenable both to the kind of logical critique so far described and also to experimental testing. This suggested explanation was that rough handling by medical students on obstetrical training in the First Division was causing the deaths. Mothers in the First Division were examined by these medical students, whereas mothers in the Second Division were attended only by midwives. Here was a factual difference between the two wards. However, inquiries and observations prompted by the hypothesis showed that birthing in the Second Division was just as rough and sometimes even rougher than in the First Division.

The midwives were no gentler in handling the mothers than were the medical students. Nevertheless, an experimental test was devised to see if the hypothesis was true. The students were trained in gentler methods and these were then put into effect. Unfortunately for the hypothesis (and for the mothers who died) this change produced no improvement in the rates of childbed fever.

Exercise 8.2

Set out in logical form the arguments which showed that the above hypothesis—rough handling by medical students causes childbed fever—was false.

Given that this hypothesis failed, Semmelweis looked for further differences between the two divisions. One such difference consisted in the fact that the priest who brought the last sacraments to those who died in the hospital needed to pass through the First Division in order to reach other wards. The priest would do so with sombre pomp. Dressed in black vestments and accompanied by an altar boy swinging an incense burner and ringing a bell, the priest was thought to have a profound psychological effect upon those who saw and heard his procession. Could this account for the higher death rates in the First Division? Well, it was simple enough to test this hypothesis. Semmelweis asked the priest to enter the hospital by another door so as to avoid the First Division. No difference in the death rate resulted.

Exercise 8.3

Set out in logical form Semmelweis's reasoning concerning the priest's procession. Identify the form of the argument and say whether it is valid.

Semmelweis worked on various other hypotheses as well, but without success. Finally, it was an incident that did not seem to be related to the problem he was working on, that gave him the vital clue. Another doctor at the hospital died with symptoms which resembled those of childbed fever. On inquiring as to what might have led to the death, Semmelweis discovered that his colleague had received a cut on the finger from a scalpel held by a student with whom he had been performing an autopsy. Given that he had already been thinking about the possible role of medical students, Semmelweis was quick to make the connection. Apparently, the students did autopsies before entering the First Division for their lessons in obstetrics and, given that the role of bacteria in transmitting disease was not understood in those days, they only washed their hands in a superficial way. Semmelweis formed the hypothesis that, in his own words, 'cadaveric matter' (from the Latin word 'cadaver', meaning corpse) on the hands of the medical students was causing the fever.

Even before he tested this hypothesis it was clear that it accorded with the known facts. Medical students did not examine the mothers in the Second Division and they did not examine the mothers who were delivered of their babies in the street. And the death rates amongst these mothers were quite low.

The deductive form of this thinking would be:

Example 8.6

1. If cadaveric matter on students' hands was causing the deaths, then there should be lower death rates where there are no students.
2. There are lower death rates where there are no students.

⇒Cadaveric matter on students' hands is causing the deaths.

The logical form of this argument is:

x ⇒y
y
⇒ x

where x = the hypothesis that cadaveric matter on students' hands was causing the deaths and y = there being fewer deaths when there are no students in attendance. But what is really interesting about this argument is that it is a logical fallacy! It seems rational enough to think this way, but the fact is that it is a case of asserting the consequent. For this reason, the reasoning involved is not conclusive. We can see that Semmelweis was on to something important (especially given our current knowledge of bacteria), but he has not proven his case. It is still possible that something else was causing the problem.

So Semmelweis needed to do more to be convincing. He devised a test. He ordered that the medical students should wash their hands in a solution of chlorinated lime before making any examinations of mothers in the First Division. Although he knew nothing about germs or microorganisms, he had a fair idea of what would get the students' hands clean. This worked. The death rates fell to rates comparable to those in the Second Division.

Once again, the form of Semmelweis's thinking would be:

Example 8.7

1. If cadaveric matter is causing the deaths, the death rates should decrease when cadaveric matter is removed by washing.
2. The death rates do decrease when cadaveric matter is removed by washing.

⇒ Cadaveric matter is causing the deaths.

And once again we find that from a strictly logical point of view, the argument has the same invalid form as before. It affirms the consequent.

Nevertheless, we feel intuitively that Semmelweis is on the right track. The fact that we have a fuller understanding of the transmission of infections today makes it even more likely that we would accept Semmelweis's explanations. However, if we try to imagine ourselves with only the background knowledge of his day, when nothing was known of micro-organisms, we can see that the matter might not have been settled. In its favour, Semmelweis's hypothesis seems to explain why the death rate in the First Division was higher than the rate in the Second. It explains why mothers who gave birth in the street were not in danger, and it explains why the students' washing of their hands should make a difference. Indeed, given that the latter procedure seemed to solve the problem we could suppose that the case was closed.

But the fact is that Semmelweis was wrong. He realised this when, on a later occasion, he examined a woman in labour who was suffering from a festering cervical cancer and then examined the other mothers in the ward. He had disinfected his hands before entering the ward but, nevertheless, eleven out of the twelve mothers died of puerperal fever shortly afterwards. There had been no 'cadaveric matter' on his hands, so what could have been the problem? With his thinking now well attuned to the idea of contamination carried by hands, it did not take Semmelweis long to surmise that the infection could also be transmitted from 'putrid matter derived from living organisms';[2] in this case, putrid matter derived from the festering cancer wound.

The logical outline of his thinking here might be shown as follows:

Example 8.8

1. (Only) 'cadaveric matter' causes childbed fever. (hypothesis)
2. Where there is no 'cadaveric matter' there will be no childbed fever. (1)
3. There was no 'cadaveric matter'. (fact)
4. There should be no childbed fever. (2,3)
   (This is a valid deduction—affirming the antecedent)
5. But there was childbed fever. (fact)
6. The hypothesis (1) is false. (4,5)

Notice that a thorough researcher would have to check the two premises labelled as facts here. She would have to be assured that there really had been no 'cadaveric matter' on the hands—that the hands had been thoroughly washed. And she would have to be assured that the illness of which the eleven mothers died really was childbed fever. If all this checked out, then the incident really did show that Semmelweis's hypothesis was false. Even though he had been on the right track, he had not correctly identified the source of the problem. This is highlighted by our formulation of the hypothesis as, '*Only* "cadaveric matter" causes childbed fever'. Today we know that lethal bacteria can be picked up from both corpses and festering wounds. Semmelweis had to discover that whatever it was that caused childbed fever could be picked up from either of these sources. He did this, under rather unfortunate circumstances, and subsequently broadened his hypothesis to include the new information.

An interesting point about science that is illustrated by this incident is that many hypotheses are fruitful and successful not simply because they solve problems, but because they suggest further lines of inquiry which allow new knowledge to be developed. Semmelweis not only solved the problem of the death rate from puerperal fever, but he also suggested a new line of inquiry. What do 'cadaveric matter' and 'putrid matter derived from living organisms' have in common? It was not till later that an answer could be found to this question, when the relevant bacteria were discovered.

Beaumont's research had a similar effect. As soon as it was realised that digestion was a chemical process, and hence that other biological processes were also likely to be chemical in nature, the science of chemistry could be brought to bear on the problems of medicine.

The Structure of Scientific Thinking

We can now summarise the logic of testing hypotheses. To do this we must introduce a new term, namely **implication**. In the deductive arguments which we described above, we substituted the symbol x for the hypothesis being tested and y for the expectation to which the hypothesis gives rise. So for example we had:

Example 8.9

1. If rough handling by medical students was causing the deaths, then the death rates would reduce when handling was gentler.
2. Death rates did not reduce when handling was gentler.

⇒ Rough handling by medical students was not causing the deaths.

or: $x \Rightarrow y$

$-y$

$\Rightarrow -x$ (denying the consequent: valid)

where x = the hypothesis that rough handling by medical students was causing the deaths, and y = death rates reducing when handling is gentler. But the hypothesis here is itself a nested deductive argument. It can be given in the following form:

Example 8.10

1. If medical students handled patients more gently, there would be lower rates of death.
2. (Let us suppose) medical students do handle patients more gently.

⇒ Death rates will be lower.

that is: $x \Rightarrow y$

x

$\Rightarrow y$

where x = medical students handling patients more gently, and y = there being lower rates of death. Another version of the argument might have x = there being no contact with rough medical students, or x = there being birthing in the street outside, and so on. In this way, we can spell out the implications that a particular hypothesis has. (Examples 8.2 and 8.3 show the nested deductions in the logical outline of Semmelweis's reasoning.)

Every hypothesis will have a number of implications. Semmelweis's successful hypothesis, in its original form, implied that where mothers were attended by people without cadaveric matter on their hands, like the midwives in the Second Division, there would be lower rates of death. And it implied that wherever there was no cadaveric matter, such as in the streets outside the hospital, there would be no fever. In this way the hypothesis did not conflict with known facts. Indeed, it was an **explanation** of those facts.

Another implication of the hypothesis is that if the medical students who can be expected to have cadaveric matter on their hands were to disinfect those hands, there would be a reduction in cases of childbed fever. This implication is in the future tense. It describes what *would* happen if certain steps were taken. In this sense it is a **prediction**. And this prediction turned out to be correct. So implications of hypotheses can yield explanations of facts already known, or they can yield predictions of facts not yet known. Experiments are procedures for testing whether such predictions are correct. In this sense, Semmelweis's ordering the medical students to disinfect their hands was an experiment designed to see if the hypothesis was correct.

In order to highlight the point we have just made, we could say that any hypothesis should be able to be put into the form: **If** it is true **then** certain facts would be explained or certain predictions would be true. Or again, **If** the hypothesis (H) is true **then** its implication (I) would be true. In its most schematic form, this could be expressed as:

$H \Rightarrow I$

In cases where the prediction proved false, as with the case of the priest's procession (the implication/prediction would have been that changing the priest's route would solve the problem), the next premise would be:

$-I$

and this would have yielded:

$-H$

as a valid deduction (denying the consequent).

But if the test results support the hypothesis, we get:

$H \Rightarrow I$
I
$\Rightarrow H$

and, as we have noted, this is an invalid deduction (affirming the consequent).

This is why researchers have to do numerous tests in order to confirm hypotheses. But, from a logical point of view, what do numerous tests or confirming facts add to the credibility of the hypothesis? We might represent numerous tests as follows:

Example 8.11

$H \Rightarrow I_1, I_2, I_3, I_4, I_5, \ldots I_n$
$I_1, I_2, I_3, I_4, I_5, \ldots I_n$
$\Rightarrow H$

Now, even though we have explored numerous implications (I_1, I_2, I_3, I_4, I_5, . . . I_n) and found them all to obtain, we still have only got numerous cases of affirming the consequent and so we still do not have a valid deduction.

But what we are getting now is a warranted **induction**. These many tests give inductive warrant to the hypothesis. The more tests or observations that confirm the hypothesis, the more assertable it becomes; the more rational it becomes to believe it. And so we see that the roles played by induction and deduction in science are both important. Deduction is at its most powerful in showing hypotheses to be false. Hypotheses can be disproven with complete certainty. But when it comes to showing hypotheses to be true, we must rely on induction. The more implications (facts that can be explained or predicted by the hypothesis) of the hypothesis which are true, the more believable the hypothesis is and the more irrational it would be not to believe it. We might never achieve logical proof but we can certainly achieve warranted assertability.

A sad footnote to Semmelweis's story illustrates the above point. Despite his success, Semmelweis's colleagues were not convinced. They judged his ideas unproven and found the hand washing routines distasteful. He was dismissed from the Vienna General Hospital and went to Budapest, where his ideas were also disregarded. Eventually, he went insane and died in an asylum.

Exercise 8.4 (Revision Questions)

1. What is a hypothesis?
2. What are some of the ways in which we can test hypotheses?
3. What is the logical form of the argument implicit in a test procedure?
4. What is the role of induction in scientific testing?
5. When would we be satisfied that a hypothesis is true?

Where Do Hypotheses Come From?

There is just one more question we need to address before we finish this chapter: Where do hypotheses come from?

It used to be thought that hypotheses could be arrived at by induction: that researchers should observe and record all the facts, then analyse and classify them, and then draw inductive generalisations from them so as to form hypotheses that would then be subject to further testing. It might be thought that Beaumont's research illustrates this. Nine years of observations and experiments adding up to a single general hypothesis.

But can *all* the facts ever be collected? To fulfil this requirement Beaumont would have had to record the colour of St Martin's clothes, whether he liked the food he ate, the number of people present in the laboratory, the names and addresses of St Martin's friends, and so on. Semmelweis would have had to record the condition of the weather when mothers died, the colour of their hair, the names and addresses of everyone present or not present, and so on. The list of facts that obtain in any given situation is infinite. Commonsense dictates that one should only record those facts which are relevant to the matter at hand.

But then how would you know what is relevant and what is not, if you have not yet made the relevant discovery? By having a hypothesis. It was because he already surmised that digestion was a chemical process that Beaumont could select which facts to record. Time taken and amount of heat generated are relevant features of chemical reactions. While Semmelweis was entertaining the possibility that the priest's procession might have been the cause of the deaths, the facts relating to the priest's procession were relevant. When he ruled out that hypothesis, those facts ceased to be relevant. Just as it takes experience, judgement and a grasp of the relevant background knowledge to form a hypothesis, so it takes the same skills to see what facts are relevant to that hypothesis. It was these qualities in Semmelweis that led him to see the death of his colleague as relevant.

The formation of a hypothesis to start with might not have played so central a role in Beaumont's research. We can imagine Beaumont simply being curious about the processes in the stomach. But he was aware of certain debates among medical thinkers about 'vitalism' as well, and this is what led him to see that his research might be relevant to this debate. It led him to ask whether the processes of digestion are chemical. Perhaps he began his research wanting to test the hypothesis that they were, or perhaps this hypothesis occurred to him during the course of the research, when he began to notice the similarity between the processes *in vivo* and *in vitro*. Either way, it would have been his familiarity with the vitalism debate which suggested the hypothesis to him.

In the Semmelweis case, we see someone who has an immediate and urgent problem that he needs to solve. He needs to look for differences between conditions in the First and Second Divisions but he has no idea what sort of things might be relevant. He cannot afford to ignore anything, not even the priest's procession which, to our ears, sounds a very unlikely explanation. But it was his ability to recognise the relevance of a coincidental event which gave him the necessary clue. His colleague's death might not have been thought of as relevant by other doctors at that hospital because their minds had not been prepared by grappling with the problem of puerperal fever.

So we see that hypotheses arise from the background knowledge that the researcher has in relation to the problem, and by intuitive insights. In fact, it does not much matter where hypotheses come from. There are even cases of scientists literally dreaming up hypotheses that have turned out to be true. The important thing is that they be tested against the facts in the ways we described above.

In summary we can say that scientists proceed by:

1. forming hypotheses
2. deriving implications from these hypotheses
3. seeing if these implications obtain as facts (in which case the hypothesis is said to explain these facts)
4. or designing experiments to see if the implications predicted by the hypothesis turn out to be true
5. and asserting that the hypothesis is inductively warranted if there are a sufficient number of confirmations of it
6. or rejecting the hypothesis if the implications turn out to be untrue.

Central to these procedures is the deduction of implications from the hypothesis. For this reason, there is a fancy name for the set of methods and procedures which we have been describing. It is called the 'hypothetico-deductive' method of science.

Exercise 8.5 (Revision Questions)

1. Where do hypotheses come from?
2. Why couldn't scientists expect to proceed effectively if they set about gathering all the facts so as to be able to make inductions?
3. What is the 'hypothetico-deductive' method of science?
4. What is 'warranted assertability', how does it differ from proof, and how is it achieved in science?

NOTES

1. Quoted by Rom Harré in *Great Scientific Experiments*, Oxford, Oxford University Press, 1981, p. 39.
2. These quotes are from Carl G. Hempel's account of the Semmelweis experiments in *Philosophy of Natural Science*, Englewood Cliffs, New Jersey, Prentice-Hall, 1966. The relevant section is reproduced in Mosedale, Frederick E. (ed.), *Philosophy and Science: The Wide Range of Interaction*, Englewood Cliffs, New Jersey, Prentice-Hall, 1979.

Chapter 9

The Nature of Explanation

This chapter explicates six models of explanation: the interpretation model, the classification model, the purposive model, the covering law model, the statistical model and the causal model. It is suggested that explanation and persuasion have a similar logical structure. The difference is that, while in persuasion we offer reasons, in explanation we look for causes.

In the previous chapter we said that if a hypothesis is consistent with known facts, then it serves to explain those facts. In this chapter we will explore more thoroughly what it means to explain something.

What Is an Explanation?

The first point that should be noted is that an explanation is a psychological event. It is an answer to a question like 'why?' or 'how come?', or 'what is it?' It is an answer to a puzzle or a problem. What this means is that people accept that something has been explained when they feel satisfied in their own minds that they have an answer to a question which they were asking.

There is a cartoon which illustrates the point very well. It shows a mother tucking her young child into bed. It is winter and it is snowing outside. The child asks its mother why it is snowing and she replies that it is cold outside.

'Why?' asks the child.
'Because it is winter,' answers the mother.
'But why?' persists the child.
'Because there is not much sun.'
'Why?'
'Because elephants have flat feet.'
'Oh.'

And the child goes to sleep happy with the thought that mothers know everything.

Of course what this little story also illustrates is that not anything will do as an explanation. That elephants have flat feet may be true but it hardly explains snow. Just why it doesn't is, however, not so easy to make clear. What we are apt to say is that elephants' feet are not relevant to meteorology. But in order to be able to say that we must already have some knowledge of the relevant matters. The child in the cartoon does not have such knowledge and hence cannot see that the state of elephants' feet is not relevant to snow.

If we can change the example slightly from snow to rain, we will be able to consider those tribal peoples who engage in various kind of religious ritual in order to produce rain at times when they need it. Anthropologists record numerous instances of such practices around the world. These tribal people seem to believe that rituals such as rain dances can affect the weather and, were it to rain soon after one of their dances, they would explain the occurrence of that rain by referring to their dance. Is this any different from explaining snow by referring to elephants' feet? From the point of view of our modern scientific culture, it may seem not. Yet, these tribal peoples are doing what we all do: using their background knowledge and understanding of how the world works to explain events. It is just that their background knowledge and understanding of how the world works includes ideas about the gods causing rain if and when it pleases them, and about how humans might influence the gods to make rain by performing certain ritual dances. This is not a body of knowledge which most of us would share but it makes the matter of ritual dances just as relevant to rain for those tribal peoples as our scientific knowledge of meteorology is for us. We can imagine these tribal peoples being satisfied with an explanation for rain which said that it was a gift from the gods in response to the rituals, or with an explanation for the absence of rain which said that the gods were not pleased and needed to be expiated with ritual dancing.

Our first point, then, is that an explanation for an event or phenomenon is an account of that event or phenomenon which is intellectually or emotionally satisfactory in the context of a body of background knowledge. Our next point is that in our culture generally, and in our professional practice as health care workers in particular, the background body of knowledge which operates to make explanations possible is science. Most frequently, the scientific knowledge which you will bring to bear on problems in your professional practice is that of medical science, or bioscience, but the whole field of modern scientific knowledge will be involved. Basic physics is involved in explaining why you can hurt your back when you lift patients wrongly, and both sociology and psychology are involved in understanding patients as whole persons.

A further point which we noted is that an explanation is an answer to a problem. Most often we seek an explanation because we are puzzled by something. We might be puzzled simply because we are curious about the matter at hand, or we might be puzzled because we have an immediate and urgent problem. We can imagine Beaumont, whom we discussed in the previous chapter, simply being curious about how digestion worked and keen to enhance the store of physiological knowledge, while Semmelweis was clearly driven by an immediate and urgent problem. He needed to explain the deaths from childbed fever because he wanted to prevent them. Thus, the intellectual or emotional satisfaction which we mentioned in the previous paragraph comes about when the perceived puzzle or problem is solved.

But what is interesting about our suggestion that in giving an explanation, a problem is solved, is that there is no requirement that an explanation be true for it to be satisfactory. The tribal peoples whom we imagined before will feel that they are solving their drought problem when they engage in their ritual dance even though we, with our differing scientific background, might think their explanation to be false. In a similar way, when a doctor prescribes a placebo and it works to alleviate suffering, the relieved patient may well explain his improvement by saying that it was the medicine that gave him relief, even though the doctor knows that it was just the psychological effect of being given the medicine which effected the improvement. The patient's explanation is false, but it is quite satisfactory. (Indeed, the placebo can only be effective as long as the patient has this false belief.) Another example comes from the Semmelweis story. Before Semmelweis expanded his explanation to include putrid matter from living bodies, it was satisfactory even though it was not true (or at least only partly true). He did reduce the incidence of childbed fever even though, in specifying 'cadaveric matter', he had not correctly identified the source of the infection.

Exercise 9.1 (Revision questions)

1. What is an explanation?
2. Why is background knowledge necessary to explanations?
3. Do explanations have to be true to be satisfactory?

Models of Explanation

There are several typical models of explanation:

1. the interpretation model
2. the purposive model
3. the classification model
4. the covering law model
5. the statistical model
6. the causal model

We will discuss each of these in turn.

1. The Interpretation Model of Explanation

We use the interpretation model of explanation when we say what something means. An everyday example of this would be when we hear someone say something in a foreign language or when we listen to someone with a speech defect. Or we might be reading a difficult text book or watching a sophisticated movie. In all these cases we may be puzzled about what is meant and our task will be to interpret what we hear or see. In this context an explanation will take the form of someone, or the speakers themselves, giving us a translation, or an account of what they were trying to tell us. In the case of a text book, your teacher might explicate what the difficult passage means.

But it is not only in relation to written or spoken language that we can find ourselves puzzled as to what something means. We often use the interpretation model of explanation in relation to the behaviour of other people. If a patient in a ward is constantly calling for a nurse to attend to trivial matters or to assist in simple tasks of which the patient is quite capable you might say that the patient is lonely and wants company. This would be an interpretation of the patient's behaviour. You are explaining why the patient is being troublesome by suggesting that they want company or attention. Again, in speaking of a person who frequently attempts suicide but seems strangely incapable of bringing it off effectively, we might say that they are uttering a cry for help. This would be an interpretation of their behaviour. This explanation is given in terms of what the behaviour means.

This form of explanation is especially important in the psychiatric field. Indeed, it is the very essence of the method of psychoanalysis in which the patient is brought by the analyst to see what their troublesome behaviour means in the light of early experiences in their lives. However, there are ongoing debates about whether these forms of explanation are ultimately satisfactory in solving psychiatric problems. If certain psychiatric problems are caused by disorders in the brain, then interpreting the meaning of the disordered behaviour might not be as effective as prescribing drugs which will prevent the behaviour.

On the other hand, for less dramatic cases such as that of the troublesome patient in the ward, having an explanation which gives us the meaning of what the patient is doing might well suggest simple and effective remedies, for example, providing more opportunity for the patient to enjoy the company of others.

2. The Purposive Model of Explanation

We use the purposive model of explanation when we say why something happened. Often, when we are confronted by a puzzling event, we are satisfied when we find out the reason for its occurrence. You will often hear patients who are suffering greatly from an illness ask, 'Why me?' A person of religious faith might answer such a question by saying that their suffering has the purpose of expiating sin. Whether or not we agree with such an answer, we can recognise that what it gives is a purposive explanation.

The way that such an explanation works is by saying that the puzzling event occurred because it served some purpose. In the case of the religious believer seeking to explain their suffering, this purpose is attributed to God. But the most obvious instances of this form of explanation are when we explain the actions of human beings in terms of the intentions that those human beings had in performing the action. 'Why did Bob close the window?' 'Because he wanted to stop the noise outside coming into the room.' This explains why Bob did something by telling us what Bob's intention or purpose was in doing it.

You will notice that this is similar to explanations which give us the meanings of actions. The difference is that in the case before us, Bob knows what his purpose is. He knows why he is doing what he is doing. It is Bob who is best able to tell us that he closed the window because he wanted to stop the noise. The troublesome patient, on the other hand, probably doesn't know that he is actually trying to overcome loneliness. If you asked him why he rang for the nurse, he will tell you that it was to get a glass of water. It would not occur to him that he had some other goal, whereas our interpretation of his actions is that they are ways of overcoming loneliness. The difference between these two forms of explanation is subtle but real.

If a purposive explanation requires the inquirer to identify some purpose for the sake of which the event occurred, then it is clear that purposive explanations are most at home in the area of human actions, or the actions of any other beings, which can have purposes. Our suffering religious believer had no trouble attributing a purpose to God and was able to explain his own suffering in this way. We have no trouble explaining the behaviour of animals by attributing purposes either. If we see a dog sniffing the ground in a puzzling way, we might say it is looking for food. This is to suggest that the dog has the purpose or goal of finding food, and this explains the behaviour perfectly well because we know that dogs are the kinds of things that can have such purposes.

But what if we use a purposive explanation for something that cannot have purposes in this way? The now discredited doctrine of vitalism which we mentioned in connection with Beaumont's research is an example of this. Vitalists believed that living organisms were made up of parts or substances which had purposes of their own, such that those purposes taken together constituted the life processes of that organism. For example, it was the purpose of the heart to pump blood and the purpose of the kidneys to clean it, and so forth. They did not just mean that it was the function of these organs to perform those tasks. We have no trouble today in accepting that certain organs have specific functions or roles to play in the life of the organism. But vitalists believed that organs had inherent tendencies or inclinations to perform these functions because they contained 'vital principles' which were like purposes, and that the organs did what they did in order to fulfill these purposes or tendencies. It was as if the organs were motivated to do what they did. The best example of this kind of thinking comes from vitalist theories of the development of the embryo. Before the development of modern embryology, it was thought that a foetus developed by way of a gradual unfolding of its own inner tendencies and potentialities. It was as if the embryo had a purpose or a plan to develop itself into the foetus. We will see in Chapter 11 why this thinking was fallacious. For the moment, it is important to see that purposive explanations are only valid in relation to beings which can act purposefully.

3. The Classification Model of Explanation

We use the classification model of explanation when, in response to a puzzle, we say what something is. When a child points to something and says, 'What's that?', she is looking for a classificatory explanation. The answer, 'It's a car', will satisfy her.

The classification model can be exemplified by those sciences which seek to understand and classify natural phenomena. Botany and zoology are good examples. Field workers in these sciences go into the field, collect specimens of plants or animals, and classify them. If a zoologist finds an unfamiliar little furry animal in a forest, she has a puzzle or a problem. She will wonder what it is. On inspecting it she may find that it has a pouch and various other features that belong to the classification of marsupials. She will note the length of the tail, the shape of its ears, and so forth, until finally her puzzle is solved. She identifies it as a marsupial rat. This may not sound like an explanation, but it has the same psychological features as an explanation: a satisfying answer to a puzzle or problem which makes use of background knowledge (in this case, knowledge of zoological classifications).

Classifications do seem more like explanations in another area where they are common, that of medical diagnosis. Suppose a person presents themselves to a doctor or a district nurse with a persistent cough and a pain in the chest. The health worker engages in the usual investigative procedures, noting the nature and severity of the symptoms, and concludes that the patient has a severe cold. For the patient this explains her cough and chest pain. That she has a cough and a pain in the chest is now explained by the diagnosis that she has a cold. This satisfies her in that she now knows what is causing her cough and pain and she also knows what she needs to do to find relief. The doctor may have prescribed an antibiotic or the patient may merely need a patent medicine from the chemist. She still has a cough and a pain, but she no longer has a puzzle.

Indeed, the explanation for her symptoms might be satisfying in a more profound way. She might have been worried that her symptoms indicated pneumonia. In this instance the diagnosis will be met with relief. It is merely a case of a cold. On the other hand, the diagnosis may have been that she had lung cancer. There will be no relief in this diagnosis. Nevertheless, this diagnosis does explain the symptoms and solves the problem of what was going on in her chest.

Now it might be said that merely knowing what something is does nothing to explain it. The child we alluded to earlier learns nothing about how cars work simply by being told that something is a car. Our zoologist learns nothing about the habits or origins of marsupial rats simply by labelling it correctly. Nor does the patient find out how she came to have a cold, or how the symptoms of the common cold are caused, simply by receiving the diagnosis. All this is true. Yet, in each case, a puzzle has been solved in a satisfactory way with reference to background knowledge. You certainly have an explanation for your cough and chest pain when you are able to say, 'It's just a cold.'

And there is another point to consider. Once you know what something is (what class of things it belongs to), you can apply your knowledge of that class of things to this individual instance. Once the zoologist knows that this furry animal is a marsupial rat, she will be able to apply to it all that she knows about that species: what its feeding needs are, what its mating habits will be, and so on. She will be able to make predictions about this animal's behaviour and other characteristics. She will expect it to have a pouch if it is female, and so forth. Similarly, the patient with a cold, once she knows that a cold is what she is suffering from, will know what to expect and what to do. So a classificatory explanation is not only an answer to the question, 'What is it', or 'What is the patient suffering from?'; it can also lead to an answer to the question, 'What features do we expect this thing to have?' or 'What is the prognosis for this patient?'.

So in a narrative description of a patient's knowledge of their problem, we might note that a number of symptoms led to the question, 'What am I suffering from?' Suppose the symptoms were earache and a sensation of fullness in the ear. The explanation was that the patient had a blockage of the eustachian tube. The next day the patient is worried that they have a partial deafness in the ear. The nurse reassures the patient by saying that partial deafness is one of the symptoms of a blockage of the eustachian tube. Given the diagnosis, such temporary deafness is to be expected. (At this point the classificatory explanation that has been given enables you to give further covering law model explanations—a type which we will describe presently.) So the narrative sequence is that symptoms lead to a classification and then the classification leads to the explanation or prediction of more symptoms which might arise.

4. The Covering Law Model of Explanation

We use the covering law model of explanation when we answer a question about a puzzling event by saying, 'This is what always happens'. Imagine a child who watches you strike a match to light the stove. He is amazed at the sudden appearance of flame and asks for an explanation. If you have plenty of matches you might strike another one, and then another, and then another. Then you might say, 'See? This is what always happens.' While the child has not learnt anything about the chemistry involved or about the role of friction in generating heat, he has learnt how flames are produced by matches and will not be surprised when he sees such an event again. He is satisfied and an explanation has been given.

The phrase 'covering law' which is used to give the technical name to this form of explanation refers to what most scientists take themselves to be producing when they devise scientific theories. Having discovered that sodium reacts violently with water on a number of occasions, and having discovered why by way of the chemistry involved, scientists conclude that, given certain conditions, sodium will always react violently with water.

There is a process of induction involved here and the conclusion can be given the rather grand name of 'a law of nature'. Once that law is known, it can be used to explain things. Suppose there is a puzzlingly violent reaction in a laboratory involving water, the laboratory worker need only discover that sodium had been in contact with the water and he will have his explanation.

A general truth which is more apt to be described as a law of nature is the law of gravity. In lay person's terms this law says that everything that goes up must come down. So if a child sees something drop to the ground and asks why, we can simply explain it by saying that that is what always happens. It is what we would expect, given our previous experience of the world. In this way, it is the product of inductive thinking. For most of us, it would only be if we saw a body not supported by anything and yet not falling, that we would be puzzled and feel in need of an explanation.

The logical form of this kind of explanation is that which we described in the previous chapter. There is a general law from which certain implications can be deduced. If a body is unsupported it will fall. This body is unsupported. Therefore, it will fall. The event which the child wanted explained is implied by (or can be deduced from) the covering law, and is therefore explained by that law. Whatever is an implication of a covering law (or of a hypothesis) is explained by it.

But covering law explanations can also occur in contexts where no 'law of nature' is involved. Observation over a period of time may have yielded (by induction) the proposition that a certain disabled person always gets angry when he is offered help in circumstances where he can manage himself. One health worker might say to another, 'Bill always gets angry when you try to help him unnecessarily.' This is background knowledge about Bill. If a person with this knowledge is surprised on a particular occasion when Bill suddenly becomes angry, it will serve as an explanation to say, 'Bill could have managed that task which you tried to help him with.' Now let us imagine a visitor to Bill's residence. She tries to help him with something and he gets angry. She is puzzled. It will serve as an explanation to say, 'Bill always gets angry when you try to help him unnecessarily.'

One reason that the covering law model is of considerable importance within science is that it allows one to think deductively. We noted in the previous chapter that one can deduce an implication from a general statement and this implication allows the general statement to be tested. You will recall that these general statements can be of the form: 'All x's are y', or 'Whenever something x's, it will y', or 'If this is an x, then it will be y.' These general statements can yield implications which take the form of predictions that can be tested, or explanations for what has taken place. If x obtains, then so will y. In logical form:

$x \Rightarrow y$
x
$\Rightarrow y$

So if y happens and it puzzles us, finding that x happened will explain it. After all, the association of x and y is what always happens. One can deduce one from the other.

5. The Statistical Model of Explanation

This model of explanation is a variation on the previous one. There are many events that are frequently associated with another, but not always. A lifetime of heavy cigarette smoking is likely to cause lung cancer but it will not always do so. We describe this by saying that cigarette smokers run a greater risk of contracting lung cancer. We can calculate this risk by the use of statistical methods. If we study a large population by using medical and other records we might find that of all the people in the sample who smoked, 25% died of lung cancer. This would mean that smokers have a 25% chance of dying of lung cancer. There would be lots of statistical and epidemiological matters that needed to be looked at here. There may be other causes of lung cancer at work amongst those who smoke. But let us leave aside these niceties. Suffice it to say that we have here a case of what we described in Chapter 7 as the relative frequency of the occurrence of an event, expressed as a probability.

Our point is simply that if it were known that smokers are more likely to die of lung cancer than non-smokers, then if someone died of lung cancer and we asked for an explanation, being told that this person was a smoker would give us an answer. It would be an answer that would satisfy us to the extent that the statistics allowed. That is, if the statistical correlation between smoking and death by lung cancer was 100% (that is, if every smoker was known to die from lung cancer), then the explanation would be thoroughly satisfactory. It would be a case of 'This is what happens every time'. But if the correlation between smoking and lung cancer was only 25%, then the explanation for this death in terms of the deceased being a smoker would be only 25% satisfactory. If the risk of getting the disease for any smoker is 25%, if only 25 out of every 100 smokers contracted the disease, then the cogency of the explanation of any one case is only 25%. One would have to do an autopsy to confirm that the lungs had been affected by nicotine, or carry out whatever other tests might be needed to confirm the hypothesis that it was the smoking that caused the death.

Nevertheless, insofar as knowing the statistical correlation between events leads us to expect one event when another occurs, that event is explained by the other. If smoking is known to increase the chances of lung cancer, then a particular case of lung cancer is to that extent explained by the fact that the victim was a smoker.

The logical form of the statistical model is similar to that of the covering law model. One can deduce an implication from a probability statement. If there is a 40% probablity that a y will follow an occurrence of x, then one can deduce with a 40% margin of probability that a given x will be followed by a y. So if y does occur and we find that an x also occurred, then we have a 40% probable explanation. This follows by deduction:

x ⇒y (in 40% of cases)
x
⇒y is 40% likely.

6. The Causal Model of Explanation

There is a sense in which the causal model of explanation is the most important of all. It occurs when, in ordinary conversation, we say, 'It happened because something else happened.' Mind you, this locution is also used in purposive explanations, as when we say that Bob closed the window because he wanted to block out the noise. The word 'because' is certainly a signpost for an explanation, but it need not always be a causal explanation.

We give a causal explanation when we indicate the mechanism by which something occurs. Such a causal explanation explains why the event always happens. We can go back to the case of the child who is puzzled about the matches to illustrate this. Suppose the child is a little older and has some rudimentary knowledge of scientific concepts. In this event, the parent might try to explain that the match has a head on it which contains sulphur and that sulphur burns at a relatively low temperature. The friction generated by rubbing the match against the rough side of the matchbox generates heat above this temperature and thereby lights the sulphur. In this way the child learns not only that 'it happens every time' but also why it does. He now learns what causes it to happen every time: what the mechanism is that makes it happen.

That this knowledge is superior to the knowledge the child had when he merely understood that it happens every time is shown by noting that the child is now also in a position to understand what happens when the match fails to light. (Notice that the claim that it happens every time is not strictly true. Certain conditions have to be met. Oxygen has to be present, for example. The fact is that oxygen usually is present and that is why we can get away with saying that it happens every time.) In the event that the match fails to light, the child might inspect the match and notice that the head is missing. He will now know why it did not light. In a more sophisticated example, he might notice that the head is wet and, remembering the point about combustion requiring a certain temperature, he might form the hypotheses that water keeps the temperature on the head too low, or that it lubricates the head so that it does not generate enough heat against the side of the box. It is because the child knows the causal mechanism involved when the match does light that he is able to form these hypotheses.

An interesting implication of this last point is that causal explanations frequently indicate further lines of research which yield further knowledge. The Semmelweis case illustrates this, as we had already noted. When he knew that morbid matter from either corpses or wounds could cause childbed fever, he contributed to a body of knowledge that would eventually yield the germ theory of disease. The discovery of bacteria and micro-organisms was the discovery of the cause of infection.

Semmelweis discovered that infection was the cause of childbed fever—later researchers discovered the cause (that is, the mechanism) of infections.

In a similar way we might note that the law of gravity does not merely say that things which go up must come down or that unsupported bodies will fall. It explains why this always happens by identifying a mechanism or cause. It postulates a force by which all bodies are attracted to one another and calculates the strength of that force as a function of the mass of that body. Once this is understood we can not only explain the falling of the apple which was said to have hit Newton on the head, by saying that it became unsupported when it was severed from the tree, we can also explain why some unsupported bodies do not fall. Man-made satellites seem to be unsupported bodies and yet they do not fall to earth. We can explain this by saying that although they do fall, their trajectory is such that they miss the earth's surface and are then pulled around the earth again by the force of gravity. Once again, knowing what causes gravitational phenomena allows us to explain odd cases as well as common ones.

In a similar way, knowledge of psychology will give us a deeper explanation of Bill's anger when people try to help him. If we know about the importance of self-esteem in people's lives and about how being able to do things for oneself enhances self-esteem, then we can readily understand why Bill gets angry when he does. When people try to help him to do things that he can manage for himself, he feels that they are assuming he is helpless, and this threatens his self-esteem. This is the mechanism, as it were, which produces his anger. This knowledge allows us to give a number of different explanations. Firstly, it underwrites the covering law explanation. We not only know that Bill always gets angry when people try to help him unnecessarily, but we also know why. Secondly, this knowledge may allow us to give an interpretative explanation. We might say that Bill is really trying to preserve his self-esteem even though he may not be aware of this himself. Thirdly, if Bill knows in his own mind why he is getting angry, we might offer a purposive explanation and say that he is getting angry in order to preserve his self-esteem.

In these cases too, knowing the cause, and not just the covering law, will allow us to explain what is going on when an exception to the law occurs. Suppose there is someone who helps Bill unnecessarily but Bill does not get angry. This could be explained by the fact that Bill and this person are in love. Love involves a degree of mutual acceptance that does not threaten, but enhances, the self-esteem of the lovers. Knowing this we can understand that being helped by someone who loves him would not threaten Bill. In this way we can explain the departure from the generalisation that Bill always get angry in such circumstances.

Causal explanations also deepen our knowledge of statistical explanations. It is important to know that there is a high correlation between smoking and lung cancer, but it is even more important to know what causes the correlation. If we knew what the causal mechanism was by which nicotine in the lungs produced cancer we would be able to explain why not everyone who smokes contracts the disease and we would be able to prevent and even cure the illness for those who did contract it.

Lastly, knowing what causes a given phenomenon allows us to intervene in the causal mechanism in order to prevent the outcome or repair the damage. If we know how matches work, then we know what to do in the event that a particular match does not light. If we know why Bill gets angry, we will know what to do in the event that we can see that he needs help even though he cannot see it. We would help him in an unobtrusive way so as not to damage his self-esteem. And most obviously, if we knew what caused cancer we would know how to develop effective treatments for it. We already know that we should avoid smoking. The statistical correlation is enough to tell us that. But if we knew what the causal mechanism was, we would be able to develop techniques for curing the disease. As soon as Semmelweis knew what the mechanism was by which childbed fever was transmitted (the unsterilised hands of the medical students) he knew what he needed to do to solve the problem.

Exercise 9.2

Identify the model of explanation used in the following cases:

1. This student studied very hard in order to pass her exams.
2. If we can repair the damaged arteries we will be able to restore the patient's circulation.
3. Spoken to a mother worried about the blotches on her child's skin: 'It's a mild case of atopic eczema.'
4. Her pupils are dilated and react sluggishly to light and she only responds to painful stimuli. She must be in a coma.
5. Ignore little Johnny's tantrum, he's just trying to get attention.
6. She went home early because her child is sick.
7. The engine stopped because the car had run out of petrol.
8. Her lips are cyanosed. Her breathing is laboured and shallow. Therefore she has respiratory disease.
9. About a woman in the outpatients department speaking in a foreign language: 'I think she is complaining of a sore stomach.'
10. Joe had heart problems because he did not do much exercise.
11. This strange looking object is a new kind of syringe used by paramedics in the field.
12. Embryos develop by way of a complex process involving the splitting and replication of cells.
13. The cylinder in the burning shed exploded because gas expands when heated.
14. It would be no use using antibiotics. I think it's a viral infection.
15. His obsessive desire to succeed in business stems from his not having been accepted as an equal by his businessman father.

16. This patient is restless, unable to concentrate and uninterested in food. He must be in pain.
17. The patient's temperature dropped following the administration of aspirin.
18. The government is reviewing its health policy because health care costs are rising too fast.
19. I wasn't surprised to find that the patient was unemployed given that he came from that poor suburb.
20. The patient's recovery was enhanced by the cheerfulness of the nursing staff.
21. As you would expect from families in the higher income bracket, Robert and Mandy only had two children.
22. The eminent biologist Theodosius Dobzhansky said: 'Nothing in biology makes sense except in the light of evolution.'
23. Karl Marx argued that all the events of history such as wars, revolutions, industrial struggles and even developments in the arts, could be accounted for with reference to the struggle between those classes who owned capital and those who sold their labour for wages.
24. The IV will not flow, the flask is not empty, therefore the cannula must be blocked.
25. I always get a headache and feel irritable when I do night duty. I was on night duty last night so that must be why I have a headache and feel irritable now.
26. A friend of mine has had irritating eczema for many years. He went to a Chinese herbalist recently, was given some strange herbs to ingest, and found that his skin problems cleared up in a matter of days.
27. I'm not surprised that that Mediterranean patient I had in here today was complaining of a bad back. They're all work-shy!
28. No wonder Judy was complaining about the rosters again. She's never happy about anything.
29. It's no wonder he had an accident. He's been driving like a madman for months.
30. Mrs Smith is in acute renal failure. That is why she is anuric.

Because explanations solve puzzles, they have a strong place in arguments. The aim of an argument is to persuade, and a good way of persuading someone of something is to offer them an explanation of it. If I wanted to persuade you not to help Bill unnecessarily, I need only explain to you why Bill gets angry when such help is given to him, and you would be persuaded. If you thought that Bill was getting angry for some other reason you would not be persuaded. Therefore, to convince you not to help Bill unnecessarily, I need only convince you that my explanation for his anger is correct. It is in this way that explanations have important persuasive and practical implications.

Exercise 9.3

Write a logical outline of the following item which is based on a letter to a newspaper. Also identify the kinds of explanation that are being used to persuade the audience.

> To say that alcohol is one of the factors that destroys Aborigines (This paper, 11/2) is to state the obvious, and it would be nice to think that their much publicised community spirit could save them from it overnight.
>
> What causes people to drink is a low self-esteem and a sense of futility, and Aborigines have plenty of both. In general, our relations with them are still power relations. We are seen as the providers and they can only respond with complete dependence and acceptance, or bad manners and irrationality. Or they can drink.
>
> Last year I was encouraged by the difference in the lives of many of the Aborigines in Carnarvon, Western Australia, since the setting up of their own medical service. They employ a white doctor and a white sister, but the rest of the staff are Aborigines, with on-the-job training. All the Aborigines in the town attend the clinic as well as some white people.
>
> They have also acquired a small tract of otherwise useless land which they are setting up as an out-station, run by themselves, in their own way. Pride in their achievements can be detected right across the community, and a new purposefulness.
>
> Throughout Australia a consistent and clear signal has been coming from Aboriginal people for a very long time—at least two centuries—give us back some of our land and the autonomy that should go with it.
>
> As for a respected leader, I nominate Pat Dodson.

Exercise 9.4 (Revision)

Refer back to the logical outline you have just written and identify the form of argument (deduction, induction, method of remainders, analogy etc.) used to draw any conclusions that you have identified. Say whether the conclusions are valid and why.

Chapter 10
Searching for Causes

This chapter argues for a problem-solving view of causality, in which what one looks for are the necessary and sufficient conditions for a given condition so that a problem can be solved. Reference will be made to the discovery of the cause of the transmission of cholera. John Stuart Mill's methods for discovering necessary and sufficient conditions are explained. These are the method of agreement, the method of difference, the joint method, the method of concomitant variation and the method of residues.

We suggested in the previous chapter that the causal model was the most important model of explanation, at least in the context of medical science. It seems clear that professional health work requires a scientific mode of thinking which helps to explain things by reference to what causes them. We want to explain symptoms by reference to the disease entities that cause them, pain and distress by reference to the injury that causes them and so on. Of course, we should not lose sight of the importance of understanding patients as whole persons and of the need for interpretative models of explanation in order to achieve this. However, in this chapter we want to focus upon causal thinking in the context of health care.

An Example of a Search for Causes

But first, we want to tell you a story. This is the story of John Snow, an English physician who was born in 1813 and died in 1858 having discovered how to prevent the spread of cholera. As with the story of Semmelweis, in order to understand the originality of his achievement in the history of medical science, we have to remember that the germ theory of disease was not yet known in his time. It was not until the later work of Louis Pasteur (1822–1895) and Robert Koch (1843–1910) that the insights of earlier pioneers like Semmelweis and Snow could be fully explained in terms of the micro-organisms which cause disease.

There were cholera epidemics in England in 1831–32, 1848–49 and 1853–54. Snow made observations on each occasion, studied the findings of previous writers on the topic and published, late in his life, a now classic study entitled *On the Mode of Communication of Cholera*. The major conclusions of this study were:

1. Cholera is contagious.
2. The mode of transmission is not 'effluvia' or 'miasma' but the ingestion of particles from the excreta of cholera victims.
3. Such excreta can be transmitted in a number of ways, especially through drinking contaminated water.

The first point refutes an ancient idea that disease could arise spontaneously. The concept of contagion was already partly understood in Snow's day because it was consistent with the fact that outbreaks of cholera occurred in clusters. The impact was on whole villages or neighbourhoods in large cities where people were crowded together, while other places were left untouched. But it was not clear how the outbreaks could occur in widely separated places if they did not arise spontaneously in those new areas. Snow demonstrated that, even in those instances where cases of cholera arose in places far removed from where the disease was virulent, some connection could be made with cases elsewhere. In one example, a victim had been visited by her son because he was suffering from it and wanted nursing. He had brought it from a distant place where the disease was present. In another case, the unwashed clothes of a victim had been sent to relatives in a distant village and these relatives had contracted the disease soon after unpacking the parcel. In his book, Snow concludes his discussion of numerous cases of this sort by saying:

> The above instances are quite sufficient to show that cholera can be communicated from the sick to the healthy; for it is quite impossible that even a tenth part of these cases of consecutive illness could have followed each other by mere coincidence, without being connected as cause and effect.[1]

Let us pause to comment on the logic of this conclusion. Firstly, we should note that in his book Snow cites numerous cases. This shows that he is using induction to draw his conclusion. But secondly, and more importantly, he suggests that it could not have been mere coincidence that there was some kind of physical contact between existing cases of cholera and new cases, even though the kinds of contact varied.

Constant Correlation

What is at issue here is that inductive thinking should only allow Snow to conclude something like, 'Whenever there is a new case of cholera, there has been some kind of contact with another case.' The form of this conclusion is that of a covering law. It describes what philosophers call **constant correlation**. This fancy phrase means merely that certain phenomena always occur with other phenomena. For example, whenever you throw an object into the air, it comes down again (unless some extraordinary circumstance prevents it). But constant correlation is just that and nothing more. All that you are saying is that certain things always go together. Whenever there is a new case of cholera, there has been some form of contact with an existing case.

But it is possible when two phenomena always occur together that it is just a coincidence. One of Snow's contemporaries used statistical data to show that cases of cholera were much more frequent amongst people who lived in low-lying neighbourhoods of London, while cases were rarer amongst people who lived on the hills or in other elevated places. This was a (relatively) constant correlation, but was it a mere coincidence? Or was there some causal link between living in low-lying places and being at greater risk of contracting cholera?

Let us imagine another case. You might notice that, in a given week, every new admission into a casualty ward is of Asian origin. This might lead you to make inquiries and you might find out that there is a gang war going on in Chinatown. This tells you that the high rate of Asian admissions is no mere coincidence: there is an explanation. But now suppose that you had discovered no such explanation. In this case, you would have to conclude that it was mere coincidence that all the admissions in that week were Asian. What this thought experiment shows is that we are apt to conclude that a constant correlation is a coincidence when we can find no causal connection to explain the correlation. If we are aware of a cause, then we do not take the constant correlation to be coincidental.

But this also leads to a further step in thinking. We might note a constant correlation, know of no cause, but reject the idea that the correlation is a coincidence. There might be just too many cases to make it plausible that they are coincidences. In such a case we are forced to conclude that there must be a cause even though we do not know what it is. This will be a puzzle needing an explanation and we will set about finding the cause. This was precisely Snow's position. He noted the constant correlation between new cases and existing cases, refused to believe that it could be a coincidence, and so concluded that 'these cases of consecutive illness [must be] connected as cause and effect'. What he must now go on to do, of course, is demonstrate what the mechanism is by which the disease is transmitted from existing cases to new ones. He will not know what the cause of transmission is until he knows this.

Causal Mechanisms

Theories of what caused transmission of disease in Snow's day included the idea that people could contract disease by breathing in the 'miasma' that was said to emanate from stagnant and putrid water such as was found in marshes and cesspools, and the idea that people could contract disease by breathing in the 'effluvia' or breath of those people who had already contracted the disease. In either case, the means of transmission would be the intake of infective matter through the lungs. Health workers in cholera-affected areas used to wear masks and carry pitchers of smoking coals in order to ward off the hidden airborn contagion. Also, during cholera outbreaks in London, people frequently commented on the foul smell of the Thames River, especially on hot days in summer, and thought this to be unhealthy.

Snow was one of the first to recognise that different diseases could be transmitted in different ways and that there was a number of diseases in which 'bad air' could not be involved. In the case of cholera he was able to show that the theory of transmission by effluvia was not correct by adducing the following considerations:

1. Not everyone who is in the same room as cholera victims, and who would therefore be breathing in their effluvia, contracts the disease.
2. Effluvia could not have been involved in cases of transmission over a distance, such as that of the parcel of contaminated clothes cited above.
3. The disease affected the intestine immediately without there first being an effect upon the lungs, or even a fever.

Exercise 10.1

With reference to material from previous chapters, identify the logic of Snow's thinking in arguing that the effluvia theory of transmission was incorrect in the case of cholera.

Snow's Solution

The first of the points noted above referred to the striking fact that doctors who made very frequent visits to cholera patients were not as likely to contract the disease as the people who lived with or near the victims. The main symptom of cholera is violent diarrhoea. The clothes, bedclothes, linen and bedding of victims were therefore frequently soiled with excreta. Snow noticed that people having physical contact with these (little being known of hygiene at the time) would eat, drink or prepare food with soiled hands. Doctors, on the other hand, hardly ever ate in the homes of their patients and, in any case, washed their hands more often.

It was these facts that led to Snow's second important hypothesis: cholera was transmitted when morbid matter in the excreta of victims was ingested by the new victim. This also explained why crowded housing conditions were associated with the spread of the disease. In such conditions, food was often prepared in the same room as that occupied by the victim.

But if this hypothesis were correct, then how did the contagion reach people far removed from the victims? One could not suppose that cases like the one in which contaminated clothes were sent in a parcel would be all that frequent. Moreover, people in distant places, or in the houses of the rich, did not eat food prepared by those who had had contact with victims. It was at this point that Snow formed the hypothesis for which he is most famous. The morbid matter in the excreta of the victims got into the open and primitive sewerage systems that existed at the time, and so infected the river water and the wells from which people got their drinking water.

There turned out to be striking evidence for this. In the case of the wells, it could be assumed that people living near them would use water from those wells, and a study of the distribution of cholera cases on maps showed that they were indeed concentrated around wells and pumps. As for the pumps, a strikingly concentrated outburst of cholera occurred in homes around the Broad Street pump in London. Snow ordered that the handle be removed from the pump and the number of cases declined sharply. Admittedly, the outbreak was already in decline by the time the handle was removed, but there were many other interesting facts that supported Snow's hypothesis.

- One woman died who, though she lived far from the Broad Street pump, so liked the water from it that she had a bottle of it brought to her house for her to drink.
- There was a brewery in the Broad Street area whose workers remained unaffected by the epidemic. The brewery had its own well.
- There were many deaths amongst customers of an ale house which was somewhat removed from the Broad Street area but where the Broad Street water was used as a mixer in drinks.
- Snow had the Broad Street pump opened and, although there was no visible evidence of sewage contamination (as there had been in many other cases), chemical tests showed the presence of chlorides at levels consistent with contamination by sewage.

Even more striking was the case of the piped water supplies. Wells and pumps supplied definite areas and seemed to explain the concentration of outbreaks around them. But could there be other explanations for such clusters of cases? In London at that time, people with similar occupations tended to cluster in particular districts. So if cholera was concentrated in particular areas, it could have been that the similar occupation of people in those areas was what was causing it. Or it could have been the low altitude, or proximity to the foul-smelling river or any other circumstance that was particular to the area. But in any given district there were people who contracted the disease and people who did not, despite their similarity of occupation and other circumstances. Snow's hypothesis would be demonstrated beyond doubt if the only difference between victims and non-victims was their water supply.

It turned out that water was supplied to various districts of London by wells and by water companies who ran pipes from the Thames and charged subscriptions. In some districts there were several companies in competition, and neighbouring houses might take their water from different suppliers. Because the receipts of subscription payments were kept, it was possible for Snow to determine accurately which household used which water supply. There was a Lambeth Water company whose subscribers were remarkably free of the disease, while users of water from the Southwark and Vauxhall Supply were nine times more likely to get the disease. The Lambeth company drew its water from the Thames at a point that was upstream and well away from where drains and sewers flowed into the river, while the Southwark and Vauxhall Supply drew its water from a point further downstream, where the river was contaminated.

The section of Snow's book where he describes these facts provides an especially striking example of what is called a **controlled experiment**. A controlled experiment is one in which all the conditions and circumstances (that is, variables) that might have an influence on the effect that you are trying to explain (in this case the outbreak of cholera) remain the same except that particular variable which you have hypothesised is the cause (in this case the presence of contaminated water). Given the nature of the water supply in these districts of London, it was possible for Snow to test his hypothesis because the only circumstance that was consistently different amongst households in these districts was the water supply. All other conditions in the households were similar. In the laboratory, an experimenter has to carefully design tests in order to exclude conditions or variables that might influence the outcome, but which are not being tested. Snow had the good fortune to find the necessary circumstances for a controlled experiment created by the contingencies of the situation.

Snow had discovered the mechanism by which cholera was transmitted. He had shown what causes cholera to spread. The authorities in London and other cities were quick to learn the lesson and new and effective sewerage systems were installed, and programs for education in hygiene and public health instituted. As a result, cholera was effectively contained. The puzzle having been solved, a means was found to fix the problem.

Exercise 10.2 (Revision)

1. How did John Snow conclude that cholera was contagious?
2. What was Snow's key insight which led to his discovery of what caused the transmission of cholera?
3. What is a 'controlled experiment' and which of Snow's observations illustrate such an experiment?
4. Why was Snow's discovery deemed a success even though he had not identified the bacterium which was responsible for cholera?

What Is Causality?

What was the logical structure of Snow's thinking in all this? To answer this question we need to digress for a while to consider what exactly is meant by the concept of causality.

But first, a brief discussion of terminology. We use the term **effect** to describe the state of affairs that we are puzzled about and which we are trying to explain when we seek a causal explanation. We use the term **condition** to describe any state of affairs which precedes or accompanies the effect. We will explain this more fully later. Another term often used in the way we use the term 'condition' is **variable**. A variable is so-called because it is a condition which can change and, in changing, cause an effect. For example, the amount of fats in our bodies can change and, if it reaches a critical level, can then increase our risk of heart disease. In this sense the condition identified as the level of fats in our bodies is a variable.

From a commonsense point of view, we might define the concept of **causality** as 'a power to produce an effect'. But the problem with this definition is that a power cannot be seen as such. We do not, for example, discern the force of gravity, we only see its effects. We feel ourselves falling when our ladder topples, but we do not feel ourselves being pulled by the force of gravity. We note the correlation between some events and others, such as contact between existing cases of cholera and new cases, but we do not observe the nature of the communication of disease from one person to another. Even if we observe the drinking of contaminated water, we do not observe the workings of the micro-organism that infects the victim. And even if, with the use of modern microscopes and research equipment, we saw the very germ that caused the disease, it would take still further equipment to see how exactly it affects healthy cells so as to produce the symptoms of the disease. (And at this point we would certainly be interpreting what we see in the light of the theories or hypotheses that we had already formed.)

Accordingly, to say that a certain condition or variable causes a certain effect is always to offer a hypothesis. Such a statement cannot be made on the basis of observation alone. You are not reporting on what you can observe when you say that something causes something else. This is one reason why scientists have to rely so much on constant correlations. If we could see something causing something else, then we would need to see only one instance to learn what the causal mechanism is. What actually happens is that we see numerous cases where certain conditions or variables are associated with a certain effect, believe these correlations not to be coincidences, and are thereby led to hypothesise what the causal mechanism might be.

Constant Correlations Again

What evidence can there be for a causal hypothesis? We have already seen the answer to this question. We need to see a constant correlation between the effect and that condition which is hypothesised to be the cause.

But not all constant correlations are causal in nature. We noted that there was a constant correlation between contracting cholera and living in low-lying districts of London, or between cholera and foul smells from the river. We also imagined a case where there was a constant correlation between being admitted to casualty and being Asian. In the absence of gang wars in Chinatown, this latter was clearly coincidental. But what are we to make of the low-lying districts and foul smells cases? It seems clear from our modern point of view that living in low-lying areas would not cause cholera, and that foul smells would not. Yet the constant correlation is undeniable and does not seem to be a matter of coincidence.

Snow's hypothesis that sewage in drinking water was the principal cause of the transmission of cholera is able to explain this correlation without suggesting that it is a causal one. The Thames River was contaminated with a lot of sewage from drains and open sewers at the time. It was this which caused the foul smells. Knowledge of geography would suggest that people in low-lying areas lived nearer to the Thames River. And people in those areas were likely to draw their domestic water directly from the river, or else their pumps and wells were likely to contain seepage from the river. This allowed sewage to get into their drinking water and this explains why they suffered a high incidence of cholera. So when we know what causes the transmission of cholera we would expect or predict that there would be a high correlation between living near the river and cholera, and living in areas affected by river smells and cholera. Living in low-lying areas near the river made it more likely you would drink contaminated water. As for the smells, these were caused by the sewage. The sewage also caused the cholera. Therefore the bad smells and the cholera were correlated; not as cause and effect, but as two effects of the same cause. The bad smell was an **incidental effect** of the sewage.

We can illustrate what is at issue here with the case of night and day. One of the most consistent constant correlations that we know about is that between night and day. Never has a day passed but that night has followed it, and been followed in its turn by day. Yet we do not suggest that night causes day or that day causes night. This is because we know both of them to be the effect of something else, namely the rotation of the earth around the sun. Day and night are correlated because they are both effects of the same condition. In the same way, bad smells near the river and cholera were correlated because they were both effects of the same condition, namely sewage, rather than because the one caused the other.

We said before that we do not observe the power of a cause to produce its effect. We should now clarify this further. John Snow had shown that what he called 'morbid matter', carried from the excreta of cholera victims into the drinking water, was what caused the transmission of cholera. But he did not know what this morbid matter was. He did hypothesise, correctly as it turned out, that it was a micro-organism which propagated itself in the stomach of the victim during the incubation period of the disease, but the laboratory techniques for observing and identifying this micro-organism did not exist in his day. It was Robert Koch who identified the micro-organism. He learnt how to use dyes to stain samples of biological material so as to be able to discern details under the microscope. In 1883 he discovered what he called the 'comma bacillus', so named because it looked like a comma. This was the micro-organism which caused cholera. We might say that this bacterium is the 'power to produce the effect', that is, the cause of cholera. (Of course it remains true that he did not exactly observe this power. Koch still did not know just how this micro-organism caused the disease and its symptoms to occur.)

But if he did not discover the 'comma bacillus' which was the very mechanism by which the transmission and infection took place, then in what sense did Snow discover the cause of the transmission of cholera? In technical terms, the answer to this question is that he discovered the necessary and sufficient conditions to produce the effect. Because we do not observe the actual power that produces the effect but only those conditions that are constantly correlated with the effect, we need to be able to distinguish those constant correlations which are coincidental from those which are causal. We have no way of knowing which conditions actually have the power to produce the effect except by noting which conditions are necessary and sufficient for the effect to occur. Let us spell out what this means.

Necessary and Sufficient Conditions

We gave a preliminary definition of causality above as 'a power to produce a given effect' but noted that powers as such cannot be observed. Only their effects can be observed, and the conditions which are constantly correlated with them. Now if we could identify that condition which was **sufficient** to produce the effect, then we would be well on the way towards locating the power that was producing the effect. A sufficient condition is a condition which, when it obtains, is always followed by the effect. If you want to produce the effect, producing the sufficient condition would do it. So, if you want to light the match (effect), strike the side of the match box with it. This will normally be sufficient to produce the effect. Friction between the match head and the box is a sufficient condition to produce the effect. It would seem that a cause is a sufficient condition.

But we know that the match does not always light. The match must be dry and oxygen must be present. These are **necessary** conditions for the effect. A necessary condition is a condition without which the effect would not occur. By itself a necessary condition is not sufficient. Dry matches lying around in oxygen do not light by themselves. But when these necessary conditions are fulfilled, and only then, will striking the match be sufficient for lighting it. Of course, we could also say that striking a match was necessary for lighting it. There are quite a number of conditions that are necessary for the match to light. But some of these will be ongoing states of affairs, like being dry and being in the presence of oxygen, and others will be events which will be sufficient to produce the effect, given these other necessary conditions. We might refer to these ongoing states of affairs which we normally take for granted as necessary **background conditions**.

Given that a number of conditions will be necessary, we might define a sufficient condition as the complete set of necessary conditions. If everything that is necessary to produce the effect is present, then it will occur. If everything necessary for the lighting of the match obtains, including the event of striking it, then it will light. So what has happened to the notion of a sufficient condition? Which of these necessary conditions is the cause? The answer to this question depends on what we are interested in. If we are that child who was curious about the match lighting, we would be interested in what makes it happen, given the other necessary conditions. We would be interested in the striking and take this to be the cause (or, as we said in the previous chapter, the explanation). But suppose we were in a teaching laboratory seeking to explain the necessity of oxygen for combustion. We might be holding the match and matchbox in a chamber that we thought was free of oxygen so that on striking it it would not light. Now suppose that it did. We would ask, 'How did that happen?' We would not be looking for an explanation for match lightings in general, but for its lighting on this occasion when we had expected that it would not. Suppose our laboratory assistant said, 'Sorry, I think I let some oxygen into the chamber.' Now we would have solved our puzzle. We would say that it was the oxygen that caused it to light. What is normally assumed to be a background necessary condition has here become the necessary condition which was sufficient (given the striking) to produce the effect. So we designate the oxygen as the cause. We designate as the cause whichever necessary condition was sufficient to produce the effect and which we hadn't known about. In other words, a cause is a **necessary and sufficient condition** for the effect to occur.

We can illustrate this rather complex terminological point with reference to Snow's discovery. Snow discovered that, provided all the necessary background conditions are met, ingesting particles of excreta from cholera victims was a necessary condition for contracting cholera. Also necessary was some means of getting these particles into the alimentary system of the new victim. Drinking contaminated water was sufficient for this. Also sufficient for this was eating food prepared by people with such particles on their hands, whether from tending the corpse of a victim or handling soiled bedding or clothing. Any of these forms of contact would be sufficient for transmitting the disease, because some such contact was necessary. So, in the particular case of someone drinking from the Broad Street pump, for example, drinking contaminated water would be a necessary and sufficient condition for contracting cholera, provided necessary background conditions were met.

And yet the matter was still more complicated. What Snow did not know at the time was that a certain kind of susceptibility to the disease was a necessary background condition. The fact was that some who drank contaminated water contracted the disease while others who drank it did not, and he needed to explain why this was so. He had some ingenious answers to this puzzle. For example, he said that morbid matter did not spread evenly in the water and so some drinkers could ingest some of it and others not. The infection did not come from a chemical reaction with the water but from a micro-organism which might be present in some parts but not in others. This answer has not stood the test of time. We now know that people can have or acquire immunity in various ways. In other words, susceptibility is a necessary background condition. If a person who had been inoculated contracted the disease, we would look for a new cause, a necessary condition such as the wearing off of the inoculation effect, which would, together with other necessary conditions such as the drinking of contaminated water, be sufficient to produce the effect.

So it is not enough to say, as people after Koch did, that whenever there is an ingested comma bacillus, there will be a case of cholera, and vice versa. All of the necessary background conditions, including that of the susceptibility of the victim, must be present also. The full cause is the complete set of necessary conditions which, when they all occur, are sufficient to produce the effect. But what we look for and call the cause is that particular necessary condition, from amongst that complete set, which we did not know about and which, given the other necessary conditions, is sufficient to produce the effect. In Snow's studies, this condition was most often the ingestion of contaminated water. In Koch's case, it was the presence of the comma bacillus. In the case just envisaged, it was the wearing off of an inoculation. In the context of the inquiry being conducted, each of these circumstances could be identified as a necessary and sufficient condition for the effect to occur, and is therefore called the cause.

The Structure of Causal Thinkng

Snow might have expressed his discovery this way: If contaminated water is ingested (and if other necessary conditions are met), then cholera will occur. Put formally (and ignoring the other necessary conditions), we can express this as:

If P, then Q   or,
P is **sufficient** for Q to happen,

where P stands for ingesting contaminated water and Q stands for contracting cholera. Similarly, eating food prepared by people whose hands had had contact with excreta from victims was a sufficient condition (if other necessary conditions were met). In this instance P would stand for eating food prepared by people whose hands had had contact with excreta from victims.

But what this last point shows is that a number of conditions can lead to the transmission of cholera. No one of these conditions is necessary. Given the necessary background conditions, each one is sufficient, but they do not explain every case of transmission. We cannot (and not just for reasons of logical validity) reason from Q to P. We cannot say that just because a person contracted cholera, they must have drunk contaminated water. They might have contracted it in some other way.

But, following Koch's work, we could say that if cholera occurred, the comma bacillus must have been present. In formal terms:

If Q, then P   or,
P is **necessary** for Q to happen

In this instance, P stands for the presence of the comma bacillus and Q for the contracting of cholera. What this formula means is that if cholera has occurred, the comma bacillus must have been present. The comma bacillus is a necessary condition for cholera. From Q we can infer P. Another way of expressing this in a formula is to say:

Q only if P

This means that Q (the contracting of cholera) will only occur if there is P (the presence of the comma bacillus).

So 'P is necessary for Q' differs from 'P is sufficient for Q' in that the first is expressed as:

If Q, then P,

while the second is expressed as:

If P, then Q.

The difference is that although contaminated water frequently causes cholera, it is not the only thing which does. Eating food prepared with soiled hands also does. So you cannot conclude from the fact that someone has contracted cholera that they drank contaminated water. In contrast, the comma bacillus is the only thing which causes cholera. Nothing else could do it. It follows that if we have a case of cholera, we must have a case of the presence of the comma bacillus. The comma bacillus is necessary in that there could not be a case of cholera without the presence of that germ.

And when all the necessary background conditions obtain, the comma bacillus is also sufficient to cause the disease. If a person is susceptible and that person ingests that germ, they will contract cholera every time. It follows that, in this case, the formula 'if P, then Q' is reversible. As we said just now, from Q we can infer P. But also, from P we can predict Q (if the background conditions obtain). Once we know what the cause of something is, we can not only predict the effect from the cause, but we can also infer the cause from the effect. After Koch, we can predict that anyone ingesting the comma bacillus will contract cholera (provided the necessary background conditions are met), and we can infer from any case of cholera that that germ was present. We can express this in the formula

If Q, then P, **and** If P, then Q.

Or in more formal terms:

$P \Leftrightarrow Q$

This formula expresses the idea that a cause is both a necessary and a sufficient condition.

This formula also expresses the idea of constant correlation in formal terms. Whenever there is an ingested comma bacillus with the necessary background conditions, there will be a case of cholera, and vice versa. But it says more. It makes clear that the constant correlation is not a coincidence. There is a mechanism to produce the effect Q and this is indicated by the fact that P is a necessary and sufficient condition for Q. Although we can identify the necessary and sufficient conditions which must obtain before the effect can take place, we still cannot observe the power which produces the effect. But, when the background conditions obtain, we can produce Q by producing P. Moreover, one can prevent Q by preventing P. If we know the necessary and sufficient condition for the effect, we have the ability to inhibit as well as produce the effect. And this shows that we have correctly identified the power which produces the effect.

Exercise 10.3

The following statements all express a relationship between two variables:

a. Where appropriate, restate the relevant relationships in terms of the notions of necessary or sufficient conditions by rewriting the statement in the form, '... is sufficient for ...' or in the form, '... is necessary for ...'.
b. Identify which of the relationships are coincidental.
c. Identify which of the relationships are causal.

1. If the number of places in nursing courses is cut, there will be a shortage of qualified nurses in the future.
2. If a patient is under great stress, aspirin will not work for pain relief.
3. Smith always goes for a walk after dinner.
4. All swans in the Botanic Gardens in Sydney are black.
5. You will not be allowed to practise nursing if you have not qualified to do so.
6. Most people who die of heart disease have had a diet too high in fats.
7. If we could destroy the comma bacillus we would wipe out cholera.
8. Staff should wash their hands carefully before entering the operating theatre so as to prevent infection.

Methods for Finding Causes

We now need to turn to a consideration of the methods for discovering causes propounded by a philosopher of the last century, John Stuart Mill. We have already pointed out that to identify a cause is to answer a pragmatic question so as to solve a problem. We know that a large number of conditions are necessary to produce a certain effect and that they are all, taken together, sufficient to produce it. But when we have a puzzle on our hands we are looking for that particular necessary condition which, given the presence of the other necessary conditions, would be sufficient to produce it. In this sense, we are looking for the unknown condition which is both necessary and sufficient to produce the effect.

By what method can we find the necessary and sufficient conditions which cause a particular effect? John Stuart Mill identified five methods.

1. The Method of Agreement

This method involves looking for a common element in a range of cases. Suppose a number of patients in a particular hospital have suffered from an attack of food poisoning. A simple way of determining the cause of the attack is to ask what they ate and, even if their various meals were different, to see if there was something that was common to all of them. One patient might have had soup, steak, and chocolate mousse; another soup, lamb, and vanilla fudge; and a third, soup, chicken, and cheese. It would be clear in this case that the soup would be under suspicion. In formal terms we could illustrate the thinking thus:

Case 1: $a, b, c, \Rightarrow E$
Case 2: $a, d, f, \Rightarrow E$
Case 3: $a, g, h, \Rightarrow E$

where E is the effect under investigation and the other letters represent courses in the meals. As this formula makes clear, a is the factor common to all three cases and is thereby identified as responsible for E . All three cases 'agree' in having a as a common factor. It is a sufficient condition in that, with it, the effect occurs.

The logic of this method applies in the same way if we deal with more than three people. It might have been groups of people who had those various meals. Or the components of those meals might have been had in various combinations. What the method requires is that one item only was common to all the cases who took sick.

We could use Snow's research to illustrate the method of agreement (and we will add some imagined conditions to make the point). Suppose, in a first case of a person contracting cholera, that person had drunk water from the Broad Street pump, worked in a brewery and lived in Wickham Lane. In a second case, the person had drunk water from the Broad Street pump, worked in a tannery and lived in Dartmouth Road. A third person worked in an office, had drunk water from the Broad Street pump, and lived in High Street. It is clear that the one condition or variable which is common to all these cases is that each had drunk water from the Broad Street pump. Of course you would need many more cases to draw a reliable conclusion, and Snow collected many hundreds, but the logic of the thinking is clear. If all the cases studied had drunk water from the Broad Street pump, and if this was the only factor which all these cases had in common, then drinking water from the Broad Street pump would be identified as a sufficient condition for contracting cholera.

2. The Method of Difference

This method involves looking for an element without which the effect would not occur. The dietician in charge of catering in the stricken hospital might decide to take soup off the menu the following evening. If no one gets sick (and if all other conditions remain the same), then the case against the soup is very strong. In formal terms we could illustrate it thus:

Case 1: $a, b, c, \Rightarrow E$
Case 2: $-a, b, c, \Rightarrow -E$

(Where '−' means 'not'. So '$-a$' means 'no soup' and '$-E$' means there was no sickness.) Therefore, a is responsible for E. It is a necessary condition in that, without it, the effect does not occur.

John Snow used this method when he had the handle removed from the Broad Street pump.

The method of difference is the logical structure of the 'controlled experiment' which we described earlier. Let us assume that, in John Snow's research, place of residence and occupation are the only variables under suspicion, apart from what has been eaten or drunk. And let us also assume that all other variables remain constant. Snow would be using the method of difference if he notes that a group of people who have contracted cholera had drunk water supplied by the Southwark and Vauxhall Supply, worked in a brewery and lived in Wickham Lane, while a second group of people, who have not contracted cholera, had not drunk water supplied by the Southwark and Vauxhall Supply, but did work in a brewery and live in Wickham Lane. If these and all other conditions relating to both groups of people remain the same, then Snow would have identified a necessary condition for contracting cholera. If the only difference between those who contracted the disease and those who did not is that the latter have not drunk water supplied by the Southwark and Vauxhall Supply, then drinking water from the Southwark and Vauxhall Supply would be a necessary condition for contracting the disease.

3. Joint Method of Agreement and Difference

This method is rather more complicated in that it combines the previous two methods. But it needs to do this because the method of agreement will only identify sufficient conditions, while the method of difference identifies necessary conditions. In order to identify the cause we need to identify conditions which are both necessary and sufficient.

One problem which the method of agreement leaves us with is that there might be another factor, from among the limitless number of factors that obtain at any time, which all the cases have in common. All the sick hospital patients may also have had a chocolate mint, or coincidentally eaten some contaminated food at lunch time, or been allergic to some substance commonly used in the hospital. To be sure that we had identified the cause we would have to argue that having soup was not only sufficient, but also necessary for the effect to occur. To this end we need the method of difference as well. Of course, in most circumstances, common sense would be content with the soup hypothesis, but in highly complex situations or in situations where the basic processes are not well understood, such as those confronting Snow, no possibility should be disregarded.

Similarly, the method of difference by itself will not tell us with complete reliability where the problem lies. It will tell us that no illness occurs when no soup has been eaten for the group that had steak and chocolate mousse, so that the soup was necessary for members of that group to get ill. But other foods might have been necessary to produce the illness in others. Among those who had steak and chocolate mousse, only those who had soup fell ill, but others might have fallen ill because they ate the chicken even though they had no soup. Such a group could be described as:

Case 2a: $-a$, d, f, $\Rightarrow E$

In short, the method of difference can only show that it is definitely the soup which causes the sickness when there are a very limited number of variables. There might be other carriers of the gastric infection on the menu and so the soup may not be necessary to cause the illness.

This kind of problem occurs frequently in epidemiological studies when it is not possible to isolate all the conditions and control each of them. It might not be possible to create two groups where only one condition varies between them. Snow was lucky with his water supply case, but most researchers do not have access to populations like this where only one condition is varied between them. Experiments can be controlled in the laboratory, but research on people in the real world has to take account of many variables. For this reason a more complex matrix for research is required.

Schematically, the combined method can be illustrated thus:

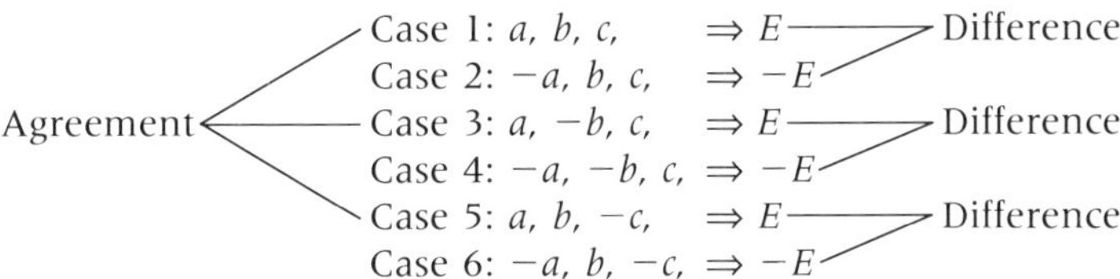

We can illustrate this with the group of patients who ate soup, steak and chocolate mousse. Cases 3 and 4 show that removing the steak from the diet makes no difference, and cases 5 and 6 show that removing the chocolate mousse makes no difference.

Exercise 10.4

A child patient has presented with symptoms of asthma. The task is to find out which of the various factors in her life she is allergic to. It could be:

a. a stuffed toy
b. getting too excited at play
c. pollen in the air.

Select which of Mill's methods discussed so far would be best to find the cause of the asthma and describe the logical structure of the reasoning involved.

There is also another way of illustrating the combined method, namely:

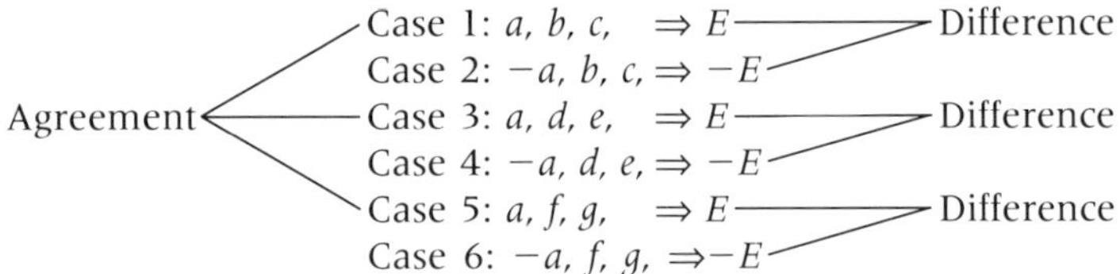

With this formula we can deal with more variables. Rather than simply playing around with three variables and whether or not they obtain, we can deal with seven, or even more. We can let the letters stand for the various courses of the meal. In this way *d* and *e* could stand for lamb and vanilla fudge respectively and so forth. The logic of the method is still the same however. Cases 3 and 4 show that it makes no difference whether you eat lamb, whereas it does if you eat soup.

Now it might be thought that, given the number of variables and hypotheses he had to deal with, Snow could have used the combined method in order to identify the carrier of the contagion definitively. However, things were not that simple. As we have seen, there were a large number of hypotheses available to Snow as to what caused a particular local outbreak of cholera, for example:

a. drinking contaminated water
b. working in the mines
c. living in foul-smelling areas
d. being a sailor
e. living in low-lying areas
f. having contact with the bodies or the property of victims
g. being poor.

To simplify things we will assume that each of these variables either obtains or not (rather than being present in varying degrees).

Following the formula for the combined method given above, if only those who drink contaminated water get the disease, then cases 1 and 2 might exemplify the method of difference in that all these cases work in the mines and live in areas affected by bad smells, but only some drink contaminated water. For this group, drinking contaminated water would be a necessary condition. But the fact is that working in the mines or living in areas affected by bad smells was associated with the disease. There were no latrines in the mines and hence, if any miner contracted the disease, it would quickly spread in the mine, and we have already seen why there was a connection between contracting the disease and bad smells. Even one case of an affected miner who had not drunk contaminated water would show that condition *a* was not necessary for contracting the disease.

The logic of cases 3 and 4 is similar. It would make it easy for Snow if, for all those who are sailors and/or live in low-lying areas, only those who do not drink contaminated water do not get the disease. But the fact is that sailors frequently picked up the disease in foreign ports where the epidemic was present, and for reasons we have already noted, low-lying areas did have more cases of the disease. Cases 5 and 6 work the same way.

What we do have in this range of cases is an instance of the method of agreement. The only variable that cases 1, 3 and 5 have in common is *a*, the drinking of contaminated water. This shows that even with variations in background conditions such as employment or place of residence, drinking contaminated water is a sufficient condition for contracting the disease. But it does not show that drinking contaminated water is the only condition that leads to contracting the disease.

What Snow needs to do is deepen his thinking and to find out what it is about the contaminated water which frequently makes it a sufficient condition for contracting the disease. We know he did this in that he postulated a micro-organism ingested into the stomach. This leads to an important point. The methods we have been describing lead to confident predictions and explanations based on correlations between certain conditions and certain effects. But we only understand the phenomenon fully when we have postulated a causal mechanism. We could reconstruct Snow's thinking with the model of the combined method if, instead of *a* being 'the drinking of contaminated water', we called it 'the ingestion of micro-organisms from the excreta of victims'. In this instance, *a* would indeed be a necessary and sufficient condition for the occurrence of the disease. It would only require Koch's work to then identify the micro-organism and the inquiry would be complete.

Robert Koch (1843–1910), who was an important pioneer in bacteriological research, discovered the micro-organism which causes cholera in 1883. His rules for bacteriological research were:[2]

1. The infectious agent of a given disease must be shown to be present in every case of that disease.
2. It must be absent from all other diseases.
3. We should be able to isolate it.
4. We should be able to cultivate it.
5. An animal inoculated with it must contract the same disease.
6. We should be able to trace the agent again in the organism of the inoculated animal.

Exercise 10.5

Specify which of Koch's rules for bacteriological research may be seen to illustrate John Stuart Mill's methods for finding causes. Which of Mill's methods are being used in these rules?

We now turn to the last two of Mill's methods for finding causes.

4. The Method of Concomitant Variation

In the cases that we have been considering so far, we have been assuming that the conditions and variables which we were inquiring into could be isolated. We could easily stop patients from having the soup and Snow could distinguish those who had drunk contaminated water from those who had not, especially in the case of the two different water supply companies. But sometimes it is not possible to isolate factors in this way. As well, it can happen that factors cannot be eliminated from test groups, but can only be reduced or increased. In cases such as this we might look for a factor which varies as the effect varies.

Let us imagine a person who is showing an allergic reaction to certain foods. We suspect that it might be sugar which is the cause. But it is not possible to eliminate sugar from one's diet completely. However, we notice that as we decrease the amount of sugar by eliminating the most obvious sweet foods, the allergic reaction decreases, while if we increase sweet foods, the reaction gets worse. We could represent our thinking here as follows, where *a* represents sugar, *b* represents dairy products, and *c* various fibrous foods. The '−' sign represents 'a reduction in', while the '+' represents 'an increase in'.

Case 1: $a-$, b, c, $\Rightarrow E-$
Case 2: a, b, c, $\Rightarrow E$
Case 3: $a+$, b, c, $\Rightarrow E+$

Therefore, *a* is causally connected with *E*.

One could use this method in a more thorough way by also varying the intake of dairy foods and fibrous foods and seeing if the effect varies accordingly.

Another variation on this method is where an increase in a variable produces a decrease in the effect, while a decrease in the variable produces an increase in the effect. One example might be where the variable is pressure on a car's brake pedal and the effect is the speed of the car. We can illustrate this as follows:

Case 1: $a-$, b, c, $\Rightarrow E+$
Case 2: a, b, c, $\Rightarrow E$
Case 3: $a+$, b, c, $\Rightarrow E-$

Therefore, *a* is causally connected with *E*.

5. The Method of Residues

This method is used to look for a missing factor when an effect is out of proportion to the known causes. For example, imagine that you stand on the scales and your weight is somewhat greater than you expected. You will look for some factor to explain this. Then you find that you are wearing your money belt and this explains the extra weight. In a more realistic case, you might have administered a drug to reduce a patient's pain. But then the patient not only experiences reduced pain, but also reduced responsiveness in perception and affect, and drowsiness. The effect is excessive given the dosage of the drug. Here you will look for some other factor which is causing the effect.

Schematically, we can represent this mode of thinking as follows. It is known that:

$a \Rightarrow E$

But in this particular case, the effect is out of proportion to the cause. Let us call this $E+$. We conclude that there must be some other factor, b, which accounts for the increased (or decreased) effect. We illustrate this as:

$a + b \Rightarrow E+$

Of course, this will not tell us what b is. We need to make further inquiries to discover this. The patient might have had an allergic reaction to the drug, or be suffering from a heart condition. But some other factor of which we were not aware before will have been identified as being present.

Exercise 10.6

For the arguments below:

a. Which factor is being said to be (or not to be) the cause and which effect?
b. Identify the method being used to support the conclusion (Method of Agreement, Difference, Joint Method, Concomitant Variation or Residues).
c. Use the formal schemas explained in the text above to outline the argument.

1. There has been a decline in the number of deaths from lung cancer since public awareness campaigns about the dangers of smoking reduced the consumption of tobacco.
2. A woman who was prone to depression experienced a grand mal seizure and continuing manic symptoms after replacing sugar in her tea with aspartame, an artificial sweetener. On reverting to sugar, her symptoms ceased.
3. The mere sight and smell of a hospital ward can fill some patients with severe anxiety.
4. In a series of experiments which would raise eyebrows in ethics committees today, Walter Reed sought the cause of yellow fever (a frequently fatal disease) amongst the following possibilities:

   a. mosquitoes which had fed on victims
   b. excreta of victims
   c. dishes and utensils used by victims for eating
   d. the clothing of patients.

   Reed built a mosquito-proof building divided into two sections. In one section he introduced mosquitoes which had fed on victims. Volunteers were put in each half of the building and only those in the mosquito side contracted the disease. Then the other possible factors were introduced, with the volunteers divided into groups such that half were exposed to the factor and the other half not. The illness did not strike any of these groups. The various factors were combined in all possible combinations. It became clear that mosquitoes were solely responsible for transmitting yellow fever.

5. Jones must have been the culprit. He was present at the scene of each of the crimes.
6. According to a nine-year study, 3% of prostitutes in Nairobi who statistically should become infected with HIV, do not. This is thought to indicate that some people have an immunity to the virus.
7. According to laboratory experiments, male and female mice use different brain mechanisms to handle extreme pain. But females react to pain in the same way as males when their estrogen-secreting ovaries are removed. It follows that there is a link between estrogen and the female pain-suppression system.
8. Researchers have identified a broad-spectrum antibiotic called squalamine which seems to be present in all shark tissue and explains the high degree of resistance to bacteria and fungal microbes shown by sharks. Pharmaceutical companies are seeking to synthesise the substance.
9. Research by the Australian Bureau of Meteorology has brought forth the surprising conclusion that perturbations in the weather can have serious effects on health. The so-called El Niño-Southern Oscillation produces climatic extremes which are associated with increased instances of vector-born diseases such as Murray Valley encephalitis.
10. The fact that the maximum life span for humans has not increased suggests that there may be built-in aging factors . . . Leonard Hayflick of Children's Hospital Medical Centre in Oakland, California, has grown cell cultures of normal human body cells taken from people of different ages. Cells from a human embryo double about fifty times before they die. Cells taken from a middle-aged human divide only about twenty times before they die.

    This control on cell aging could be in the DNA of the nucleus or in the cell body outside the nucleus. Hayflick exchanged nuclei from human embryo and adult cells and found that the primary control is in the nucleus. Whether the cell bodies were from the embryo or the adult, if the nucleus was from an adult the cell only divided about twenty times. If the nucleus was from the embryo, the cell divided about fifty times.[3]

NOTES

1. Quoted in Goldstein, Martin & Goldstein, Inge F., *How We Know: An Exploration of the Scientific Process*, New York, Plenum Press, 1978, p. 31.

2. Quoted in Starobinski, Jean, *A History of Medicine*, London, Leisure Arts Limited, 1962, p. 79.
3. Ornstein, Robert & Thompson, Richard F., 'The amazing brain', in Kelley, David, *The Art of Reasoning*, New York, W.W. Norton and Co., 1988.

Chapter 11
Fallacies of Causal Thinking

In this chapter we discuss errors in the attribution of necessary and sufficient conditions. Some links are drawn with the errors in inductive reasoning discussed in Chapter 7. Errors in statistical reasoning are also illustrated. Detecting such fallacies helps to distinguish genuine science from pseudo-science and to recognise quackery in the field of health as well as instances of superstition and wishful thinking.

Just as there are a range of errors in reasoning which one can commit in the context of debate, so there are a range of errors which can occur in the context of scientific reasoning and other forms of explanation. Here we are not talking about fallacies in logic, such as affirming the consequent or denying the antecedent in deductive arguments. Rather, we are talking about sloppy thinking in causality that often (but not always) leads to error.

Most causal thinking begins by noting a constant correlation between two events (let us call these A and B respectively) and then goes on to postulate, on the basis of this correlation, that A causes B. In the previous chapter we studied the several rigorous methods that can be used to show that these correlations are not just coincidental but rather identify necessary and sufficient conditions. When these methods are followed, the move from constant correlation to causality is most often a sound form of reasoning. Nevertheless, it is subject to many risks of error. The major types of such error are the following:

1. The 'Post Hoc' Fallacy

The full name of this fallacy is the 'post hoc ergo propter hoc' fallacy. This Latin phrase means, 'after this, therefore because of this'. What this means is that A is said to cause B simply because B follows A in time. An example that frequently occurs is that of the person who catches a cold and then takes a heavy dose of vitamin C. When the cold abates the person says that it was because of the vitamin C. The fact is that he has no way of knowing whether the vitamin C caused the cold to go away or whether the cold just ran its natural course. Colds are known not to last very long and so whatever remedy you use, the cold is bound to lift soon after. It would be a mistake to suppose that, just because the cold disappeared soon after you took the remedy, it disappeared *because* you took the remedy. The improvement might have occurred because of the vitamin C, or it might not.

You need to make an independent study to see whether this was the cause or not.

John Snow might have been tempted to commit this fallacy when he had the handle taken off the Broad Street Pump. The number of cases of cholera in the Broad Street area certainly reduced after he had the handle removed, and he might have concluded that it was the lack of access to this water that had caused the reduction in rates of infection. But he was careful enough to notice that the rate of incidence was already declining when he had the handle taken off.

The 'post hoc' fallacy can be seen to be a particular version of another fallacy which we have already identified, namely the fallacy of hasty generalisation. To conclude that your taking of vitamin C has cured your cold involves an induction from a sample which is too small. You are thinking only of your own case. If you were a medical researcher, however, this experience might lead you to form the hypothesis that vitamin C can cure the common cold and you might test this hypothesis with a suitably large sample of cases and with a control group of similar people. You give your test group vitamin C when they have a cold, while you give your control group nothing (or a placebo that looks like vitamin C). You ensure that your groups are large and varied and you compare the length of time that it takes the colds to clear up in the two groups. If the test group gained relief more quickly, you have evidence in favour of the hypothesis. Now it is true that your test group gained relief after taking the vitamin, but because it is a large and varied group, and because you are comparing it to a control group which has not taken the vitamin, you have avoided the post hoc fallacy. You will have shown that the correlation between the alleged cause and the effect is not a coincidental one.

But the best way of all to avoid the post hoc fallacy is to identify the causal agent which is producing the effect. If pharmacologists were able to say what it was about vitamin C that countered the symptoms of the common cold and how it did so, then we would not have to rely on the mere temporal correlation of the two phenomena to ground the hypothesis of a causal relationship. In the same way, John Snow's research was brought to completion, as it were, when Koch discovered the comma bacillus, the actual causal agent of cholera infection which was carried in the contaminated water.

2. Confusing Cause and Effect

The thinking that leads to a causal hypothesis frequently begins with a constant correlation. But if A is correlated with B, how do we know whether it is A that causes B rather than B that causes A? Constant correlation by itself will not tell us. The error of confusing cause and effect consists in suggesting that the effect is the cause and vice versa: that is, saying that B causes A, when A causes B. For example, a nurse might notice that when visitors bring flowers to patients in hospital, those visitors often seem more cheerful. The nurse might conclude that bringing flowers makes the visitors cheerful. But it is equally possible that when the visitors are cheerful they are more likely to bring flowers. Rather than the flowers causing thc cheerfulness, it might be the cheerfulness which is causing the flowers to be brought.

3. Ignoring a Common Cause

With this error, we once again have a constant correlation between A and B. This time the error consists in failing to see that both A and B might be caused by something else: C. Their having a common cause, C, would certainly explain why A and B always occur together. A case of this which we have already mentioned in a different context is that of night and day. There is a perfectly constant correlation between these two events, but one does not cause the other. Both are caused by the rotation of the earth around the sun.

A more interesting example arises from debates about the effects of television violence on children. Experts around the world continue to disagree about whether the portrayal of violence on television causes children to behave more violently towards one another and to grow up into adults who are prone to violence. That there is a correlation between the amount of television watched (and there is no question that there is a large amount of violence portrayed on television) and increased violent behaviour or increased tolerance of violence seems unquestionable. The question is whether the television violence is causing the real life violence. There may be something which causes both. There may be a common cause. It may be that our individualistic and competitive culture implicitly teaches us (through its admiration for ruthless businessmen, violent sports heroes and vigorous law enforcement) that violence is an acceptable way to resolve conflict. This being so, television producers will make programs that portray this because they imagine that that is what the audience wants, while children will learn from a variety of sources within this same culture that violence is acceptable. If this hypothesis is right, then it is our cultural ethos as a whole which is to blame for both the increased portrayal of violence on television and also for the increased violent activity of children. (Of course, TV violence may also reinforce the causal influence that is coming from our culture.)

4. Overlooking Complexity

This error consists in falsely concluding that A causes B directly, when there are intervening necessary conditions or processes. To understand this error we need to distinguish a **proximate cause** from a **remote cause**. A proximate cause is the immediate necessary and sufficient condition for something's happening. In the case of lighting a match, the proximate cause is the striking of the match against the box. The remote cause of something is a cause that is removed from the effect by several necessary and sufficient steps. So the curious child in the kitchen might ask what caused the eggs to cook. The answer to this is that they were put into boiling water for a sufficient length of time. If the child continues to ask how this comes about, his father might answer that the pot of water was put onto the gas burner and the gas lit. And this came about because the gas was turned on and a lighted match held to it. And this came about because the match was struck against the side of the box. In this way the striking of the match is a remote cause of the cooking of the eggs. Rather than A simply causing B, A causes B which causes C which causes D and so forth until we describe a causal chain which links A, the striking of the match, to E, the cooking of the eggs.

Now this sort of thinking can get out of hand. We have already noted that every causal process can be analysed into constitutive steps. We can analyse the match lighting into the generation of heat, the combustion of sulphur and so on. And we can analyse these processes down into their chemical causes and move on to fundamental physical explanations. In this sense, every cause is a remote cause at some level of explanation. It is also true that the chain of effects never stops. In fact, the matches may not have worked because the box was wet and the father had to go out and buy more, which had the effect of delaying the father from picking up his other child at school, and this caused that child to be subject to some bullying, and this caused the child to be traumatised and to have an unhappy life. Is all this caused (remotely) by the fact that the match would not light? It would be absurd to require explanations that follow causal chains this far.

We must remember that causal accounts are given in the context of practical and diagnostic tasks. We identify causes in order to solve problems. It serves no purpose to analyse every process down to the deepest detail or to trace every causal chain through to its most remote effects. So the terms proximate cause and remote cause are relative to the pragmatic context in which they are used.

Now suppose that a patient comes into a clinic complaining of persistent bouts of headache. Talking to the patient, the nurse discovers that he works in a situation of great pressure and concludes that the headache is being caused by stress. Using the above terminology, stress is deemed to be the proximate cause of the headaches. However, it turns out on further investigation that the patient is in the habit of responding to his occupational pressures by having a number of stiff drinks when he gets home from work. It now appears that his headaches are hangovers caused by these drinks. But he is having these excessive drinks because of his stress, so his stress is still causing his headaches. Only it is causing the headaches as a remote cause rather than as a proximate cause. The nurse is correct in identifying the stress as a cause of the headaches but incorrect in thinking that it is the proximate or immediate cause. The stress is causing the drinking and the drinking is causing the headaches.

5. Extrapolating Beyond an Appropriate Range of Cases

This error consists in thinking that A will cause B every time, no matter what changes might have occurred in the relevant circumstances. Nurse Jones might have planted roses in the hospital garden and, knowing that water (along with other necessary background conditions) causes flowers to grow, he waters the roses three times a day every day of the week. The roses die. Jones has extrapolated from the fact that water is necessary for flowers to grow to the idea that any amount of water will do so, or perhaps to the thought that the more water you use, the more growth will occur. Nurse Jones incorrectly thinks that if A causes B, then more A will cause more B.

Another example might be Nurse Rodoupolous, who sees a former patient in the shopping centre. When this person was a patient, Nurse Rodoupolous spoke to him in a very caring way and asked after his state of health in a very solicitous tone of voice. This seemed to cheer him up and help his recovery. So Nurse Rodoupolous now proceeds to talk to the former patient in the same solicitous tones about his health. But now the former patient is embarrassed and angry. He is with his football team friends and does not want them to know that he was ill or that he is in any way lacking in manly vigour. Nurse Rodoupolous was correct in thinking that her caring speech had caused the patient to have a speedy recovery in the clinical setting. But it does not follow that talking to him in this caring way would be helpful in a different setting. Although A causes B in one context, it might not in another.

6. Ambiguous Variables

If causal hypotheses arise from correlations between A and B, then A and B had better be terms that are well defined and consistently used. The fallacy of ambiguous variables consists in making correlations (including statistical correlations) between items or groups which are ill-defined, or whose definition changes between cases.

To avoid this fallacy it is necessary that there be appropriate forms of classification for the variables. Indeed, this is also necessary for cases of classificatory explanation. But classifications are not given in nature. They are invented by researchers and may be more or less effective in picking out what is relevant to a given case. And they may vary over time. Zoologists have worked for many years to develop classificatory systems that are adequate to the variety of animals that they find, and yet group them in useful ways. There are subtle reasons why we call one group of animals by the name 'dog' even though they display a great variety of shapes and sizes and can be very different from each other. It took a great deal of research and subtle observation to develop the classifications used in medical and psychiatric diagnosis. There was a time when any instance of fever plus diarrhoea was taken to be a case of the same disease. It took medical science many years to develop the current distinctions between cholera, typhoid, dysentery, bacterial food poisoning, colitis and others.

This point can be even better illustrated by considering the classification of schizophrenia and of manic-depressive disorders. It was found that during the 1950s and 1960s the pattern of diagnosis for these psychiatric illnesses differed greatly between the United States and Great Britain. Schizophrenia seemed to occur much more frequently in the United

States, while the rates for hospital admissions for manic-depressive psychosis in Great Britain were twenty times higher than those of the United States.[1] Given that the social, cultural and economic conditions of these two nations were quite similar, it seemed odd that so many more Americans should be schizophrenic, while so many more English people should suffer from manic-depressive syndromes. After exhaustive and rigorous study of this apparent discrepancy it was found that the difference was due to the differing diagnostic practices of psychiatrists in the two countries. When the diagnoses were checked by mixed groups of psychiatrists from both countries, it was found that the nature of the mental illnesses which people in both countries suffered did not differ very markedly, only the diagnoses did. American psychiatrists were more prone to use the classification of schizophrenia, while their British counterparts were more inclined to describe their patients as suffering from manic-depressive disorders.

What this shows is that diagnoses and other classificatory explanations use categories which are created by scientists and applied in ways that reflect the conventional practices of that scientific community. So when a puzzling event or pattern of events is explained by saying, 'It is a case of . . .', we are applying knowledge which reflects our background understanding and systems of classification rather than an objective and absolute category which must be true for everyone and at all times. Of course, these classifications are necessary and useful conventions and we cannot do without them or apply them arbitrarily. But neither are they absolute facts. As a result, errors can arise if the classifications are used inconsistently when correlations are reported.

We have already referred to this matter when we were discussing statistics in Chapter 7. We said then that when we are comparing statistics we should be careful to check that the classifications used in gathering those statistics are the same in all cases being compared. One example of this might be a set of statistics which purports to show an increasing rate of success in treating cases of cancer over time. Let us imagine that medical authorities are claiming success in treating cancer by showing that the number of deaths from cancer as a ratio of the number of diagnosed cases of cancer has been steadily decreasing over a ten-year period. Money allocated to cancer research has increased over this period. These statistics would seem to indicate that there is a positive correlation between money spent on cancer research and success in treatment of diagnosed cases.

But it may be that there has been a qualitative change in the cases of diagnosed cancer as well as a quantitative change. Since the growth in awareness of cancer and the growth in willingness on the part of people to have health checks, many cases of cancer are diagnosed much earlier, including those that do not turn out to be malignant. As a result, the statistics relating to diagnosed cases of cancer may have increased without there being a similar increase in morbidity as a result of cancer. Previous figures might have reflected cases of cancer with less positive prognoses and therefore more likely to result in death, while more recent figures show a total number of cases which includes those with more hopeful prognoses. As a result, the proportion of deaths in the earlier figures will be relatively higher than in the later figures. But the groups being compared should not be classified in exactly the same way. The earlier groups contained people with relatively advanced cases of cancer, while the statistics gathered later in the ten-year period reflect cases that were diagnosed at earlier stages of the disease. The apparent improvement is not due to the funding of cancer research, but to other changes in the populations that are being studied. As a result, the wrong causal inference has been drawn.

There are a number of further errors associated with causal thinking, and with explanatory and scientific thinking in general, which should be discussed. These errors do not arise from faulty thinking about correlations, but from other methodological mistakes.

7. Postulating an Undiscoverable Cause

This error is not an error that arises from thinking about constant correlations. Indeed, with this error we do not have correlations between events A and B at all, we only have event B which is the phenomenon to be explained. The error consists in postulating a cause, A, for which there is no, or cannot be, any evidence. A celebrated example of this fallacy occurs in a play by the French writer Molière. A somewhat pompous physician is asked why a rather lazy character in the play is constantly drowsy and he answers that it is because this character suffers from an excess of the 'principia dormitiva'. Now 'principia dormitiva' is Latin for 'principle of sleepfulness' or 'power to produce sleep'. So the physician has answered the question, Why is this person sleeping all the time? by saying that he is subject to a power to produce sleep. But this is no explanation at all. It simply refers to the phenomenon which needs to be explained—that the person is prone to sleep—and uses that same phenomenon to explain it by saying that the person has too much of whatever it is that produces sleep. And this simply means that the person is prone to sleep. So the answer is a circular one. It is an answer that begs the question.

The methodological rule that is being flouted here is that in any causal explanation, the cause must be identified separately from the effect. The physician in the play is using the effect, sleepfulness, to identify the cause, a power to produce sleepfulness. What he should do is point to something, as the alleged cause, that can be observed separately from the sleepfulness of the patient, which is the effect. Using the effect to identify the cause is a circular procedure which does not add any information and so does not explain what needs to be explained.

Although we have illustrated this fallacy with an example from literature, the fallacy occurs very frequently in real life. There is a body of ideas and theories which goes under the general name of sociobiology which frequently commits this error. Sociobiology claims to be able to explain human behaviour and cultural practices on the basis of our genes and Darwin's theory of natural selection. For example, it explains altruism and ethical behaviour by suggesting that at an earlier stage of evolutionary history there would have been proto human beings who had genes for being selfish and also proto human beings who had genes for being altruistic. The latter would have protected one another in times of danger while the former would have looked only to their own safety. As there is greater security to be derived from cooperation, the altruistic ones would have survived longer, reproduced more, and gradually come to outnumber the selfish ones. Indeed, the selfish ones would have died out altogether over time. And so the human race would gradually have become altruistic in nature.

This is an interesting story but it depends on the hypothesis that there are identifiable genes for altruism and selfishness respectively. How could we identify such genes? At the present time we cannot. We do not know enough about the genes and how they affect behavioural traits. So the only way of identifying the genes is by noting the behaviour (altruistic or selfish) which they are said to cause. But this offends against the methodological principle that cause and effect must be separately identifiable and so the argument is circular.

Another methodological principle that this way of thinking offends against is the **principle of falsifiability**. A well known philosopher of science, Karl Popper, first articulated this principle. The idea is that for an explanation to count as genuinely scientific (as opposed to being a piece of pseudo-science), there must be a way of showing that it is false. This is another way of saying that it must be testable. The idea is not that you have to show that it is false—only that there must be some test available so that if it were false, it could be shown to be so. We could return to Semmelweis's research to illustrate this. His hypothesis that the priest's procession was causing the deaths in the First Division could be tested by asking the priest to take a different route through the hospital. Although it seems rather superstitious to us, this was a genuinely scientific hypothesis because it could be (and was) falsified. In the same way, the hypothesis that putrid and cadaveric matter was causing the deaths was genuinely scientific because it could be (and was not) falsified. If Semmelweis had postulated that the deaths were being caused by a secret death wish on the part of the patients themselves, what could he have done to test the hypothesis? No test could have shown this hypothesis to be false. On the contrary, every death could have been taken as a confirmation of it. For every mother who died, Semmelweis could have said, 'See, there's another case of a mother with a secret death wish. My hypothesis must be right!' And of any mother who did not die, he could have said, 'That mother did not have a death wish.' But this shows that this hypothesis cannot be falsified. Any outcome is consistent with it. And the reason that it cannot be falsified is that the hypothesized cause cannot be identified separately from the effect.

8. Inappropriate Purposive Explanation

This fallacy consists in applying purposive explanations to things when such explanations are not appropriate. You will recall that purposive explanations are given in terms of the purposes that the thing being explained is said to have. Such explanations are sometimes called **teleological**. This term comes from the ancient Greek word 'telos' which means 'purpose'. There is nothing wrong with teleological explanations when they are applied to appropriate entities. As we saw when we discussed purposive explanations, such explanations are appropriate when they explain the behaviour of human beings and other beings that can act purposefully, such as animals.

One of the odd features of purposive explanations is that it is the result which explains the cause. But it is implicit in the whole idea of causality that a cause must precede the effect. If a car accident has caused an injury, then the car accident must have occurred before (even if only by a split second) the occurrence of the injury. If a drug has caused an improvement in a patient's condition, then that drug must have been administered before the patient's condition improved. Now in the case of Bob who closed the window in order to block out the noises from the street, the blocking of the noise is the result of Bob's action. It comes after Bob's forming the intention to close the window and his closing it. Yet in this case we cite the blocking of the noise as the explanation for his closing the window because this was his purpose. Blocking the noise explains (or causes) Bob's closing of the window. This would seem like saying that the injury explains (or causes) the accident. And this seems absurd.

The solution to this puzzle is easy to find. Bob is able to imagine or anticipate the blocking of the noise and it is his thought of this future event which motivates him to act. This thought precedes the action in time. But it is a thought about the result of the action, an anticipation of it, and hence a thought about the future. This is what makes it seem as if a future event is explaining or causing a present one. Another way of expressing this idea is to say that what causes Bob to open the window is his desire to block the noise. This desire is a state of Bob's that obtains before he closes the window. The desire is a desire for a future state of affairs but it is a presently existing condition of Bob's. In this way a purposive explanation applied to a rational agent like Bob, who can have thoughts about the future, does not offend against the principle that the future cannot cause the present or past. It follows from all this that purposive explanations can only be valid in the case of human beings or other conscious beings who have future-directed desires or intentions.

Some social scientists use purposive explanations to account for social and historical phenomena. For example, some anthropologists explain the rain dances of certain tribal peoples by saying that those dances occur because they produce cohesion amongst the people. But here it is not suggested that these tribal people intend to weld their tribes together by engaging in a ritual activity in which everyone takes part and which everyone will find important. Their intention is to make rain. But (given that from the anthropologists' point of view, this intention is silly because dancing doesn't cause rain) the real purpose that is served by the dance is the maintenance of social cohesion and harmony. It is the achievement of this goal (of which the people know nothing) which explains the ritual activity. The ritual activity exists for the purpose of creating social and cultural cohesion in the tribe. Social scientists spend much time debating whether this form of explanation is valid. It certainly seems like a case of the effect explaining (that is, causing) the cause.

Yet another example of this apparently back-to-front form of explanation is frequently found in explanations of natural events given in the context of evolutionary theory. If you watch nature programs on television, you often hear such statements as, 'This species of moth developed its darker wings in order to be able to hide from predators on the dark bark of trees.' What this seems to be saying is that these moths consciously thought up the idea of darkening their wings. This would be absurd, of course. Yet the statement does imply that the outcome of the process of evolution—in this case the creation of camouflage through having darker wings—is a purpose pursued by that process. It is as if nature had a purpose in creating darker moths and this purpose explains the phenomenon.

But we know that nature does not have purposes. The processes of nature are not things which can have future-directed desires or intentions. In nature, what happens happens. We also know that evolution works by a process of natural selection. Moths which are born with lighter wings (that is, have genes for lighter wings) will be more easily seen and destroyed by predators. They will reproduce less often. In this way, genes for light wings will start to die out and the moths with dark wings (that is, having genes for darker wings) will come to dominate in a given population. These moths will reproduce more often and gradually the whole moth population will have genes for dark wings. This may seem like an outcome that has been designed for some purpose, but there is nothing purposive in the process. It is just what happens. And so it is an error to explain it by way of a purposive or teleological explanation.

9. Using an Inappropriate Explanatory Model

The fallacy which we have just discussed was a case of using an inappropriate explanatory model. A purposive model was being used when a causal model was the appropriate one. But there are other forms of this mistake. The most common is to use a causal model when an interpretative or purposive model is appropriate. And this happens most frequently when we are dealing with people.

Suppose that a nurse is dressing a wound. The patient flinches. It would be easy for the nurse to think that his touching the wound had caused the pain reaction in a direct and quasimechanical way. Lessons in physiology will have taught him that nerve ends located at the wound are connected through major nerve fibres in the spine into the brain and various pain centres, and that these react in various ways so as to cause pain. This seems like a classic case of a causal mechanism. As such it is what would be expected to happen and would occasion no surprise. Moreover, insofar as the reaction is simply caused by touch, there is nothing that can be done about it except to be more gentle. As an account of what happened this is not incorrect. It is an application of the causal model to this patient.

But it is also possible to use the interpretative or purposive model to understand this event. After all, it is always possible for a patient not to flinch. One could imagine a patient with very strong self-control not flinching in a situation like this. So if the patient does flinch it may be that she is trying to tell the nurse something. She may be wanting to ask the nurse to be more gentle. Or she may be expressing her fear of the whole procedure that she is undergoing. Or she may want the nurse to notice that she is there as a person and not just as a body that needs bandaging. In short, the flinch may have a meaning.

Although we say that the patient flinched because the nurse touched her wound, the signpost 'because' can be misleading. This signpost is ambiguous as to the kind of explanation being offered. Very often it indicates a causal explanation, as in, 'The match lit because it was struck against the side of the box.' But it can also indicate an interpretative or purposive explanation, as in, 'The patient flinched because she wanted the nurse to say something comforting to her.' This latter statement is an interpretation of the patient's reaction rather than a causal explanation of it.

To understand that flinch in purely causal terms prevents the nurse from trying to understand it as a willed expression of how the patient is feeling. That the patient is a person in need of care requires that we understand the events surrounding that patient in appropriate ways. Often this will mean that the causal model is not the only explanatory model that we use. It is part of the art of nursing to be sensitive to this and to be able to judge what sort of explanation is required in various settings.

Exercise 11.1

Identify which of the fallacies in causal thinking is being committed in the cases below. Explain the fallacy or indicate what more would need to be done to identify the cause correctly.

1. The people of a certain island had observed perfectly accurately over the centuries that people in good health have body lice and people in poor health do not. They had traditionally concluded that lice make a man healthy.[2]
2. Aspirin relieves headaches. So if you have a very severe headache, take lots of aspirin.
3. Jones works very hard at his studies. He must have a burning ambition to succeed.
4. The number of women who fail to gain places in the School of Nursing at Deakin University is much higher than the number of men. Therefore, Deakin University discriminates against women.
5. Bacteria invade healthy cells in order to feed off them and multiply into malignant growths.
6. You are bound to be a happy personality because you were born under the sign of Capricorn.

7. Statistics have shown that children from Aboriginal families are three times as likely as children from white families to die from infectious diseases and twice as likely to die from accidents. Aboriginality is an 'invisible killer' more deadly than cancer.
8. The *Medical Tribune* of 13 May 1993 has urged doctors to look out for 'Beauty Parlour Stroke Syndrome'. The neck rotation and hyperextension involved in professional shampoos can reduce vertebral artery flow and cause other injuries that may lead ultimately to stroke, especially in older clients.
9. The meetings of the Nurses' Union have had hardly any significant items on their agendas for months. Perhaps the meetings are only occurring in order to maintain the commitment of the membership.
10. One night a lady in a private ward switched off her television. Suddenly there was darkness in the room and outside (as seen through the glass panel in her door). There was a sound of commotion in the corridors and the word 'black-out' could be heard. The lady burst from her room and explained to the first nurse in sight that she must have blown the hospital's fuses.
11. Being single increases the likelihood of eating chocolate. Statistics show married persons eat less chocolate than single persons. (A second look at the data showed that if married and single individuals of equal age were compared, the correlations vanished.)
12. The government found that by reducing the number of staff and reorganising work practices in the administrative branches of the public service, it could reduce costs but maintain efficiency. Encouraged by this success, it decided to cut its funding to public hospitals.
13. The *New England Journal of Medicine* (25 March 1993) recently reported a case of 'Margarita photodermatitis'. The patient presented with 'burning, severe swelling, and blistering of his left hand'. The diagnosis of photodermatitis was made following revelations that two days previously the patient had squeezed some five dozen limes in the course of making a large quantity of margaritas, whereupon he had spent the rest of the afternoon sunbathing. The condition is usually described as an occupational hazard of citrus workers and celery harvesters.[3]
14. Naturopathy really seems to work. A friend of mine went to a naturopath recently complaining of stomach pains. He was given a herbal infusion to drink and his pain disappeared soon after.
15. Give that child an aspirin. She is crying because of pain.
16. A nurse found that whenever she went round the wards to administer prescribed medicines (which included analgesics) the patients complained of their symptoms less and became more cheerful soon after. She took great pride in this, thinking that her very presence in the ward was of help to the patients.
17. A counsellor was dealing with a nurse client suffering from anorexia nervosa. She noted that the nurse suffered severe depression and concluded that the depression caused the anorexia.

18. Any scientific study of religion should take account of the fact that a central theme of religion is the attempt to maximize human 'goodness'. I speculate that religious practices have in part a genetic basis, involving genes linked to potential for goodness. Societies in which this potential is actualized in a sizeable proportion of its members will tend to function more harmoniously and more efficiently, so that natural selection will tend to favour the presence in human societies of genes of this type. (From a letter to *Nature*, April 1992.)
19. Perhaps we should give patient Roberts, who is in pain because of a leg fracture, some morphine. Morphine certainly helped control Mrs van Graaf's pain while she was dying of cancer.
20. A psychotherapist noticed over a considerable period of time that his clients were more decisive and determined to overcome fear and nervousness when they came for their regular consultation than when they missed their appointments for any reason. The therapist congratulated himself for increasing the self-confidence of his clients.
21. Early researchers on schizophrenia, using patients in psychiatric hospitals as research subjects, argued that the disease was characterised by an increasing lassitude and listlessness over time. Schizophrenic patients seemed to lose all interest in things around them and to just mope around. A cause for this was thought to be some kind of degeneration of the brain cells.
22. A recently published study has determined that 'lacking health insurance is associated with an increased risk of subsequent mortality, an effect that is evident in all socio-demographic health insurance and mortality groups examined.' The prospective study of 4694 patients between 1971 and 1987 found that 9.6 percent of insured patients twenty-five and older died, compared to 18.4 percent of uninsured patients.[4]

NOTES

1. These figures and their explanation are discussed in Chapter 5 of Goldstein, Martin & Goldstein, Inge F., *How We Know: An Exploration of the Scientific Process*, New York, Plenum Press, 1978.
2. Taken from Huff, Darrel, *How to Lie with Statistics*, New York, Norton, 1954, p. 98. and quoted in Walton, Douglas N., *Informal Logic: A Handbook for Critical Argumentation*, Cambridge, Cambridge University Press, 1989, p. 216.
3. Reported in *The Hastings Centre Report*, September–October 1993, p. 2.
4. Reported in *The Hastings Centre Report*, November–December 1993, p. 2.

Suggested Further Reading for Part Two

The literature on the philosophy of science is vast and the list that follows includes only books that the authors have judged to be useful and accessible to students.

Chalmers, A.F., *What Is This Thing Called Science?* (2nd edition), Brisbane, University of Queensland Press, 1982.
This is a very popular book amongst students and gives a good overview of current theories about science and its claims to truth.

Giere, Ronald N., *Understanding Scientific Reasoning* (3rd edition), New York, Holt, Rinehart & Winston, 1991.
This is a very useful book in that it focuses on the logic of scientific reasoning without getting distracted by philosophical questions about the epistemological status of scientific truth. It includes sections on conditional thinking, statistical reasoning, the nature of theories, the logic of testing and the interface between scientific thinking on the one hand and values and decision making on the other.

Goldstein, Martin & Goldstein, Inge F., *How We Know: An Exploration of the Scientific Process*, New York, Plenum Press, 1978 (Paperback edition, 1981).
Very readable and with case studies, including the one about cholera which we used.

Harré, Rom, *Great Scientific Experiments*, Oxford, Oxford University Press, 1981.
A very readable history from which our example of the process of digestion was taken.

Madden, Edward H., *The Structure of Scientific Thought: An Introduction to Philosophy of Science*, London, Routledge & Kegan Paul, 1960.
An older but very useful anthology covering the philosophical issues.

Miller, Richard W., *Fact and Method: Explanation, Confirmation and Reality in the Natural and the Social Sciences*, Princeton, Princeton University Press, 1987.
A more difficult book, with a very technical discussion of causality.

Mosedale, Frederick E. (ed.), *Philosophy and Science: The Wide Range of Interaction*, Englewood Cliffs, New Jersey, Prentice-Hall, 1979.
A very useful anthology embracing a large range of issues, including the relation of science to religion. It includes the article by Carl Hempel from which our Semmelweis example was taken.

Riggs, Peter J., *Whys and Ways of Science: Introductory Philosophical and Sociological Theories of Science*, Melbourne, Melbourne University Press, 1992.
A good overview of current theories about science and its claims to truth.

Starobinski, Jean, *A History of Medicine*, London, Leisure Arts Limited, 1962.
An illustrated history with good examples written at a popular level.

Susser, Mervyn, *Causal Thinking in the Health Sciences: Concepts and Strategies in Epidemiology*, New York, Oxford University Press, 1973.

A very thorough treatment of statistical methods in health research.

Toulmin, Stephen, *The Philosophy of Science: An Introduction*, London, Hutchinson & Co., 1953.

Somewhat dated but still a classic and very clearly written.

Winslow, Charles-Edward Amory, *The Conquest of Epidemic Disease: A Chapter in the History of Ideas*, New York, Hafner Publishing Company, 1967.

Exhaustive treatment of the topic including a discussion of Snow and cholera.

Ziman, John, *Reliable Knowledge: An Exploration of the Grounds for Belief in Science*, Cambridge, Cambridge University Press, 1978.

A good general introduction with a keen awareness of the social context of science.

PART THREE: THE LOGIC OF ETHICAL THINKING

Chapter 12
Introduction to Ethical Argument

This chapter begins with an explanation of what ethics is. It then introduces the basic structure of ethical argument and indicates how to write logical outlines of ethical arguments. The fundamental methods of critically evaluating ethical reasoning are explained. The need to understand the meaning of ethical concepts is noted.

Although a commonly used term these days, 'ethics' does not always mean the same thing to everyone. So it will be useful to begin with some sort of definition.

What is 'Ethics'?

Ethics is about moral right and wrong (rather than factual correctness and incorrectness). That is, it is about how people *should* behave, what they should do in certain circumstances and how they should treat other people. The 'should' involved has a special quality and sense of importance—if something is morally wrong, then I should not do it, even if I want to, even if it would be advantageous to me, even if someone would pay me to do it. Put more formally, one defining feature of moral right and wrong is that it makes a special demand which takes precedence over other reasons for acting. For this reason, many expressions of moral or ethical value, whether employing the term 'should' or not, either are or imply exhortations. Ethics is not a neutral matter: a statement that killing is wrong also urges people not to kill.

Sometimes a distinction is made between morality and ethics. Morality refers to the beliefs about right and wrong which we grow up with. The ideas are not well-organised or carefully thought about, and we usually don't know why we have them: we just do. Ethics, on the other hand, refers to a system of ideas about right and wrong, which has been thought about and consciously adopted. Thus, ethics tends to be connected with professional life, and morality with everyday life. This distinction is sometimes helpful, but it is important not to exaggerate it: morality and ethics are both about the same sort of right and wrong, and often it makes sense to use the terms interchangeably.

The Role of Ethical Discussion in Nursing

The need for nurses to engage in ethical discussion at all, let alone have an understanding of ethical reasoning, has been questioned in the past.[1] If nurses are seen as wholly subservient to doctors, acting only on doctors' orders, then it can appear pointless for nurses to worry about the rights and wrongs of what they are doing. This perception is not entirely correct, even for the 'doctor's handmaiden' model of nursing, but fortunately the debate about nursing and ethics has moved beyond this stage. Now that nursing is seen as a profession in its own right, the need for nurses to understand and engage in ethical discussion is obvious. As professionals, nurses have scope to make their own decisions, and are accountable for them. They have ethical obligations to their patients, quite independent of any doctor's obligations, and must make their own decisions about what these obligations are, and how to carry them out in situations of conflicting values or competing claims.

Individual nurses need the ability to engage in ethical reasoning in many different settings. Most commonly, nurses need to make decisions about how to nurse their patients. If Mr Jones refuses to have a shower, should he be forced to? If Mrs White is restless at night, should she be restrained? Nurses also need to participate in inter-disciplinary team discussions about patient management. Here they need to be able to formulate and express their views clearly, and give reasons for them which will be comprehensible and compelling to health professionals from other disciplines. For example, Mr Tran has been in intensive care for 12 days and his condition has improved only slightly—should we comply with his family's request to withdraw treatment? If so, does this include tube-feeding?

Ethical reasoning is also important in situations other than direct patient care. Nurses need to make or participate in policy decisions in their workplaces where ethical values are at stake, and there will be important implications for patient care. For example, consider a hospital which routinely has orthodox Jewish patients. According to orthodox Jewish beliefs, women are not permitted to touch dead bodies, and there have been a number of difficult times in the hospital when uncertainty and dispute have arisen over what to do when an orthodox Jewish patient dies, and no rabbi or other suitable person is able to come immediately to clean up and lay out the body. Should the hospital adopt a policy of leaving the body exactly as it is, with drips still connected and so on, for however many hours it takes for the rabbi to arrive (by which time the body will be too stiff to be moved), or should it allow some preliminaries to be done by the nurses (the vast majority of whom are women) to ensure the body will be in a reasonably acceptable state?

At a more abstract, but nonetheless very important level, nurses are also involved in formulating codes of ethics for their profession or area of specialisation. Understanding of ethical reasoning is vital here for producing a workable document which will actually be of assistance to nurses in their daily decision making. Should a code of ethics contain a series of rules which nurses must follow, or a set of ideals for nurses to aim for, or should it be expressed in terms of patients' rights instead? And *which* rights, rules or ideals should it embody? What role should a code of ethics play in the thinking of individual nurses anyway?

For all these reasons, nurses need to understand the basic logic of ethical thinking. Ethics is certainly a complex area, and difficult decisions cannot be made to disappear by a sweep of the magic wand of critical thinking. However, a critical understanding of ethical reasoning can go a long way towards avoiding some of the major pitfalls of ethical discussion. The questions raised above can be dealt with in a clear and reasoned way, which will minimise personal conflict and maximise the chances of coming to an ethically sensitive decision which is acceptable to all parties.

Common Misapprehensions about Ethics

Nurses, and others, often experience ethical discussions as frustrating and pointless. It seems that everyone is simply putting forward their own personal opinions, no one is going to change their mind, and no resolution will be possible. Not infrequently, such discussions degenerate into personal conflict, as people become more passionately attached to their own views, and angry with those who have a different view. Although many ethical discussions are indeed like this, they do not have to be. There are a number of common misapprehensions about ethics which cause discussions to turn out this way. Once these are cleared up, and a better understanding of the nature of ethics and ethical reasoning is acquired, these sorts of discussions can become more cooperative, calm and fruitful.

One common, but mistaken, view is that ethics is simply a matter of personal opinion. We might call this the 'chocolate icecream' view of ethics: my belief that, for example, abortion is wrong, is just like my preference for chocolate icecream. It is just a matter of personal taste. And if you happen to think abortion is not wrong, or happen not to like chocolate icecream, then that is just your personal taste. Neither of us is wrong or mistaken, and there is nothing to discuss between us.

People often express this sort of view of ethics, without thinking through its full implications. The 'chocolate icecream' view has some clear attractions: it defuses ethical conflict (by suggesting that everyone is right in their own terms), and explains why differences on ethical matters are so difficult to resolve (people's tastes are arbitrary and unlikely to change). But it also has some very grave difficulties. On this view of ethics, a person could have ethical values that were racist, sexist and cruel, but there would be nothing wrong with this—it would be just like a preference for an odd flavour of icecream. For example, it implies that there is nothing wrong with a view that disabled people over the age of ten should be killed, or that people from non-English speaking backgrounds should be denied medical treatment, or girls should not be allowed to go to school. All of these ethical views would just be someone's unchallengeable personal opinion, no worse than a preference for seaweed-flavoured icecream. However, this seems an absurd position to be in. As ethical views, these seem to be just plainly wrong: it is obviously wrong to deny education to girls, or kill disabled people. If you agree that these views are unacceptable, then what you are saying is that there *are* some limits to what we can believe to be right and wrong. Ethics is not purely a matter of personal taste: there are some standards by which we can evaluate ethical views.

A related misunderstanding is the belief that there is no true or false in ethics—any conclusion or decision is as good as any other, and it makes no sense to say that any view is more or less correct than any other. This belief is clearly connected to the impression that there is nothing to go on but personal opinion. But the mistake also lies in ignoring the role played by argument (in the critical thinking sense, as defined in Chapter 3). Ethical discussion actually involves a large number of arguments, or lines of reasoning. These may not be obvious because of the way in which the discussion is carried on, but they are there nevertheless. (This will be demonstrated in the next section.) If reasoning is taking place, it is possible that mistakes of all kinds are being made (see Chapters 5, 6 and 7 for a reminder of errors in formal and informal logic). So even if we were to say that a person's ethical values are beyond criticism and evaluation (which in fact we do not), we could still evaluate the reasoning process which was used to move from a general ethical value to an ethical decision about a particular situation. In between the general value and the particular decision lie many possible errors of fact, and errors of reasoning, which could make that particular decision incorrect.

The next section will set out more clearly the structure of ethical reasoning and the following chapters will discuss some of the errors which can occur in that reasoning. Armed with this understanding, you will be much better placed to make sound ethical decisions yourself, and to evaluate the ethical opinions of others.

The Structure of Ethical Argument

Example 12.1

> It is our obligation to protect the residents of this nursing home from coming to harm. Residents who use walking frames are at risk of falling in the corridors. Therefore, a nurse must accompany these residents to and from the day room, rather than allowing them to walk by themselves.

The paragraph above contains an argument. It is a text that 'supports a point of view with reasons'—the definition of an argument which we gave in Chapter 3. As with any argument, a logical outline of this argument can be written. Here, the conclusion is easily identified by the signpost 'therefore'. Two different premises, offering reasons in support of the conclusion, can clearly be seen in the first two sentences. So the logical outline of this argument would be:

POC: Nurses must accompany residents who use walking frames in the corridors.

1. It is our obligation to protect residents from harm. (ethical exhortation)
2. Residents who use walking frames may come to harm walking in the corridors. (fact)
3. Nurses must accompany residents who use walking frames in the corridors. (1,2, ethical exhortation)

The feature which makes this an ethical argument is the first premise, which expresses an ethical value, rather than giving any information about facts. This distinction between different types of premises was made in Chapter 3. Some premises are informative, in that they aim to give information about how the world is: in a logical outline they are labelled as either facts or assertions, depending on whether they are uncontroversially true, or asserted without support. Other premises are not informative—they express attitudes or, more strongly, urge others to act: in a logical outline they are labelled as values or exhortations. (If this is not clear, you may wish to turn back to Chapter 3 to refresh your memory). In ethical reasoning, there is always a premise which refers to or expresses an ethical value. This premise may be in the form of an exhortation (urging others to act) or a value (expressing an attitude). Either way it is an ethical premise if it refers to moral right and wrong, as was explained at the start of this chapter. In this argument, the ethical premise is in the form of an exhortation, as many ethical premises are. And since the argument contains an ethical premise, it also has an ethical conclusion, again in the form of an exhortation.

So the first step in understanding ethical reasoning is recognising the structure of the argument and the type of premises it contains. Informative premises are usually fairly easy to pick out. They are making some sort of claim about the way the world is—a claim which could be checked or tested in some way. The correctness of the claim does not depend on anyone's attitudes, but on what the facts are. For example, in the argument above, the second premise makes the claim that residents who use walking frames are at risk of falling in the corridor. We have labelled it as a fact because it does not seem contentious. But if we doubted its truth, we could easily check it, for example by examining the incident reports in the nursing home's records. A factual claim in an informative premise could turn out to be false—to say that it is factual or informative does not mean that it is true, but rather that it is about facts or aims to inform. When writing logical outlines, you may wish to label informative premises which look dubious (unlikely to be true) as assertions rather than facts. But remember that assertions and accepted facts belong to the same broad group of informative premises, and are quite different from ethical exhortations and ethical value claims, which both belong to the broad group of ethical premises.

Ethical premises can usually be recognised by the type of language used, but they also have a special type of meaning which sets them apart from informative premises. There are a number of words and phrases which are characteristic of ethical premises expressed in the form of exhortations. These signposts include:

- it is wrong / right
- it is our duty / obligation / responsibility
- we are required to . . .
- it is ethical / unethical to . . .
- should / must / ought.

The signposts for ethical premises expressed in the form of values include 'good/bad', 'praiseworthy/blameworthy', and reference to virtues (morally good character traits) such as 'courageous', 'generous' and so forth.

It is important to keep in mind that not all exhortations and values are ethical: they may express or spring from some other sort of attitude or evaluation. For example, many values are based on personal taste, as we pointed out earlier in this chapter. Preferences for icecream or sunny weather are examples of this sort of value. Another common type of non-ethical evaluation is a **prudential** evaluation. A prudential value or exhortation expresses an attitude about what is sensible, or in one's own best interests to do. For example, a person looking for a new job may be told by her friend 'You should not let the boss know that you are looking for another job.' This is a prudential rather than an ethical exhortation, because it is based on what will be best for the person concerned, not on what is morally right or wrong. In fact, the person looking for the new job may well feel that, although it might harm her own interests if she tells her boss (perhaps she will be sacked before she actually finds another position), she has an ethical obligation to tell the truth anyway. Another type of evaluation is **aesthetic** evaluation, which expresses an opinion about how beautiful or ugly something is. For example, a person might have an aesthetic objection to boxing. This would mean that he or she objected to boxing because it looked ugly or unpleasant (not because it was dangerous or immoral).

Exercise 12.1

All the following sentences contain signposts which could indicate an ethical premise. Which of these sentences is expressing an ethical exhortation or value, and which some other sort of value or rightness?

1. I hope I used the right sling on that man's broken collarbone.
2. It is not right to leave residents sitting on the toilet with the door open.
3. Children shouldn't swim for an hour after eating.
4. A district nurse should not enter an elderly person's home without permission from that person.
5. Nurses should not wear coloured shoes with a white uniform while on duty.

6. Dr Rhodopoulos is very handsome.
7. Nurse Braasten acted very sensitively with that frightened young patient.
8. It is wrong for parents to deprive their children of food as a form of punishment.

When properly formed, an ethical argument has (at least) one ethical premise, expressed in the form of an exhortation or value, and an ethical conclusion, expressed in the form of an exhortation or value. (From now on we will use the terms 'ethical premise' and 'ethical conclusion' to refer to these.) It also has at least one informative premise. The type of reasoning used in most ethical arguments is **deductive**. (Go back to Chapter 6 if you need to remind yourself of the meaning of this term.) This means that the conclusion really just spells out what is already implicit in the general statement in one of the premises. For example, in the argument above, the ethical premise, 'It is our obligation to protect residents from harm,' is a general statement. The conclusion, that residents on walking frames must be accompanied when walking in the corridors, simply spells out one of the things that this general statement implies. This simple form of deductive argument is sometimes called a **syllogism** (again, see Chapter 6), so what we have in this sample argument is an ethical syllogism. This is the standard structure of ethical reasoning.

One extremely important point to note here is this: an argument which has an ethical conclusion *must* have an ethical premise. That is, an ethical conclusion cannot spring from nowhere. An ethical conclusion cannot be drawn from informative premises alone—it must be drawn from either an ethical premise alone, or from a combination of informative and ethical premises. This is a fundamental feature of the logic of ethical reasoning; facts and values are distinct entities, and a fact cannot by itself imply a value. This is often called the 'fact-value distinction', or, referring in particular to exhortations, the 'is-ought' distinction. It is vitally important to be aware of it when first analysing and then evaluating ethical arguments.

Exercise 12.2

Write out a logical outline for each of the following ethical arguments. Label the premises and conclusion 'fact' or 'ethical value/ ethical exhortation'. Remember that you are not being asked to evaluate these arguments, so labelling a premise as 'fact' does not imply that you accept the premise as true, or that you agree with the conclusion of the argument. If you prefer, you can label informative premises which you think are false or dubious as 'assertions'.

1. It is wrong to kill innocent human beings. Abortion involves killing an innocent human being. Therefore abortion is wrong.

2. Not telling Mrs Kee that she has cancer is just the same as lying to her. But lying is wrong, so we must tell her.
3. These patients should not be used as subjects in a trial of a new drug. This is because people should be asked to give their informed consent before becoming part of a clinical trial, and given that these patients will be unconscious, they will be unable to give their consent.
4. Sometimes it takes courage to be a good nurse. When you were confronted by that aggressive patient, you should have stood your ground.

Assumptions in Ethical Argument

Unfortunately, the standard structure is often not easy to see in 'real life' ethical arguments, both verbal and written. The problem is that often either the informative or the ethical premises are not stated, usually because the author thinks they are so obvious that they do not need to be spelt out. This does not mean that these premises are not part of the argument. On the contrary, the argument cannot work without them, because the structure would not be complete. They are **hidden** premises; or, to use the terminology introduced in Chapter 3, **assumptions**. Remember that assumptions are not necessarily incorrect or unreasonable—just unstated. Assumptions, as hidden premises, can be informative or ethical.

In ethical argument it is very important to identify assumptions, because they frequently play a crucial role. Often, if people disagree with each other over an ethical issue, it is because they are not aware of the assumptions which the other person is making, or they disagree with these assumptions. But if the assumptions remain unstated, the argument on both sides will remain unclear, and the source of disagreement will remain hidden.

Example 12.2

Here is an ethical argument:

> Mrs Garcia has a tendency to leave the gas stove on in her kitchen, and she has had several falls in her backyard. She ought to be moved out of her home and placed in some sort of assisted accommodation.

A logical outline of this argument as it stands would be:

1. Mrs Garcia tends to leave the gas stove on. (fact)
2. She has had several falls in her backyard. (fact)
3. She ought to be placed in assisted accommodation. (1,2, ethical exhortation)

Here we have an ethical conclusion drawn from two informative premises. Since it is not logically possible to draw an ethical conclusion from informative premises alone, this alerts us to a hidden premise which is needed to make the argument work. And since an ethical premise is needed for an ethical conclusion, we know that the hidden premise will be an ethical premise.

The role of the hidden ethical premise here is to provide a connection between the fact of Mrs Garcia's behaviour and the ethical value-judgement that she should be placed in assisted accommodation. Usually an ethical premise is quite general, rather than specific, because of the nature of ethical values. (Check back to the first section of this chapter if this does not make sense.) So we can expect it to be about people in general, rather than Mrs Garcia in particular. A common first suggestion might be this: 'Mrs Garcia is not safe in her own home.' However, this is not the hidden premise that we need. For a start, it is too specific but, more importantly, it is another informative premise. (In fact, this is really a summary of the first two fact premises.) We need an ethical premise. But at least this will help us on the way to the ethical premise, by giving us a general idea—that of people at risk—to work on. Putting the idea of risk into a general ethical premise, we would get something like this: 'People who are at risk in one place should be moved to a safe place.' Again, the exact form of words is not vitally important: if you thought something like, 'People should be protected from risk', this would also be appropriate.

So the logical outline of the expanded argument would be:

1. Mrs Garcia tends to leave the gas stove on. (fact)
2. Mrs Garcia has had falls in her backyard. (fact)
(3. People should be moved from risky places.) (ethical exhortation)
4. Mrs Garcia should be placed in assisted accommodation. (1,2,3 ethical exhortation)

Now the argument is in a logically acceptable form. It has an ethical premise to support its ethical conclusion.

However, it is not only hidden ethical premises which are important in ethical argument. Hidden informative premises are also frequent, and also need to be identified. In the above argument, there are also a number of assumptions (hidden premises) about factual matters. These, too, form part of the structure of the argument, because they provide (unspoken) reasons in favour of the conclusion. In some circumstances, hidden informative assumptions can turn out to be crucial (in the sense defined in Chapter 4—that is, if they were removed from the argument, the conclusion would be left without strong support). For example, one factual assumption is that leaving the gas stove on is potentially harmful to Mrs Garcia. Another is that Mrs Garcia would be safe from harm in assisted accommodation. If either of these hidden premises turned out to be false, the argument would be seriously weakened. There would be no reason to conclude that Mrs Garcia should be moved if she was not actually in danger in her own home, or if she would still be at risk in the place she was moved to.

Making hidden premises explicit in this way is vital for evaluating the argument, as will be shown in the next section. Evaluation of an argument, ethical or non-ethical, cannot begin until the structure has been correctly analysed. This is why identifying premises and conclusions, and especially hidden premises, is such an important step in understanding ethical argument.

Exercise 12.3

Keeping in mind the rule that if there is an ethical conclusion, there must be at least one ethical premise, find at least one assumption or hidden premise in each of these arguments. Write out the logical outline of each one, indicating the hidden premise by writing it in parentheses (brackets). Label the premises (including the assumption) and the conclusion 'fact/assertion' or 'ethical value/ethical exhortation'.

1. The results of Mrs Raka's pre-natal testing show that her foetus has haemophilia. She ought to have the pregnancy terminated.
2. It is wrong to kill people. Therefore abortion is wrong.
3. Mr Wilson, the resident with advanced Alzheimer's disease, keeps pulling the feeding tube out of his nose. Since we have no right to continue treatment which patients have refused, we should not put the feeding tube back in.
4. Karl is a good nurse because he is generous with his time.
5. This woman already has two children from a previous marriage, so she should not be allowed on the IVF programme.
6. It is wrong to frighten people before they have an operation, so they should not be given any information about the surgery until after it has been done.

Evaluating Ethical Argument

The basic method for evaluating ethical argument is no different from that used for ordinary, non-ethical argument. There are two main questions to be asked:

1. Are the premises true?
2. Does the conclusion follow logically from the premises?

Thus, evaluating an argument means critically examining two facets: the content of the premises, and the reasoning process which is used to make the leap from the premises to the conclusion. If one (or more) crucial premise is false, or if the reasoning is faulty, then the conclusion is not warranted (which means 'not sufficiently supported by the premises'). Note here that we cannot say for sure that the conclusion is false—we don't actually know this. All we know is that this particular argument is not good enough to show that it is true. But perhaps some other argument, using different premises or a different method of reasoning, could show that it is true. To the critical thinker, this is an extremely important distinction. When evaluating an argument, use the correct terminology: the conclusion is unwarranted, or the argument is invalid. Avoid saying that the conclusion is false, because this is not, strictly speaking, correct.

Evaluating the Premises

The process of evaluating the content of the premises of an ordinary argument was described in Chapter 4—you may wish to look back there to refresh your memory. The process is just the same when you are dealing with an ethical argument. Remember that both the informative and the ethical premises must be examined, since either type could be the crucial premise in a particular argument. Indeed, conclusions in ethical arguments rely just as much on informative premises as on ethical premises. So, to make a thorough evaluation of an ethical argument, you first need to write a logical outline of the argument, showing the hidden premises (assumptions) as well as the stated premises, and carefully labelling them 'fact/assertion' or 'ethical value/exhortation'. Then you can proceed to look critically at the content of the premises.

This critical evaluation is fairly easily done for informative premises. We need to ask whether the factual claims are true or false, and usually there will be quite straightforward evidence about this. If the factual claims are general ones (for example, about the cause of a disease, or the cost of a hospital bed for a day), there may well be written sources where their truth can be checked—textbooks, encyclopaedias, journal articles, government reports and so on. If they are specific, perhaps about a particular patient, there will be other ways of checking—medical records, personal observation, confirming with the patient or relatives and so on.

Of course, as you will be aware from your reading so far in this book, often we cannot be absolutely certain that some factual claim, especially a claim about scientific knowledge, is true. There might be a good deal of evidence in favour of the claim, but not absolute proof. For example, suppose an ethical argument contained this premise: 'Exposure to high voltage power lines causes leukaemia in children.' If you check to see whether this factual claim is true or false, you will not find a conclusive answer one way or the other. Instead, there will be some studies showing an increased level of leukaemia in children who live close to power lines, and other studies showing no increase at all. That is, the evidence is conflicting. In this situation, we cannot say for sure that the factual claim is true, nor can we say it is false. But this does not leave us unable to say anything. What we can do is talk about degrees of probability, or likelihood. In between the extremes of definitely true and definitely false, a factual claim might be 'very probably true', 'possibly true', 'well-supported by evidence', 'unlikely to be true' and so on.

When the informative premises of an argument have been evaluated in this way, each such premise can be given a rating somewhere on the spectrum of true to false. This is only part of the first step of evaluating the argument (we still have to look at the value premises to complete the first step, and then the next step is to look at the reasoning), but already it may be possible to make some evaluation of the argument as a whole. Let us look at an example, already written in logical outline form, to see how this is so.

Example 12.3

1. Aspirin provides the best relief from back pain in any situation. (assertion)
2. We should relieve suffering wherever possible. (ethical exhortation)
3. Therefore we should give aspirin to all patients who suffer from back pain. (1,2, ethical exhortation)

In this example, the first premise is informative. If the factual claim turns out to be definitely false, we can say even at this early stage that the conclusion is totally unwarranted.

One complication in checking the truth of informative premises is that some 'factual' claims are actually definitions—that is, the truth of the premises really depends on the meanings of the words involved. So there is actually another way to label premises in addition to those identified in Chapter 3, that is, as definitions. The abortion debate provides a classic example of this sort of premise. Those opposed to abortion may put forward the following argument:

1. It is wrong to kill human beings. (ethical exhortation)
2. A foetus is a human being. ('fact'—definition)
3. Therefore it is wrong to kill a foetus. (1,2, ethical exhortation)

The second premise appears to be an informative premise: it seems to be a claim about facts which can be checked. However, whether or not this premise is true actually depends on the definition of the term 'human being'. If 'human being' means 'a being which has the genetic make-up characteristic of the human species', then the premise is true. But if 'human being' means 'a person, a being able to think and feel and experience the world', then (as far as we can tell at the moment) a foetus is not a human being in this sense, and so the premise is false.

This makes definitional premises hard to evaluate. Before you can say whether the premise is true or false, you must first clarify what meaning is being given to the key terms. Consulting a dictionary to establish the 'correct' meaning of a word may occasionally be helpful, but most often it will not be. This is because a dictionary simply describes or explains the range of meanings that are currently in use for a particular word. It does not specify one meaning as the correct one—on the contrary, it aims to be as vague and general as possible. In the argument we have just looked at, for example, two quite specific and different technical meanings are being attached to the term 'human being'. But a dictionary, if it gets this specific, will probably give *both* these definitions, since both are common meanings for the term. So a better strategy is to try to establish a definition which is accepted by the different parties to a debate, or is standard in relation to a particular issue. If this cannot be done, then the truth of a premise can only be assessed in a **relative** sense. That is, a premise may be true relative to one definition of a key term, but false relative to another definition.

When an argument contains this sort of contentious (disputed) definitional premise, one cannot come to a final judgement about the conclusion. But it can correctly be said that whether or not the conclusion is warranted depends on the definition of a key word or term. This is an important observation to make, because it indicates that the conclusion is to this degree precarious. The argument will not be as persuasive as one where the conclusion is based on informative premises which are straightforwardly true and do not depend on definitions.

What we have seen, then, is that in most cases informative premises can easily be evaluated by checking on the claims involved. In some areas, there may be uncertainty (such as in definitional premises) or matters of degree (such as the claim about high voltage power lines and leukaemia, discussed above), but at least in factual matters we know what counts as evidence for or against a factual claim, and how to assess it.

However, this is not so for ethical premises—they are not true or false in the same the way that informative premises are. It is not easy to see how to evaluate an ethical value claim, such as 'artificial contraception is wrong'. You might begin by saying 'I agree' or 'I disagree', but this is not the sort of evaluation that is required in critical thinking. An **objective** evaluation is needed—one that appeals to standards or criteria which everyone will accept. Personal agreement or disagreement with a value claim is only a **subjective** evaluation, based on one's own personal criteria. How can an objective assessment of ethical value claims be achieved?

At this point, we need to turn from the discipline (subject area) of critical thinking to that of moral philosophy. Moral philosophy is the branch of philosophy that studies the nature of ethics and morality. One of the main questions which moral philosophers try to answer is the one we have just asked above—how can we objectively evaluate value claims, or claims about what is right and what is wrong? A small number of philosophers have taken the view that it is impossible to objectively evaluate value claims—they are just personal, subjective opinions and that is that. However, this is not the standard position in moral philosophy. The great majority of philosophers today hold that ethical values are not immune from rational evaluation or criticism—they can be assessed as reasonable or unreasonable according to objective standards, independent of the tastes and preferences of particular individuals.

The standards that moral philosophers refer to include human rights, human flourishing and fundamental ethical values. These will be explained in some detail in following chapters; the point to take note of here is that these standards provide a way of evaluating an ethical premise that is used in an argument. So, just as informative premises can be assessed as lying somewhere on the spectrum of true to false, so ethical premises can be assessed along the spectrum of reasonable to unreasonable. And just as a false factual premise can make the conclusion of an ethical argument unwarranted, so an unreasonable ethical claim can make the conclusion unwarranted. To see how this can be so, let us consider an argument where the ethical premise can be seen to be unreasonable, even without referring to technical discussions of moral philosophy.

Example 12.4

1. It is immoral for women to do paid work outside the home. (ethical exhortation)
2. Nursing involves paid work outside the home. (fact)
3. Therefore, women should not become nurses. (1,2, ethical exhortation)

In this argument, the ethical premise is clearly unreasonable. For this reason, the conclusion of the argument is unwarranted, even though the factual premise (that nursing is a paid job) is definitely true.

So keep in mind that the first step in evaluating an argument, that is, evaluating the content of the premises, needs to be performed thoroughly. This means evaluating both the informative and the ethical premises. Usually, evaluating ethical premises is more complex than in the example we have just considered, and you will need the information contained in the following chapters to do it properly.

Evaluating the Reasoning

Questioning the premises is only one part of the process of evaluating an argument. The second part is to critically evaluate the actual reasoning, or line of thinking, which leads from the premises to the conclusion. This means asking the question, 'Does the conclusion follow logically from the premises?' Before we consider possible ways in which the reasoning process can go astray, note the importance of the reasoning itself in the overall structure of an argument. It is not enough to have true premises—the reasoning must also be sound. Even if all premises in an argument are true, a faulty line of reasoning will still produce an unwarranted or invalid conclusion.

It is not always easy to see whether a line of reasoning makes sense or not, so we suggest two strategies which can be of help. The first is an informal technique, drawing on your own past experience and knowledge. The basic idea is to try to cast doubt on the conclusion, or to ask yourself if the conclusion is plausible. Can you think of any situation in which the conclusion would be false, even if the premises were true? Can you think of some reason or evidence, different from what is referred to in the premises, which goes against the conclusion? (Asking yourself *why* the conclusion might be wrong could help.) If you can, then you may have exposed a flaw in the reasoning. The second strategy is a more formal one. The basic idea is to be familiar with the standard types of errors in inductive and deductive reasoning, which were explained in Chapters 6 and 7. Then look for these patterns of mistakes in the particular argument which you are evaluating. Whilst it is helpful to know, recognise and name specific types of errors in reasoning, the basic skill lies in recognising that something has gone wrong. This skill can be cultivated by always asking why the conclusion should be believed, and whether there is a reason to think it is false.

It was noted earlier in this chapter that most ethical reasoning is deductive. That is, it proceeds from a general claim to a particular conclusion, where the conclusion is somehow already contained in the general claim. Although, in principle, there is less room for error in deductive reasoning than there is in inductive reasoning, mistakes can still be made. (Some of the common mistakes were explained in Chapter 6—you may wish to go back and refresh your memory of them.) The following example shows an ethical argument in which a mistake in reasoning (rather than a mistake in the premises) leads to an invalid conclusion.

Example 12.5

1. It is wrong to mutilate living human beings. (ethical exhortation)
2. A cadaver is not a living human being. (definition)
3. Therefore, it is not wrong to mutilate a cadaver. (1,2, ethical exhortation)

Let us evaluate this argument fully. The first step is to ask, 'Are the premises true?' Take the informative premise first, since this is the easier one to evaluate. Is premise 2 true? Usually, we would look for evidence that the factual claims are true, but what we have here is actually a definitional premise, rather than a claim about facts. Here, the definition of 'cadaver' is not in dispute—checking in a dictionary will show that a cadaver is a dead body, so clearly a cadaver is not a living human being. So this premise is true. Now consider the other premise, that it is wrong to mutilate living human beings. This is an ethical premise. On the face of it, this looks like a reasonable value claim and there does not seem to be any obvious reason to disagree with it. For the sake of keeping things brief, we will accept it without further investigation here. However, a thorough evaluation of the argument would require that this value claim be checked against the standards, such as human rights or fundamental principles, which are described in the following chapters.

Having established that the premises are true (or reasonable), the next step is to look at the reasoning. Does the conclusion that it is not wrong to mutilate cadavers really follow from the premises? Using the strategy of trying to cast doubt on the conclusion, we can see some reasons for thinking that the conclusion might be false. For example, the wrongness of mutilating bodies might be quite independent of whether or not the body is alive. Perhaps mutilating bodies is wrong because it shows a lack of respect for the dead person, or because it will upset relatives and friends. These ideas indicate some problem with the logic, or line of reasoning. The conclusion does not seem plausible, given the premises as they stand. We are basically saying that the truth of the premises is not sufficient to make us accept the truth of the conclusion.

In fact, if you are familiar with the formal fallacies of deductive reasoning, you will easily be able to see what is wrong with this argument. Let x = being a living human being, and y = being wrong to mutilate. In this way, the argument in example 12.5 could be formulated as:

1. $x \Rightarrow y$
2. $-x$
3. $\Rightarrow -y$

This is clearly the formal fallacy of denying the antecedent.

If you are still unsure about this, consider another example of exactly the same problem, this time involving very ordinary matters. Suppose that somebody put forward this argument: 'If it has been raining, then the footpath will be wet. But it hasn't been raining. So the footpath won't be wet.' It is pretty clear that this conclusion is shaky. Even if it has not been raining, the footpath could still be wet, for any number of reasons—somebody has just washed their car in the driveway or watered their lawn too heavily and so on. Technically, the author has denied the antecedent (that is, said that the first part is false) and then mistakenly believed that this proves that the consequent (the second part) is also false.

So now we have completed the two steps in evaluating an argument. We have looked at truth of the premises and the soundness of the reasoning. We have found that the premises are true (reasonable), but that the reasoning is unsound. On this basis, we can say that the conclusion is invalid. It is not enough to have true premises—the reasoning must also be sound.

Exercise 12.4

Look back at the logical outlines which you wrote in Exercise 12.3 and evaluate each of the arguments. Note whether:

a. each of the premises is true (reasonable)
b. the reasoning is sound
c. to what degree the conclusion is warranted.

Just before we conclude this section on evaluating reasoning, it is important to note another source of mistakes in reasoning, especially deductive reasoning in ethical arguments. Mistakes can come about through a misunderstanding of concepts used in value premises. Some ethical concepts have their own logical properties, which means that they can only be used in certain ways in argument. If you do not understand these logical properties, then you will make errors of reasoning when you use them. The following chapters explain these concepts and their logical implications.

Ethical Reasoning and Sensitive Ethical Decision Making

Analysing and evaluating ethical arguments are important skills. Having these skills will enable you to understand arguments put forward to persuade you to act in certain ways, or hold certain opinions. They will help you to decide whether or not there is good reason to be persuaded by these arguments, and this in turn will significantly influence the way you practise as a nurse. The same skills will also help you to formulate and put forward sound and reasonable arguments of your own. The next two chapters explain in detail the process of understanding and evaluating arguments which use the common ethical concepts of principles and rules, and rights and duties.

However, in the course of reading those chapters, you will become aware of a complicating factor which limits the power and scope of individual ethical arguments. This is the problem of conflicting values. The issue of euthanasia provides a graphic and well-known example of this problem. Using one line of reasoning, we might argue, 'Killing is wrong, and since euthanasia is killing, it is therefore wrong also.' However, a different line of reasoning is possible, 'Allowing people to suffer against their wishes is wrong, so if a person is suffering and requests euthanasia, it is wrong to refuse the request.' The ethical premises in the two arguments are in conflict with each other, at least in the context of euthanasia. So we have two competing arguments, one which shows that euthanasia is wrong, another which shows that it is not.

We could look at this situation in a rather rigid way and say, 'These two arguments have different conclusions. One must be wrong—so which is it?' This approach would work if there were only one true ethical value or principle which applied to all situations. We could then see which argument had an incorrect value premise and say that its conclusion was unwarranted. However, despite attempts by some very well-regarded philosophers to work out what this single value might be (or to work out a set of ethical values which can never come into conflict with each other), there has been no agreement on this matter. Many philosophers now accept that there are actually a number of different ethical values, which can and sometimes do conflict with each other. A way needs to be found to resolve these conflicts, but they cannot be made to disappear.

Thus, sensitive ethical decision making in a practical context needs to go beyond individual pieces of ethical argument and look at the whole picture. Focusing on one specific argument in isolation can lead to a misunderstanding of the wider issue. Many disputes are generated, and many poor ethical decisions are made, when people do not manage this. Sensitive ethical decision making involves taking into account the arguments both for and against a particular position, and trying to come to a balanced overall position. The skill of ethical decision making will be discussed in Chapter 16.

Conclusion

An ethical argument can thus have a number of different problems. Firstly, it may not be logically complete in the form in which it is first stated—that is, it may be missing crucial premises which you will need to supply as assumptions in the logical outline. In particular, if an argument with an ethical conclusion does not have an ethical premise, then one must be supplied. Ethical conclusions cannot be drawn from informative premises alone.

Once in logical outline form, ethical argument is evaluated in the same way as any other sort of argument, by looking at:

1. the truth of the premises (or reasonableness of the ethical premises)
2. the soundness of the reasoning.

The most straightforward flaw in an ethical argument is an incorrect factual premise. If this premise is crucial, then the argument collapses. Next, the argument could have a dubious or contentious ethical premise. This does not cause the argument to completely collapse (since we cannot say that the premise is 'false' as such), but the conclusion is seriously called into question. But even if the premises are quite acceptable, this does not guarantee a warranted conclusion, because the reasoning from premises to conclusion must also be examined. Faulty reasoning will produce an unwarranted conclusion, even if the premises are true.

Finally, individual ethical arguments usually do not completely cover all considerations relevant to difficult ethical issues. This is due to the problem of conflicting values. So when trying to make an ethical decision, it is important to consider arguments both for and against particular outcomes, in order to come to a balanced conclusion.

NOTE

1. Johnstone, Megan-Jane, *Bioethics: A Nursing Perspective*, 2nd edition, Sydney, Harcourt Brace Jovanovich, 1994, Chapter 1.

Chapter 13
Rules and Principles

This chapter introduces rules and principles, and explains how they work in ethical argument. Four types of rules and principles are identified: absolute, prima facie, universal and relative. The emphasis is on developing a critical evaluation of ethical argument, by being aware of the way in which these different types of rules and principles affect the nature of the conclusions which can be drawn from a set of premises. There is also a brief discussion of how to assess whether the ethical value-claims contained in specific rules and principles are reasonable.

As we saw in the previous chapter, ethical values can be expressed in a variety of ways. Take, for example, the negative ethical value attached to killing. It might be said that 'killing is wrong', or alternatively that 'every human being has a right to life', or again 'thou shalt not kill'. The precise method of expression can depend on the author's belief about the nature of ethics and what makes actions right or wrong, or it can simply reflect a common or convenient terminology. Either way, the terms used are technical ones. That is, they have specific meanings, which are based on fundamental views about the nature of right and wrong. These views determine the **logical properties** of the terms and how they can be used in ethical reasoning. This is important because it means that ethical terms like, say, anatomical or pharmacological terms, cannot be used in whatever way happens to suit people. So the next step in developing a critical understanding of ethical reasoning is to become familiar with the precise meaning and logical properties of standard ethical terminology. In this chapter, we will discuss **principles** and **rules**, concepts which are widely used in ethical reasoning. The following chapter will discuss two other influential and widely used concepts, **rights**, and the closely connected idea, **duties**.

Of all the terminology used to express ethical values, that of 'principles' and 'rules' is potentially the most confusing. The problem is that these terms are somewhat slippery—they do not have strictly fixed meanings, even in their technical senses, and are used by different people in different ways. This does not make the use of principles and rules impossible. Indeed, this is still one of the most common and popular ways of framing an ethical argument. However, it does mean that extra caution is needed in evaluating arguments which use these terms, or the ideas behind them.

In this chapter we will set out a fairly standard and sensible way of understanding the meanings of the terms 'principle' and 'rule', as well as indicating other ways in which the terms are commonly used. This should enable you to develop a sensible usage for yourself, and also to follow the intended meaning of others.

The structure of this chapter will reflect the two questions which need to be asked in order to evaluate any argument. That is, 'Are the premises true?' and 'Does the conclusion follow logically from the premises?' In the context of rules and principles, the question of whether the conclusion follows logically from the premises is both important for ethical reasoning, and simple to answer. So this will be the topic of our first section. It will explain the logical form of principles and rules, and the sorts of conclusions that may validly be drawn from premises using or drawing on these concepts. It will set out the different types of principles and rules, and explain the significance of the differences. The second section will sketch some ways of tackling the question of the truth of premises containing principles or rules. As we saw in Chapter 12, this is not a straightforward task where ethical premises are concerned, because they cannot be checked against an agreed body of facts in the way that informative premises can. So this section will provide some suggestions as to how to decide whether a particular premise containing a reference to a rule or principle is reasonable. This will require a brief dip into moral philosophy to learn something about the basis or foundation of rules and principles (and thus factors which might make a particular premise reasonable or unreasonable).

Does the Conclusion Follow Logically from the Premises?

For ethical arguments which have premises containing rules or principles, the first step in evaluating the argument is to know the meaning of these terms, or more particularly, how they work in a logical sense. The reason for this is that the rule or principle forms the logical link between the premises and the conclusion, so everything depends on what these concepts actually mean. The examples given below will show how this is so. But first we need to be more specific about what rules and principles actually are.

What are Rules and Principles?

On one standard view, the terms 'rule' and 'principle' are interchangeable—they both have the same meaning. The easiest way to explain the meaning of 'principle' or 'rule' is to give an example, as giving a definition requires more words than is helpful. One example of a principle/rule, taken from the list of possibilities mentioned right at the start of this chapter, is 'Killing is wrong'. It is essentially a statement of an ethical value (or here, a negative value, or dis-value) in a simple, straightforward way.

It is general and usually impersonal (in contrast to claims about rights and duties, which are attached to particular people).

Note that the principle/rule could be expressed in a number of different ways. It could be in the form of an exhortation, such as 'One ought not to kill' or 'Do not steal'; it could be a value statement referring to virtues or character traits, such as 'A good person does not kill' or 'Patience is vital'. All these versions count as a principle or rule. Note also that statements which are (or contain) principles or rules do not have to include the word 'principle' or 'rule' as such—in fact they usually do not. Again, this is different from rights and duties, which are expressed in quite particular words ('right', 'duty/obligation'). The way to tell if something is a principle/rule is to look at the idea it expresses, not just the form of words used. If it is a general, fairly simple and impersonal statement of an ethical value, it is a principle/rule.

Exercise 13.1

Which of the following sentences are (or contain) ethical principles or rules?

1. Dermatology is the study of skin diseases.
2. It is wrong to treat patients without their consent.
3. James did the right thing by refusing to search the patient's locker.
4. Australian nurses believe that health professionals should uphold and work for the just distribution of health care to all persons.
5. Safety must always be the primary principle.
6. Bacteria cause infection in open wounds.

So far we have considered principles and rules together, and given a very general account of what they are. But often there is a subtle difference in their meanings, and so it is helpful to be aware of this. The distinction is as follows. A principle is a fundamental idea, a name or a description of some feature of human life or interaction which is held to be profoundly ethically valuable. For example, a draft version of the current Code of Ethics for Nurses in Australia refers to the 'ethical principles of beneficence, non-maleficence, autonomy, justice and veracity', principles which are widely accepted in the field of bioethics. These principles name the values of promoting benefit, not harming, self-determination, fairness and truthfulness. As you can see, they are very general in nature and do not immediately spell out what types of actions are right or wrong. A rule, on the other hand, is more specific, and is derived from (or based on) one of these general principles. Some examples of rules might include 'Do not treat patients without their informed consent' (derived from the principle of autonomy), 'Give men and women equal access to education' (derived from the principle of justice) and 'Telling lies is wrong' (derived from the principle of veracity). It may seem that there is very little difference between the principle of veracity (truthfulness) and the rule about not telling lies. However, if you think carefully you will see that the principle is broader and more general than the rule. Not telling lies is one way of being truthful, but it is not all that truthfulness amounts to. It also involves, for example, telling the *whole* truth without being asked, and not giving evasive or misleading answers. In this sense, rules seem to depend on the precise wording much more than principles (it is easier to see a way of avoiding the rule about telling lies than of avoiding the principle of veracity). For this reason, thinking in terms of rules is sometimes regarded as excessively legalistic: that is, too dependent on the letter of the rule rather than its spirit.

A second distinction that is sometimes made between rules and principles concerns whether or not they are always binding. 'Rule' is sometimes used to refer to something which must always be followed, without exception, whereas a 'principle' is something which usually applies, but may not be binding in all cases. On this view of rules and principles, the rule 'Killing is wrong' would be exceptionless and would have to be followed on every occasion; but the principle of respect for life, while stating an important ethical value, could be set aside or overridden in unusual circumstances. When rules are thought of in this way, the criticism is sometimes made that thinking in terms of ethical rules is too narrow and rigid, and cannot hope to meet the complexities of real life.

As noted above, these distinctions are not universally made—different people use 'rule' and 'principle' in different ways. There is not one set usage which is correct, and all others wrong. In this book we will not make a strict distinction between rules and principles, although we will have a tendency to use 'rule' when referring to specific value statements or exhortations, and 'principle' when referring to more general ones. But for all other contexts, an important step in analysing an argument is to clarify precisely what an author means when stating a rule or principle. A later part of this chapter will help you to do this by introducing some technical terminology which is used to designate different types of rules and principles. For the moment, the main points to keep in mind are firstly, the basic idea of rules and principles, and secondly, the fact that the precise meaning of the two terms varies.

Principles and Rules in Ethical Argument

Now that we have clarified the idea of rules and principles, we are in a position to look at how they function in ethical arguments. Our aim is to determine whether or not the conclusion follows logically from the premises, when one of the premises contains or states a rule or principle.

There is a fairly standard way in which principles and rules are used in ethical argument. The argument runs from the general to the particular, and is a form of deductive (rather than inductive) reasoning. (You may wish to go back to Chapter 6 to refresh your memory of deductive reasoning.) Because the reasoning is deductive, everything depends on the precise meaning and application of the words and concepts in the premises. The following example shows how this is so.

Example 13.1

Take the following ethical argument:

Killing is wrong. Therefore nurses should never administer drugs for the purpose of capital punishment.

In logical outline, the argument looks like this:

1. Killing is wrong. (ethical exhortation)
(2. Capital punishment is a form of killing.) (definition)
3. Therefore, nurses should never administer drugs for the purpose of capital punishment. (1,2, ethical exhortation)

Note that the second premise is an assumption. It is not stated in the original form of the argument, but is needed in the logical outline to fill out the logic of the reasoning. Let us grant for the moment that both premises are true, and examine the reasoning which leads from the premises to the conclusion. The reasoning starts with a general principle (killing is wrong) and from it concludes that a particular action (nurses killing for the purpose of capital punishment) is always wrong. Is this conclusion valid? It may seem obvious that it is—if killing in general is wrong, then any particular type of killing must also be wrong. But in fact the answer depends on the precise meaning of the principle stated in the first premise. If one assumes a particular meaning for the principle, namely that it applies to all people, and all instances of killing, and can never be overridden, then the conclusion is obviously valid. But this is not the only possible meaning for the principle: it may be the sort of principle that only applies in most instances, or to most people. Thus, before we can come to a definitive answer about the validity of this conclusion, we need to know more about the different types of principles and rules, and what sort of principle this one is meant to be.

Absolute Versus Prima Facie Rules and Principles

We mentioned above that some people distinguish between rules and principles on the basis that rules must always be obeyed no matter what, whereas principles may sometimes be overridden or set aside. In fact, this is a fundamental distinction which can apply to both rules and principles: it is the distinction between **absolute** and **prima facie**. Absolute rules or principles, as the name suggests, absolutely always apply, and must always be obeyed. There are no exceptions. Prima facie rules or principles, on the other hand, may sometimes be broken if the circumstances require it. The phrase 'prima facie' is Latin, and means 'at first glance', or 'on the face of it'. It is used in ethics to describe a rule/principle which must be followed, *all things being equal*: that is, unless there is a compelling ethical reason to do otherwise. Take the example of a prima facie rule against lying. In the normal course of events, this rule should be followed; this is what it means to say that it is a rule. But in exceptional circumstances we may need to take a second look, and ask whether there are other ethical considerations which might outweigh the wrongness of lying. If, for example, a lie must be told in order to prevent an innocent person from being murdered, it may be ethically acceptable to tell a lie. This is what it means for the rule against lying to be prima facie.

The term prima facie is undoubtedly an unfamiliar one: you would probably prefer a simple English word for this idea, rather than a Latin phrase. However, 'prima facie' is the standard term in ethics, partly because there is no appropriate English equivalent. Thus it is important to be familiar with it and that is why it is used in this chapter. You may feel more comfortable to translate it to yourself as you read it. You could try substituting 'non-absolute', 'overrideable' or 'all-things-being-equal' to remind yourself of its meaning.

The distinction between absolute and prima facie rules/principles is vital in ethical reasoning, because, as we suggested above, it affects the conclusion that can validly be drawn from a given set of premises. Consider again the argument in Example 13.1, which concluded that nurses should never administer drugs for the purpose of capital punishment. If the principle that killing is wrong is an absolute principle, then the conclusion is fully warranted: all forms of killing, including capital punishment, are always wrong and must never be done. But if the principle is a prima facie one, then the conclusion is not warranted: from a prima facie principle against killing, all we can conclude is that killing is wrong, all things being equal (that is, unless there are other ethical values which might take precedence in this situation). It may be the case that for capital punishment all other things are not equal, that there are other values which override the wrongness of killing. So, as the argument stands, the conclusion cannot be so strongly asserted. We would need a lot more information about the other values which might override the dis-value of killing before we could make a definitive judgement about capital punishment.

So, is the principle against killing in this argument an absolute principle or a prima facie one? This is obviously the vital question. Now we need to be careful, because there are actually two questions here:

1. What sort of principle did the author intend it to be?
2. What sort of principle is it really?

Answering the first question is necessary in order to understand what the author was trying to say. It is part of the preliminary step of clarification, along with, for example, spelling out the important assumptions in the argument. The best way to answer it is to read (or think) carefully over what the author has written (or spoken), to see which interpretation would make most sense. Of course, this is not always conclusive as the author may be vague or undecided on this matter. In this case, the best you can do is come to a qualified assessment of the argument, such as, 'Assuming that the principle is intended to be absolute, the conclusion of the argument is warranted.' The following exercise will give you some practice in working out which sort of principle/rule the author had in mind.

Exercise 13.2

Each of the following pieces of text contains or refers to a principle or rule. Is the principle or rule meant in an absolute or prima facie sense? (Or is it not possible to tell?)

1. The federal government has formulated 11 information privacy principles to protect people against disclosure of information held by commonwealth agencies such as the Bureau of Statistics and the Child Support Agency. Nurses wishing to use data from a Commonwealth agency as part of a research project must obtain approval from an Institutional Ethics Committee if the research design involves the breach of any of these principles. IECs are empowered under the *Privacy Act* to approve such projects providing that certain guidelines are met.
2. I have made it a rule never to conceal the truth from anyone, so if a patient or relative asked me about their diagnosis or their chances of survival, I would always tell them—even if the truth were painful or distressing.
3. Clients who do not speak English must be given the services of an interpreter, and no physical examination may proceed until an interpreter has been consulted. No departures from this rule will be tolerated.
4. According to the BMA Code of Ethics, a doctor must preserve absolute secrecy on everything he knows about his patients, even after they have died.
5. Whilst it is normally wrong to deliberately inflict pain on a human being, we must recognise some exceptions. Otherwise, we could never even give a vaccination, or dress a wound.
6. A nurse is required to have a commitment to the welfare of clients.

Whilst some judgement is required to work out what sort of rule/principle is meant by an author, this is usually not too hard. However, answering the second question above—'What sort of principle is it really?'—is very much more difficult. Take the principle about killing in the argument above. Is it really the case that killing is absolutely wrong, or is it just usually wrong? This is clearly not a matter which pure logic can decide. In fact, it is an issue over which philosophers and theologians (and lots of other people as well!) have argued for thousands of years. We cannot hope to give a simple solution to it here. The best we can do is look at some of the reasons why moral philosophers and others have believed in or rejected absolute rules and principles, and some of the implications of taking the absolutist position. This will give you some idea of whether to regard a particular principle or rule as absolute or not. But it will be easier to postpone this discussion for later in the chapter, and move on to another category of rules and principles which again affects the conclusion which can validly be drawn in an ethical argument.

Universal Versus Relative Rules and Principles

It is fairly natural to assume that ethical rules and principles apply regardless of time and place. It would seem that if killing is wrong, it is wrong no matter who you are, or where or when you live. Rules or principles which apply regardless of time, place and identity are termed **universal**. There is a tendency to think of all rules and principles as universal. However, it is also possible for them to be non-universal, or **relative**. For example, you may have heard it said that slavery is wrong now, but was not wrong in the time of the ancient Greeks and Romans; or that female circumcision is wrong in Australia, but not in some Muslim countries. Both of these views rely on the idea that ethical rules and principles are related to the time and place, rather than being universal.

Again, it is clear that this distinction has a significant effect on ethical reasoning. Look back again to our example about capital punishment. If the principle that killing is wrong is a relative principle, rather than a universal one, then the conclusion that nurses must never commit acts of capital punishment is not warranted. The most we could conclude is that nurses must never perform capital punishment in societies where the no-killing principle applies. We cannot legitimately draw a conclusion about *all* nurses in *all* societies. On the other hand, if the principle is universal, then the conclusion does indeed apply to all times and places.

As with the absolute vs prima facie distinction, it is important to know which type of principle is intended by the author of the argument. Careful reading of the argument is, as before, the best way to discover this. If there is no indication in the argument, it is probably fair to assume that the principle/rule is intended to be universal. This would be the most common interpretation, both among moral philosophers and lay people.

Then there is also the question of whether the author has got it right, so to speak—is the principle really universal or relative? Like the question of whether a principle is really absolute or prima facie, this is not a question to be answered by pure logic, but by moral philosophy. For this reason, we will not attempt to deal with it here: it is a complex and ongoing debate which we could not sensibly cover in a short space. However, it is an important debate for nurses to be aware of, since nurses often care for patients from different cultural backgrounds and encounter value systems quite at odds with the one they have acquired through their own culture. The list of suggested reading at the end of this part of the book indicates some further reading on this topic. For now, the important point to grasp is that an argument can legitimately be couched in universal or relative terms: not all principles/rules are automatically universal.

Exercise 13.3 (Revision)

1. Are rules and principles the same?
2. Is there a single fixed and precise meaning for the term 'rule', and the term 'principle'?
3. What is the difference between an absolute rule and a prima facie rule?
4. What is the difference between a universal principle and a relative principle?

Exercise 13.4

Write a logical outline for each of the following arguments (supply any assumptions that are needed). Then comment on whether or not the conclusion is warranted. State how your assessment would alter, depending on whether the principle/rule in the premise is taken to be absolute or prima facie, universal or relative.

1. Genital mutilation is an abhorrent practice. Health workers should play no part in it, and should report any instances which come to their attention.
2. Mr Jones is going for surgery tomorrow and he hasn't even been told what his diagnosis is. Someone ought to get his doctor to come and talk to him.
3. We know that Jack has epilepsy and might injure himself if he has a fit while he's working on the production line, but because of the principle of confidentiality, we must not reveal this to his employer.

Are the Premises Really True?

So far we have looked at the logical implications of premises containing rules and principles, to see what sort of conclusion logically follows from these premises. The key to this was to be aware of the different categories of principles (absolute versus prima facie, universal versus relative). But the other important step in evaluating an argument is to ask whether the premises are actually true. For premises containing principles and rules (and indeed any other expressions of ethical value), it is not a straightforward matter to determine this. Ethical premises are not the sort of things which can be called true or false in the usual sense of these words. Instead, we need to ask whether the claims are reasonable or justified.

With regard to principles and rules, a chain of justification or explanation can be given, with specific rules being justified by reference to more general principles. However, at some point the chain of justification runs out, and we have no real way of explaining why something is right or wrong, or ethically valuable, except to say that 'it is obviously so'. So absolute justification in this sense is impossible for ethical value claims; but before the chain of explanation runs out, we can go a long way in sorting out reasonable from unreasonable claims.

Example 13.2

The following is an example of a chain of justification, starting from a very specific rule and ending with a very general principle. After each statement of principle, the question 'why?' is asked, to elicit the next stage of justification.

1. Patients who do not speak English should be offered the services of an interpreter. (Why?)
2. Because patients should be informed of their diagnosis. (Why?)
3. Because patients should be assisted to exercise their autonomy. (Why?)
4. Because autonomy is an essential characteristic of human beings—we cannot be truly happy if we do not have autonomy.

The question 'why?' could be asked after step 4, but at this point we have really reached the end of sensible justification. It just seems obvious that autonomy matters and that human happiness is of great value: if someone thought that human happiness had no value, it would be very hard to see how to convince them otherwise.

The style of thinking involved in step 4 (and beyond, if there is a way to go that far) is characteristic of moral philosophy, and would very rarely be called for in discussions of ethical issues in nursing. For practical ethical reasoning, the level of justification represented by step 3 would normally be quite sufficient. At this level, the principle or rule referred to needs to be very general and also widely accepted within the nursing community (as shown, for example, by being endorsed in a code of ethics). If a specific rule can be explained by reference to a general principle in this way, then it is reasonable to accept it. Further justification of the general principle may be possible, but this is part of the task of philosophical ethics, and need not be attempted for every argument put forward in the field of nursing ethics.

Related to the issue of the justification of premises containing rules or principles is the question of whether particular rules or principles are properly considered to be absolute or prima facie. One way to approach this question is to look again at the chain of justification. Take for example the rule that killing is wrong. Is this rule reasonable? It can be justified by reference to a more general principle, in this way: 'Killing is wrong because it harms people by taking away the good things which they would otherwise have experienced.' This mode of justification indicates that the rule against killing is properly regarded as prima facie. This is because the explanation given for the wrongness of killing shows why killing is wrong in most instances, but it does allow for the possibility that killing is not wrong in those special circumstances where continued life would in fact not hold any good experiences which the person could miss out on. (A patient in a deep and irreversible coma due to extensive brain damage might well be in such circumstances.) However, a different type of justification would suggest that the rule against killing is absolute. For example, if the explanation for the wrongness of killing was 'Human life is so precious that it must always be preserved', then there is clearly no room for exceptions or special circumstances. The explanation shows that the rule must be followed in every situation.

One other important issue in the debate over prima facie and absolute rules/principles is the problem of conflicting ethical values. Although some very notable moral philosophers (for example Immanuel Kant and John Stuart Mill) have argued that there is only one ultimate value, the trend now is towards accepting that there are a number of different ethical values, which may come into conflict with one another. If this is so, then difficulty is involved in taking all the values to be absolute rules or principles. Consider, for example, the principles of not-harming and truthfulness, which clash in a situation where telling the truth to a person would cause harm to him or her. If both principles are absolute, then both must be followed without exception: but that is impossible in this situation. Although some moral philosophers and theologians have devised complex ways of getting around this difficulty, the current consensus is closer to the view that this just demonstrates a good reason why rules and principles cannot be regarded as absolute. Rather, they are prima facie, and the real problem is to decide which takes precedence when a clash occurs.

Again, thinking at this level of abstraction about ethical rules and principles belongs primarily in philosophical ethics or moral philosophy, rather than in practical ethics. A critical evaluation of an argument in nursing ethics would not normally involve construction of a new argument to prove that a principle was absolute rather than prima facie; recognition of the significance of the difference would normally be sufficient. If the matter needed to be pursued, then it would be appropriate to turn to the writings of moral philosophers or specialists in ethics for guidance. The reading list at the end of this part of the book offers some suggestions for this.

Exercise 13.5 (Revision)

1. What is a chain of justification for ethical rules or principles?
2. What two sorts of reasons could be given for thinking that a rule or principle is prima facie rather than absolute?
3. Provide a chain of justification for the following ethical exhortations:
   a. Students must not go home and tell their families about these patients.
   b. If subjects in a drug trial are to receive a placebo, they must be told.
   c. Toilet doors are to be shut when residents use the toilet, even if the residents do not request this.

Chapter 14
Rights and Duties

This chapter explains what it means to have a right, and how rights are connected to duties. Positive and negative rights are distinguished, and the significance of the distinction for the conclusion of rights-based arguments is explained. The foundations of both types of rights are briefly examined, and suggestions are made for assessing the reasonableness of rights-claims.

Talk of 'rights' is very popular these days. It is probably fair to say that for most people, the standard way in which to discuss ethical issues of almost any kind is to refer to rights, especially so-called 'human rights'. Likewise, reference to rights is common in relation to ethical issues in nursing (although, as the next chapter shows, it is by no means the only frame of reference in nursing ethics). One of the great problems in ethical discussions conducted in terms of rights is that people seem to be able to assert a right to anything and everything: the resultant competing claims seem impossible to resolve, and the discussion draws to a frustrating dead end. Some common examples of this include the debates over gun control (the right to carry arms versus the right to safety) and smoking (the right to smoke versus the right to clean air).

However, use of the term 'rights' in ethical reasoning can be productive and helpful, provided that due care is taken. **Right** is another technical term with a specified meaning and definite logical properties. If the logic of rights-talk is properly understood and used in ethical reasoning, warranted conclusions can be drawn, and perhaps more importantly, progress can be made in reaching a decision about an ethical issue.

At the outset, it is helpful to introduce a distinction in terminology which will make the subsequent discussion easier to follow. This is the distinction between a right and a **rights-claim**. The term 'right' will be used to refer to the fundamental concept or idea that is involved when people talk about rights. The term 'rights-claim' will be used to refer to a claim or statement that someone has some particular right. An ethical argument, if couched in terms of rights, will contain one or more rights-claims in the premises or conclusion. Using the term 'rights-claim' is a way of referring to the proposition about rights, without actually agreeing that the person really does have the right that is claimed.

This chapter, like the previous one, is divided into two main sections. Again, this reflects the two steps in assessing an argument: are the premises true, and does the conclusion follow logically from the premises?

The first section will help you to answer the question about whether the conclusion follows logically from the premises. It will explain the logical form of rights-claims, and the sorts of conclusions that can validly be drawn from premises involving rights-claims. It will also set out the technical meaning of the concept of a 'right', and explain the logical and ethical limits of this concept. The second section will help you to answer the question about whether the premises are true. Again, this is not a straightforward task, since ethical premises cannot simply be checked against an agreed body of facts in the way that factual premises can. Instead, we need to ask if the value-claim is reasonable or supportable. This section will explain how to decide whether a particular rights-claim is reasonable, given the standard understanding of rights and their origins. It will discuss the basis on which rights can be claimed (and thus factors which might make a particular rights-claim unreasonable), and examine some ways of understanding conflicts between rights-claims.

Does the Conclusion Follow from the Premises?

For ethical arguments which have premises containing rights-claims, it is vital to know the precise technical meaning of the term 'right', in order to be able to assess whether the conclusion really does follow from the premises. The reason for this is that it is the concept of a right which forms the logical link between the premises and the conclusion—everything depends on this concept, as the examples below will show.

What is a 'Right'?

When people say 'I have a right to . . .', they are in essence making a claim to be treated in a particular way. The claim is an ethical one—it is not simply that they would *prefer* to be treated in this way, but rather that they *ought* to be treated in this way. The implication is that it would be wrong not to treat them in this way. So a rights-claim is actually an ethical exhortation, since it urges people to act in a certain way, even though it lacks the usual signpost of 'should' or 'ought'. But this is only a general explanation of the concept of a right. Now the precise technical meaning needs to be spelled out.

The first point about the technical meaning of the term 'right' is that it constitutes a claim that one is ethically entitled to be treated in a certain way. The second point is that a right is something that a person chooses to exercise if he or she wants to. If I claim a right, I am making a claim to be treated in a certain way, if that is what I want. I am certainly not saying that there is any compulsion on me to be treated in this way. Having a right leaves me entirely free to do as I please. However, the third point about the meaning of a right is that it involves a compulsion (an obligation or duty) on *other people* to act in a certain way towards me. When I claim a right to something, this amounts to saying that other people must treat me in a certain way, whether they want to or not. If I have a right to something, part of the meaning of this is that other people have an obligation to act (or refrain from acting) in whatever way is necessary for my right to be fulfilled.

Example 14.1

An example will help to show what all this means. Consider this rights-claim, which might well form a premise of an ethical argument: 'I have a right to an education.' Using the explanation of the meaning of the term 'right' given above, the meaning of this rights-claim is as follows: 'I am entitled to an education if I want it, and other people have a duty to act in such a way that I can receive this education.'

In summary, then, here is a definition of a right: a right is something I am entitled to, if I want it. My right to something puts others under a duty (or obligation) to treat me in such a way that my right can be fulfilled.

It is vital to distinguish a right from a duty. A right is something I am entitled to, if I want it. A duty is something that I must do, whether I want to or not. Rights and duties are different, indeed opposite, concepts, but they are related. My right imposes a **correlative** (related) duty on other people; likewise, other people's rights impose a correlative duty on me. One of the common mistakes in ethical reasoning is to confuse the concept of right and duty. In particular, a common error is to reason as if a person's right to something meant that they were obliged to have it or do it. As should be clear from the above discussion, this is entirely incorrect. A person's right to something means that they have an entitlement to it, not that they are obliged to use it. For example, a right to education means that I am entitled to an education, not that I have to stay at school after I turn fifteen, or have to go to university.

How does all this relate to ethical reasoning? The example below shows how the meaning of the term 'right' determines what sort of conclusion it is valid to draw from a premise containing a rights-claim.

Example 14.2

Consider the following piece of ethical reasoning:

I know the patient is refusing the medication, but patients have a right to the best medical care, and so they must take their medications.

This reasoning can be set out as follows:

1. Patients have a right to the best medical care. (ethical exhortation)

(2. Medication is part of the best medical care.) (fact)

3. Therefore, they must take their medication. (1,2, ethical exhortation)

The first premise is an ethical premise—a rights-claim. The second premise is an informative premise, which was not actually explicitly stated in the original form of the argument. It is an assumption, as is indicated by the use of parentheses, and has been added here to make the argument clear. The conclusion is an ethical exhortation: it states what patients must do.

Is this a sound argument? We need to consider the two steps involved in answering this question. First, we assess the truth of the premises, and secondly, we ask if the conclusion follows logically from the premises. Let us simply accept that the premises are true (they certainly don't appear to be obviously false), and go on to examine the logical link between the premises and the conclusion, since that is what is of concern here. The logical link is carried by the term 'right'. In this argument, an inference is made from a claim that patients have a right to something, to a conclusion that they have an obligation to do something else. Whether or not this conclusion is warranted depends entirely on the meaning of the word 'right'.

As explained above, a 'right' is an entitlement to have or do something if one wants to. From a true rights-claim it can validly be inferred that a person is ethically permitted to have or do X, and that other people have an obligation to do what is needed for the person to have X. It is *not* valid to infer from a person's rights-claim to X that the person has an obligation to do or have X. This would be a serious misunderstanding of the term 'right', and the inference would produce an unwarranted conclusion.

In this example, the conclusion is based on exactly this mistake. The author of the argument has used the term 'right' incorrectly. She thinks it involves an obligation on the patient who has the right, whereas it really only involves a permission to the patient—the obligation lies on other people. For this reason, the conclusion of the argument is unwarranted. Using the correct meaning of right, the only warranted conclusion which can be drawn from these premises is that patients must be allowed to take their medications if they want to, and everyone else must not try to stop them.

The following exercise will give you practice in distinguishing correct from incorrect usage of the term 'right' (and 'duty'). Before you start, look back to the definitions of right and duty given above.

Exercise 14.1

a. Which of these usages of the terms 'right' and 'duty' is correct, and which incorrect?
b. For the correct ones, spell out precisely what is meant by the claim.
c. For the incorrect ones, explain why they are incorrect.

1. You may not like helping residents to go to the toilet, but it is your duty to do so.
2. Patients have a right to seek alternative health care therapies, so we must not try to prevent them from doing so.
3. Everyone has a right to vote, and so anyone failing to vote will be fined.

4. I may not agree with your opinions, but I support your right to express them if you want to.
5. Nurses have a right to be pleasant to clients who are personally offensive.
6. Nurses have a duty to be pleasant to clients who are personally offensive.

Positive and Negative Rights

We have said that a right is an entitlement to something, but to what? Rights fall into two broad categories, depending on what sort of entitlement is being claimed. One category is **negative rights** (sometimes called 'liberties'), where the entitlement is simply to be left alone, to be allowed to do what one wants without interference from others. This sort of right is called negative because it imposes only a negative correlative duty on others: that is, a duty *not* to act, *not* to interfere or hinder. An example of a rights-claim involving a negative right is the following: 'I have a right to smoke.' This is a claim that I am entitled to smoke if I want to, and other people have a correlative (negative) duty not to interfere—they must leave me alone to do what I want. (Of course, the right expressed in this example may not always apply, as in a no-smoking area.)

Since the correlative duty just requires other people to do nothing, it is a duty that everyone can easily fulfil. With negative rights, there is no problem about who must fulfil the corresponding obligation—it is clearly every other person.

The second category is **positive rights** (also called claim-rights or welfare rights), where the entitlement is to be provided with something or have something done for one. This is called a positive right because it imposes a positive correlative duty on others: they must act in a specific way to give me something or do something for me. For example, the claim 'I have a right to health care' involves a positive right. It is a claim that I am entitled to health care if I want it, and other people have a positive duty to provide that health care for me.

Whilst the idea of positive rights is clear, there is some difficulty in practice in determining who has to fulfil the correlative duty. Who is it that has a duty to provide me with health care, or whatever else I have a positive right to? Do people whom I meet on the street have an obligation to provide me with health care? Does absolutely everybody have this obligation? Or is it only some select group? This practical problem will be discussed further in the next section. The important thing to note for the moment is that, in regard to positive rights, there can be a dispute about who must act to fulfil my rights, whereas with negative rights, it is clear that everyone incurs the obligation to refrain from interfering with me.

In most cases, commonsense will make it clear whether a rights-claim is intended in a positive or a negative sense. In the example of smoking, it would be nonsensical to interpret a right to smoke as a positive right. If my right to smoke were a positive right, it would mean that other people had a duty to provide me with cigarettes and whatever else I needed in order to be able to smoke. But this seems absurd. It makes much more sense to construe it as a negative right, which imposes on other people only the negative duty to not interfere with my smoking. Likewise, commonsense suggests that a right to health care is a positive right, requiring others to actively provide me with health care. There would be little point in a negative right to health care, which would only require others not to prevent me seeking health care, if any happened to be available. As a general guide, it is sensible to regard rights as negative, unless there seems to be some very good reason to think that they are positive.

However, commonsense does not always reveal whether a particular rights-claim is to be interpreted as a positive or negative one. In fact, great controversy often surrounds the interpretation of rights-claims when they seem able to fall into either category. A well-known example is the right to die, or the right to die with dignity. This right is widely accepted in our community today, but there is great controversy about what exactly it means. Some people think that the right to die implies that active euthanasia (or mercy killing) should be available to those who request it, but others think that it simply means that people should be allowed to die in peace, free from unwanted treatment. The controversy is really about whether the right to die is a positive or a negative right. If it is positive, then it imposes a correlative duty on others to actively provide help in the dying process, for example by supplying or administering lethal drugs. But if it is a negative right, then it only imposes a negative correlative duty on others not to hinder the dying process. This would mean only that others should not try to prevent me from committing suicide, or should not force me to have medical treatment that I do not want. This difference is very significant indeed.

In cases like this, where it is not clear whether a right is intended to be positive or negative, it is necessary to have some understanding of the ethical basis of rights-claims. The second section of this chapter will explain the different foundations of the two different categories but, for the moment, the important thing to grasp is the basic difference in meaning between positive and negative rights.

Exercise 14.2

Which of these rights is positive, and which negative? For each one, write down the correlative duty which the right imposes on others. If you think it is unclear which type of right is meant, explain why.

1. the right to education
2. the right to strike
3. the right to information about your medical treatment
4. the right to a family
5. the right to practise your own religion

6. the right to food and shelter
7. the right to watch X rated videos

The distinction between positive and negative rights has vital importance in ethical reasoning. The conclusion which it is legitimate to draw from a positive rights-claim is very different from the conclusion that can be drawn from a negative rights-claim. As we have seen above, from a negative right it is only valid to conclude that other people have an obligation not to interfere. However, from a positive rights-claim it is valid to conclude that other people have an obligation to step in and provide whatever is needed. The following example shows how this works in practice.

Example 14.3

Consider the following argument:

1. Everyone has a right to have a family. (ethical exhortation)
2. Infertile couples need medical help to have a family. (fact)
3. Therefore, the government has an obligation to provide whatever medical help they need. (1,2, ethical exhortation)

The conclusion of this argument is only warranted if the right to have a family is a positive right. If it is, then it is correct to conclude that someone has an obligation to provide infertile people with a family. However, if the right to have a family is a negative right, then the situation is entirely different. The conclusion of the argument would not be warranted because a negative right only imposes a negative duty on others to not prevent people from having a family if they want to. It does not impose an obligation on anyone to step in and provide assistance.

Thus, it all depends on knowing whether this right to have a family is negative or positive. The second section of this chapter indicates how to go about deciding which sort of right is involved in a particular instance, when commonsense is not able to adjudicate. For the moment, the thing to note is how the assessment of an argument can depend entirely on what sort of right is being claimed in the ethical premise.

Limits on Rights-claims

It is commonly but wrongly believed that rights-claims are conclusive, and cannot be restricted in any way. It tends to be felt that if I have a right to something, then I have an unlimited right—I cannot be denied anything. Indeed, many ethical discussions involving rights grind to a halt on exactly this assumption. However, a conclusion affirming an unlimited right to something cannot validly be drawn from a rights-claim in a premise. This is due to an ethical constraint on the meaning of the term 'right'.

Moral philosophers have always recognised that rights, by their very nature, have limits. Claiming a right to something does not give you an unlimited entitlement to it. This is because of the ethical concept of **equality** which is closely associated with the idea of rights, and which arises when we are talking about individuals who live in a community. In moral philosophy, the idea of rights only makes sense if the rights are equal; that is, if everyone has equal rights. The reason is that rights are conceived of as deriving from fundamental features of human nature, which everyone shares equally, or from universal ethical principles, which apply equally to everyone. So any particular rights-claim is limited by the equal rights of others to the same thing. The sort of limitation imposed by the requirement of equality depends on whether the right is positive or negative.

The limitations imposed by equality are most easily seen in relation to positive rights. As is explained more fully in the second section below, positive rights are based on human needs: things which are required for a minimally decent human life. My positive right to these things is limited by everyone else's equal right to the same things. In practice, this means that my entitlement is limited to my fair share of the good things that are available, since there will inevitably be a limited supply of them. For example, if I have a right to health care, what I actually have a right to is an equal or fair share of the health care resources provided by this society. I have a right to my fair share of a GP's time, a stay in hospital, drugs, surgery and so on. I do not have a right to an unlimited amount of health care—I cannot legitimately claim that I am entitled to have all the resources of the hospital and all the time and expertise of the nursing and medical staff devoted solely to me.

Negative rights are also limited by the equal rights of others. However, the kind of limitation involved here is somewhat different, because negative rights are simply rights to do as we please, not rights to be given some goods or services which are necessarily in limited supply. As is explained below, all negative rights derive ultimately from the fundamental right to freedom. But my right to freedom is limited by everyone else's equal right to freedom. So I have a right to do as I please without hindrance from others, but only to the extent that I do not interfere with their right to do exactly the same.

In practice, for a group of people living together in a community, this means that no one has a right to absolute freedom. Everyone's freedom is limited to some extent—and so everyone's negative rights are limited to some extent. For example, I might claim a right to play loud music in my backyard. This is a negative right to do as I please. But it does not mean I can play my music as loudly as I like for as long as I like, because my right to do as I please is limited by everyone else's right to do as they please. My neighbours may want to sleep peacefully in their backyards, or have a conversation with their friends. If I play my music too loudly, then they will not be free to do as they please. So in fact I only have a right to play music at a volume which will not prevent them from doing what they want to do. Compromises must be reached when negative rights conflict.

Again, the fact that there are limits to rights is extremely important in ethical reasoning. If you are not aware of these limits, you will be led to draw unwarranted conclusions from premises which involve rights-claims. The following example shows how this can happen.

Example 14.4

Consider the following argument:

> As a nursing student, I have a right to a good education. If I had my own personal tutor for bioscience, I would learn a lot more than I am now. So I have a right to my own personal tutor.

This argument can be set out as follows:

1. I have a right to a good education. (ethical exhortation)
2. A personal tutor in bioscience would help give me a good education. (fact)
3. Therefore, I have a right to a personal tutor in bioscience. (1,2, ethical exhortation)

Is this a sound argument? The two steps are to ask firstly if the premises are true, and then if the conclusion follows logically from the premises. Let us accept for the moment that the premises are true (they seem quite reasonable). Let us also accept that the right to an education is a positive right—it means a right to have an education provided for me. But we still need to take into account the limit on positive rights. The limit, of course, is that I only have a right to my fair share. So the conclusion to this argument needs to be more carefully stated in order to be warranted. It should read: 'Therefore, I have a right to a personal tutor in bioscience, provided that this doesn't consume more than my fair share of the available resources.' Given the current state of funding for tertiary education, it is extremely unlikely that any budget would stretch to a personal tutor for every student! In this case, the conclusion of the argument is not warranted. You can only see this if you are aware of the equality limitation to rights-claims.

Exercise 14.3

How could you respond to the following arguments put to you by patients or their relatives?

1. My visitors have a right to come whenever they like. You have no business telling them that they have to leave!
2. My mother has the right to the best care. When I come in here, I find her sitting in the day room doing nothing. You must provide her with something to do or someone to talk to, so that she is never lonely or bored!

Are the Premises True?

Suppose that a nursing student were to claim 'I have a right to a job', as part of an argument to the conclusion that her school of nursing had an obligation to guarantee her employment when she graduated. In the first section, we were concerned with the question of whether or not this conclusion follows logically from the rights-claim in the premises. But the other important question is, of course, whether or not the premise is true. Is it true that the student has a right to a job? In this section, we will examine the basis for rights-claims, in order to sort out which rights can reasonably be claimed, and which cannot.

The basis of positive and negative rights

We noted earlier that one of the frustrations of discussions involving rights is that people seem to be able to claim a right to anything and everything. Now it is time to ask whether this is in fact really so. Where do all these rights come from? Do people really have a right to everything that they say they do? The short answer is yes and no. To explain this more fully, we need to consider positive and negative rights separately. The reason for this is that positive and negative rights have quite different foundations.

Negative rights (rights to do as we please without interference) all come from one source—the basic right to freedom. Freedom is widely regarded by moral philosophers as being one of the most important ethical values. Our whole understanding of human beings, and the way that they should live, rests on the idea that each individual has the freedom to make choices and act upon them. Indeed, it is hard to imagine how we could be truly human if we did not have this freedom.

Each particular negative right that a person may claim is really just a specific version of this general underlying right to freedom. For example, people may claim the right to take risks, make mistakes, drink alcohol, bet on horses, wear unusual clothes, climb mountains and a host of other things. All of these are simply specific ways of asserting the general right to be free to do as one pleases. So in this sense, if people are claiming a negative right, they do indeed have a right to everything that they claim. That is, they have a right to do what they want, no matter what this happens to be. However, it is important to bear in mind that even all these negative rights to do whatever one wants are not unlimited. As the previous section explained, negative rights can only be exercised within certain constraints.

Positive rights have quite a different source from negative rights. They are not based on freedom at all. Instead, positive rights are based on universal ethical principles like the ones referred to in the previous chapter, or on particular things which are believed to be good in themselves, or needed for a human being to live a flourishing life. Many of the rights in the United Nations Declaration on Human Rights are positive rights, and it is easy to see how they are based on fundamental human needs. For example, the Declaration includes the right to food and shelter, the right to education, the right to health care and the right to employment. These rights are based on the things that people need if they are to have a physically comfortable life, and an opportunity for happiness or self-fulfilment: things like adequate food and water, protection from harsh weather, treatment for diseases, the ability to read and write and to earn a living. These needs are regarded as universal—that is, needs which all human beings have, no matter who they are or where they live. That is why they can form the basis of universal rights which every human being can legitimately claim.

Because positive rights are based on these fundamental and universal human needs, they are often called 'welfare rights'. This term indicates the meaning (they are the things that people need in order to 'fare well') and also gives a clue about who ends up with the obligation to make sure these rights are fulfilled. The obligation to meet individuals' rights to food and shelter, education and health care, and so on, is usually regarded as lying with the government, rather than with other private individuals. This is because the government is the representative of the people as a whole, and has the resources to provide what private individuals cannot provide for each other.

From this account of the basis of positive rights, it is clear that only certain things can legitimately count as positive rights. They must be things which are based on some fundamental and important human need. If, for example, I claimed a positive right to go sailboarding, it would be fairly easy to argue that I have no such right, at least in a positive sense. The need to go sailboarding is not a universal and fundamental human need (indeed, most people happily and comfortably live their whole lives without ever going sailboarding): it is just something that I happen to like doing. So I can have no positive right to it, and the government has no positive obligation to provide me with a sailboard and a nice stretch of water to sail on. However, I could legitimately claim a negative right to go sailboarding—this would be a specific instance of my general right to freedom. But in this case, all that my right would require of others is that they did not get in my way. This is a much less significant right to possess.

Just before we conclude this section on the foundation of rights, it is worthwhile to note the status of 'patients' rights'. It is sometimes thought that patients' rights are different from ordinary rights or general human rights, but this is a misunderstanding. Patients' rights are simply ordinary rights as they apply to the specific situation of being a patient. Documents like so-called 'patients' bills of rights', as well as some codes of ethics for nurses, assert quite specific rights of patients, such as the right to a second opinion, the right to a detailed account from the hospital, the right of access to ministers or counsellors of their own choice, the right to the most effective treatment for their condition and so on. These are not special rights. Rather, they are simply some specific positive and negative rights derived from more general rights. For example, the right to a minister or counsellor of one's own choice is just a specific application of the general right to freedom; the right to the most effective treatment is just the right to health care; and the right to a detailed account is based on the right to autonomy. The basis for patients' rights is the same as the basis for any other rights.

Conflicts of Rights

The final complication of rights-based arguments which we will consider here is conflicts of rights. There are essentially two different types of conflict which can occur: conflicts between the same rights of different people, and conflicts between different rights of different people. We have in fact already dealt with the first type of conflict (although you may not have realised it) in our discussion of limits on rights. Let us take an example. If patients as a group have a positive right to health care, but there is only a limited amount of health care to go around, each patient's right is in competition with the others' right. This conflict is to be resolved by application of the associated ethical principle of equality which we explained earlier. This applies likewise to conflicts of the same negative right.

Conflicts of the second type, where different rights are involved, need to be approached differently, because it does not make sense to say that everyone should be given an equal share when they are claiming different things. Let us take the apparent deadlock over smoking as an example. One person says 'I have a right to smoke'; another says 'I have a right not to be subjected to a smoke-laden environment.' These rights are obviously in conflict: whose should win out? To resolve this conflict, we need to appeal to what might be called a 'hierarchy of rights'. The basic idea is that some rights are more important than others, so that when there is a conflict, the more important one takes precedence. The arguments used to show which rights are more important are quite complex, and belong in moral philosophy rather than in critical thinking. We cannot explain them in detail here. However, the general approach is to try to show which particular rights are more closely tied to the foundations of all rights, namely the fundamental human needs or significant freedoms which we mentioned earlier. So, in the smoking example, it could be argued that the right not to be subjected to cigarette smoke is derived from a fundamental positive right to a healthy environment, whereas a right to smoke is derived from the negative right to freedom, which, although vital to human flourishing in some contexts (such as freedom of religion or freedom of speech), is not so important here. After all, it really amounts to a right to be foolish, or to harm oneself, which is surely less ethically significant than a right to good health.

Note that both of these types of conflicts are interpersonal conflicts, involving the question of what duty is owed to one person when there is a competing duty apparently owed to another. There is only a limited sense in which it is possible for a conflict of rights to occur for the one individual. Let us say a patient has a right to health care, and also a right to refuse treatment. These rights are in conflict in the sense that the patient cannot have both at the same time. However, as we pointed out at the start of this chapter, people are not obliged to exercise their rights—they are free to decide which rights they want to take up and which they do not. So here there is no real problem: the patient simply chooses whether he wants treatment or not, and exercises the appropriate right. Difficulty only arises when the patient is not able (due to lack of mental capacity) to make a choice for himself, and yet nurses and other health professionals still have to decide how to act towards him. Based on his rights, they have a duty both to treat him (if he wants treatment) and not to treat him (if he doesn't want it). The key here is the patient's desires: the first step in resolving the problem is to ask which of his rights the patient would have wanted to exercise. If this can be determined, that is the end of the matter. If there is no way of knowing with enough certainty, the next step is to use the idea of a hierarchy of rights, and to fulfil whichever right seems most important, just as in the case of the competing rights of different people.

Exercise 14.4 (Revision)

1. On what are negative rights based?
2. How can one decide whether a claim to a negative right is reasonable or not?
3. On what are positive rights based?
4. How can one decide whether a claim to a positive right is reasonable or not?
5. How can conflicts between different rights be resolved?
6. What is the difference between patients' rights and ordinary rights?

Conclusion

The main points to keep in mind when dealing with ethical arguments involving rights-claims are as follows:

1. A person who has a right is not obliged to exercise that right.
2. One person's right imposes a duty on others to fulfil that right.
3. Negative rights impose a duty on others merely to refrain from interfering, whereas positive rights impose a duty to do or provide something specific.
4. Both negative and positive rights-claims are limited by the principle of equality.
5. Not all positive rights-claims are reasonable—they need to be checked against the legitimate foundations of such rights in fundamental human needs.

Awareness of these points will enable you to critically evaluate rights-based arguments, and avoid accepting conclusions derived from misunderstandings of the meaning and logical properties of the term 'right'.

Chapter 15

Current Concepts in Nursing Ethics

This chapter critically examines a number of terms and concepts which are commonly used in contemporary discussions of ethical issues in nursing. Amongst these are duty of care, dignity, accountability, advocacy and caring. The emphasis is on ambiguities in meaning which may cause confusion and disagreement in ethical reasoning. Suggestions are made for specific questions to ask in order to avoid some of the characteristic pitfalls associated with these terms.

Although many discussions of nursing ethics use the language of principles, rules, rights and duties, there are some other key terms and concepts which are frequently used. Some of these terms are directly related to the principles or rights which we have discussed earlier, whereas others are quite different. In this chapter, we will examine some of these terms and concepts to see how they work in ethical reasoning. We will look at two main areas: problems in assessing the truth of ethical premises, and potential faults in reasoning. In doing so, we may seem to be asking more questions than we answer. This is because our aim is to enable you to be on the lookout for characteristic pitfalls and (sometimes hidden) sources of disagreement in ethical reasoning.

Terms and Concepts Related to Beneficence and Non-maleficence

Best Interests, Well-being and Welfare

Ethical reasoning in nursing very frequently makes reference to the well-being, welfare or best interests of patients. This is hardly surprising, since nursing is a helping profession, but these ideas are not as straightforward as they may appear. All three ideas are related to the principles of beneficence (benefitting) and non-maleficence (not harming), which we mentioned briefly in Chapter 13. Benefit and harm, although they seem very simple ideas, can easily cause problems in ethical reasoning, as the following discussion shows. The reason is that these simple ideas can be interpreted in different ways. Further explanation is needed to see how this is so. This can be done in terms of the concept of interests. Interests, in the ethical sense, are not things which people find interesting. Rather, we speak of something being in a person's interests, meaning that it is good for them in some significant way. One way to understand interests is to think of them as basic needs: whatever will meet a person's basic needs will promote his or her interests. Benefiting people means promoting their interests, while harming them means retarding (or hindering) their interests. To say that something is in my best interests means that overall it is the most beneficial and least harmful to me, and will thus promote my interests to the greatest extent.

This term 'best interests' is a common and very important one in ethical discourse, and in this section we will consider some of the questions which need to be raised when it is used. Exactly the same questions apply to the terms 'well-being' and 'welfare', which in ethical contexts have a meaning very similar to best interests. The first of these questions relates to the problem of how to determine what counts as a person's interests or needs. We need to know this in order to determine whether a premise referring to well-being or best interests is true or not. However, the matter is somewhat complicated by differing interpretations. On the one hand there is the objective interpretation: a person's interests are determined by what human beings as a species need in order to survive (or to live well—depending on how high we set the standard). These could be social or emotional requirements, as well as physical, but they do not depend on what individuals happen to want or prefer—they are fixed by human nature. On the other hand there is the subjective interpretation, that a person's interests are not fixed in this way, but vary according to the desires and preferences of the person. In between these two positions, there is a middle ground which says that some of a person's interests are determined by universal human needs, but others depend on individual preferences. For example, every person has an interest in an adequate food supply, since no human being can survive without food. But only some people have an interest in artistic expression: some people need to be able to express themselves in this way to survive psychologically, but others do not.

The importance for ethical reasoning of this debate over subjective and objective interpretations of needs and interests lies in its implications for truth of premises which make claims about what is in a person's best interests, or what will promote his or her well-being or welfare. Suppose that a nurse decides to change a dressing on a patient's wound because it is in the best interests of the patient to do so. This involves an ethical argument containing the premise, 'Changing the dressing is in the patient's best interests.' Is this premise true? If interests is an objective concept, then the truth of this premise can be checked against knowledge about what all human beings need for survival (here physiological requirements will be at stake). However, if interests is a subjective concept, then the truth of the premise depends on the patient's own values and preferences. If the patient prefers a non-septic wound, then it is in his best interests to change the dressing; if he doesn't care about the wound, then it isn't. Exactly the same would apply to any claim about what would promote the patients's well-being or welfare.

This example may make it seem obvious that best interests, well-being and welfare are objective concepts. Surely it is nonsense to say that a dressing change is not in a patient's best interests just because he doesn't mind having a septic wound. However, this idea does not seem so nonsensical in situations which are not very different. Take for example a 94-year-old patient with various complications of diabetes, who has just had an above-the-knee amputation. Is it in her best interests to have a prosthesis fitted and go through a physically demanding rehabilitation program to learn to walk with it? Here it seems much more plausible to say that this depends on her preferences and values, and specifically on how important the ability to walk is to her, in terms of how she lives her life and sees herself. To simply assert that mobility is a basic need of every person does not really seem to answer the question here.

We do not propose to resolve the objective versus subjective question here, but rather to bring it to your notice as a vital one in any discussion of best interests and related concepts. The main message is a warning against assuming that you can always know what is in someone's best interests, without considering their outlook and preferences. Even if this is so in the case of some types of interests, it is not necessarily the case for *all* interests.

Another important issue for ethical reasoning is that of the relative priority of autonomy and best interests. Assuming that interests (and thus welfare and well-being) depend at least partly on people's needs rather than their preferences, it is possible that patients will make an autonomous choice which is in conflict with their best interests. If the patient refuses to have his dressing changed, should the nurse follow her obligation to respect autonomy or her obligation to promote his best interests? We do not intend to give an answer to this question here, but rather to point out that it is a legitimate question which needs to be asked whenever best interests or related concepts are appealed to in ethical argument. It is not obvious that promoting best interests is ethically more important than respecting autonomy, so it is important to be wary of an unspoken assumption to this effect, which will pre-determine a decision about what to do in a particular situation. The view that best interests must always take precedence over autonomy is known as paternalism, and under this name it is widely rejected in nursing. In fact, nurses often take the opposite position—that autonomy is the supreme value. However, it is also not obvious that autonomy *always* outweighs best interests—so it is best to keep an open mind when approaching any situation where there appears to be a conflict between autonomy and best interests.

In summary, when 'best interests' and related terms are used in ethical argument, there are two potential sources of disagreement or uncertainty to watch out for. One is disagreement over whether a course of action does or does not promote a patient's best interests; the other is disagreement over the relative priority of best interests and autonomy. So an argument that something must be done because it is in a patient's best interests should be critically examined rather than accepted without thought as obviously correct.

Safety

'Safety' is a word frequently used in discussions of ethical problems in nursing. An ethical concern for safety is derived from the principle of non-maleficence (not harming). Earlier we defined harming as hindering or retarding a person's interests. For this reason, the comments made above about best interests and related terms also apply to safety. When reference is made to a patient's safety, there are two questions to ask. One is whether safety is to be assessed objectively or subjectively, and the other is whether safety or autonomy is to take priority if there is conflict between them. The issues at stake here are the same as those discussed above, and the implications for ethical reasoning are the same: do not simply assume that you know what counts as safe, and do not assume that safety must always trump autonomy.

Three further issues specific to the concept of safety need to be raised. The first concerns the matter of risk. Providing safety is basically a matter of reducing the risk of harm, but careful thought is needed when assessing the amount of risk. There are two factors to consider: *how bad* the harm would be if it occurred, and *how likely* it is to occur. Risk is a function of both factors—a high-risk situation can only be said to exist if the anticipated harm is high in both degree and likelihood. So be wary of assumptions that the potential for extremely bad harm automatically brings about an excessively risky situation; the likelihood of the harm actually occurring must also be taken into account.

The second issue concerns the relationship between risk and overall well-being. We mentioned above that concern for well-being is derived from the principles of beneficence and non-maleficence: promoting well-being involves reducing harm and increasing benefit. But reducing *risk* of harm, as opposed to actual harm, does not always promote well-being. This is because a certain amount of risk is often needed for psychological well-being. A person who is protected from all risks may benefit physically from such an environment, but may well experience feelings of limitation, confinement and even boredom, which reduce psychological well-being. So another pitfall to avoid is the assumption that reducing risk always increases well-being.

The third issue concerns the place of considerations about safety, or degree of risk, in a decision about what is best to do. Riskiness is only one factor involved in deciding on whether some procedure or course of action is in a patient's best interests. The expected benefits must also be taken into account. Surgical procedures are an obvious example of this. All surgery involves a very high magnitude of risk (death is a very rare, but nevertheless possible outcome of any surgery performed under general anaesthetic), and some surgery also involves a reasonably high likelihood of a very bad outcome, especially when the patient is critically ill. But surgery continues to be performed because, in the vast majority of cases, the benefits far outweigh the risks. So be wary of arguments which focus exclusively on risks or threats to safety, without considering potential benefits. Such arguments lack balance and can be seriously misleading.

Quality of Life

Another extremely common term in ethical discussions, especially in relation to euthanasia and decisions to cease active treatment, is 'quality of life'. As a simple descriptive term, 'quality of life' means something like 'level of well-being'. So, like well-being itself, it is ultimately based on the idea of interests, but it has the added dimension of an assessment of the extent to which interests are being met. Because of this connection with interests, the now-familiar questions about objective and subjective interpretations also apply to quality of life. So the first question to keep in mind whenever you encounter the term 'quality of life' in an ethical discussion is whether the author (or speaker) means it to be something which is assessed by external, objective standards, or something which is determined by the subjective values, goals and preferences of the person concerned.

In relation to best interests, well-being and welfare, we left the subjective versus objective question fairly open (that is, we suggested that either interpretation is possible and reasonable, depending on the context), but with quality of life we can be more definite. The change of focus from well-being to life, although subtle, indicates that the subjective interpretation is the appropriate one. 'Life' is a global term, taking in all a person's experiences, and so an assessment of the quality of that person's life must be based on how their life seems to them. And this in turn will depend on many subjective factors, including whether the person feels they are able to achieve their goals, do the things they enjoy, gain satisfaction from their personal relationships and have hope for the future. This suggests that attempts to measure patients' quality of life against objective standards, such as which activities of daily living they are able to perform, are misleading—they only present a small part of the picture. What matters more is whether people actually care about being able to perform these activities and how their functional state affects their state of mind.

So far we have looked at what quality of life means, but we also need to consider how it functions in ethical argument. Arguments based on quality of life usually involve the value assumption that it is *quality* of life rather than *quantity* of life that matters, ethically speaking. Thus, lying in the background in many arguments about euthanasia and withdrawal of treatment, is an unspoken ethical principle that 'Medical treatment should only be continued when it provides an acceptable quality of life.' Behind this is an even more general principle that it is not mere biological life that is valuable, but the personal experience of life (in others words, that life is only in a person's best interests when that person values his life and wants to continue it). It is very important to note that although ethical principles of this kind can be well supported by argument in moral philosophy, and are widely accepted in the community, they are not self-evidently or undeniably true. Some people (including some patients and their families) hold an opposite view, and are also able to support their position by argument. In fact, deep disagreement over these sorts of general principles is a major source of conflict over what should be done in specific circumstances.

Another source of disagreement lies in the question of how much quality of life is enough. What is an 'acceptable' quality of life? Here it is important to avoid the pitfall of switching back to an objective perspective and trying to set some general standards or criteria for determining when quality of life falls below an acceptable level. If quality of life is truly a subjective concept, then 'acceptable' must mean 'acceptable to the person whose life it is'. What counts as an acceptable quality of life will inevitably vary from person to person.

This point leads us to the use of quality of life considerations in decisions to withdraw treatment. (Note that such decisions are never purely clinical—they always have an ethical component.) What we have said so far indicates that it is for the patient herself to decide if her quality of life has fallen so low that she no longer wishes to have her life prolonged. This is all very well where the patient is physically and mentally able to make her own decision, but what about patients who are physically unable to communicate or mentally unable to think about such matters? We have not totally ruled out the possibility that someone else could make an assessment of a patient's quality of life—we have simply pointed out that the assessment must be based on the patient's own values, perceptions and goals. Clearly the patient herself is best placed to do this, since she knows herself best, but if she is unable to do so, then someone who knows her very well may be able to give an opinion about how she would have felt. So it is not impossible to make quality of life assessments about other people, but it requires quite intimate knowledge of that person, and it is inevitably an educated guess.

The difficulty of assessing the quality of another person's life gives rise to an ethical question about whether it is right to withdraw treatment and allow a patient to die, solely on the grounds that someone else thinks that their quality of life is too low. This is not a question which we can resolve here (again it is question for ethics, not critical thinking), but it worthwhile to point out what is at stake in this matter. There are two problematic issues—is the patient actually able to experience benefit and harm, and is it better to err on the side of prolonging life or avoiding harm? If a patient is unaware of her own existence, and cannot experience pain or pleasure, then does it really matter if her life is prolonged or not? This ultimately comes back to the question of the value of biological life, unaccompanied by any psychological life. And if a patient is able to experience suffering and pleasure, but not able to make or communicate a choice about continuing treatment, which sort of mistake is it better to make? For there are two different mistakes that could be made. A decision to continue treatment, when the patient is actually suffering and does not want her life prolonged, would cause avoidable harm. On the other hand, a decision to withdraw treatment, when the patient is either not suffering or does want her life prolonged, would at the very least shorten life unnecessarily, or at worst harm the patient by depriving her of life which she wanted. This is really a question of which sort of harm is worse, suffering unwanted life or losing wanted life. Different views on these issues are another source of disagreement over what should be done in the case of a particular patient. However, it requires some effort in ethical discussion to bring such views to the surface where they can be explicitly considered—sometimes people are not even aware of these issues, let alone what their own position is.

To sum up: quality of life is most reasonably viewed as a subjective concept referring to an assessment of a person's global well-being, based on that person's own values, preferences and goals. The use of this concept in ethical reasoning raises unresolved issues about the ultimate value of life, and indisputable conclusions are not really possible. This suggests that caution needs to be exercised when making decisions about patient management on the basis of quality of life judgements.

Duty of Care

Strictly speaking, 'duty of care' is a legal term, rather than an ethical one. Nevertheless, it frequently appears in what are intended as ethical discussions, or in discussions where the ethical and legal aspects of a situation have not been clearly differentiated. In the interests of sensible ethical decision making, it is best to separate the ethical and legal facets.

As a legal term, 'duty of care' relates especially to the law of negligence. Since nursing is one of those professions where things are apt to go wrong every now and again, the risk of being sued for negligence is always present. This is why the phrase 'duty of care' is so often heard in nurses' discussions about how to manage situations. For negligence to be proved in law, the following three conditions must be met:

1. A duty of care must exist.
2. A failure in that duty must have occurred.
3. A harm must have been caused by that failure.

Having a duty of care means being in a particular type of relationship, such that one has an obligation to exercise a certain standard of care and expertise in one's dealings with the other person. Nurses are typically in this position in relation to the patients directly under their care. What counts as a failure in duty of care is determined by the standards of care and expertise accepted in the profession at the time. Importantly, the mere occurrence of some mishap or bad outcome does not mean that someone has failed in their duty of care. Instead, it very much depends on what the nurse could reasonably have been expected to do in the situation. For example, if a patient is accidentally given the wrong medication, it is fairly easy to determine what the nurse should have done. There are very specific procedures for dealing with Schedule 8 drugs, which involve checking the medication and dosage, confirming the identity of the patient, and recording the details of what has been done. A nurse who did not follow these procedures could clearly be held to have failed in her duty of care. On the other hand, imagine that a patient in a hospital ward falls out of bed during the night and breaks her arm. Has the nurse on the ward failed in her duty of care to this patient? Not necessarily. If she has taken the steps that are normally taken to prevent this happening (such as assessing the patient's physical condition and mental state), and done all that a reasonable nurse would do in that situation, then she has fulfilled her duty of care. If a reasonable nurse would not physically restrain every patient, just on the off-chance that one might fall out of bed for no foreseeable reason, then it is not part of this nurse's duty of care to do so.

In summary, then, duty of care as a legal term means a duty to take *reasonable* care, not a duty to prevent all possible accidents. Unfortunately, this is not well understood by all nurses and, as a consequence, a fear of being sued for negligence is ever-present in some nursing workplaces. As well as causing unnecessary stress, this can also result in overly defensive nursing practice, where a concern for the safety of patients or residents overshadows reasonable concern about providing a pleasant environment and allowing some freedom of choice.

The ethical ideas which lie behind the legal concept of duty of care are the principles of beneficence and non-maleficence. The law relating to negligence is in essence saying that there is a duty to safeguard the well-being of others. When duty of care is used as an ethical concept, it refers to these same principles. That is, it is used to indicate a nurse's obligations concerning the safety, welfare and best interests of patients, often implicitly in contrast to any obligations under the principle of autonomy. For example, concerns about duty of care are often expressed in a context where patients want to do things which might put them at risk. The discussion about how to deal with the situation contrasts the patient's right to make his own choices (based on the principle of autonomy) with the nurse's duty of care (to provide help and protect from harm). We have discussed in previous chapters the problem of conflicting ethical values and different ways of dealing with it, but here the problem is very readily obscured by the legal overtones of the term 'duty of care'. When this term is used (and especially when its legal application is misunderstood in the way described above), it tends to be assumed without any further thought that it is an absolute rule, or a principle which always has top priority—presumably because of the feeling that it is *the law* and so must always be obeyed. However, if the terms 'best interests', 'welfare' or 'well-being' are used (or beneficence and non-maleficence directly), this assumption is not so easily made. In this case, the autonomy side of the argument is much more easily seen, and is not so readily dismissed out of hand. It becomes a matter for open discussion as to whether the principle of autonomy or the principle of beneficence/non-maleficence should be followed here. So one pitfall associated with using 'duty of care' as an ethical term is that it tends to introduce unseen bias into ethical decision making.

A second pitfall in using 'duty of care' as an ethical term is that the distinction between law and ethics is obscured. This distinction is important in ethical decision making for at least two reasons. Firstly, there is no legal sanction against *everything* that is unethical. The law of negligence provides a good example of this. As we said above, for someone to be found negligent, a judge must be convinced that some harm has been caused as a direct result of a failure in duty of care. If a nurse fails to provide a reasonable standard of care, but by luck no patient comes to harm as a result, then no legal wrong is done under the law of negligence. However, we may very well still want to say that the nurse has done something ethically wrong if she has failed to uphold the principles of beneficence and non-maleficence. So, working out that some course of action would not attract any *legal* penalty is not enough to show that it would be *ethically* acceptable. Secondly, even if it did turn out to be the case that some course of action were legally wrong, it is still a separate question as to whether it is ethically wrong. It is possible for laws to be unethical: laws in Nazi Germany or in South Africa before the abolition of apartheid would be two fairly uncontroversial examples. A current, but more controversial, example are laws which prohibit euthanasia. Supporters of euthanasia law reform commonly argue that laws against euthanasia are wrong because they cause suffering, and surveys of both nurses[1] and doctors[2] have shown that a small but significant number have actually disobeyed the law on this matter, presumably because they believe that their ethical obligations to their patients outweigh their obligation to obey the law. So finding out that some course of action is legally wrong is not in itself enough to show that it is ethically wrong.

To sum up: 'duty of care' is a legal term, and is best reserved for use in that context. When it slides across to become a quasi-ethical term, it can lead ethical decision making astray by obscuring important issues.

Dignity

Dignity may well be the most commonly affirmed ethical value in nursing. It is, for instance, explicitly referred to in the first value statement in the Code of Ethics for Nurses in Australia. The difficulty with dignity lies not in knowing whether to endorse it as a value, but in knowing how to define it and how to respect it. 'Dignity' is not a straightforward term with a single, obvious meaning, as the controversy over 'dying with dignity' shows. It would be very difficult to find someone who was not in favour of dying with dignity, but there are quite divergent views about what is actually required for a person to die with dignity. So thinking or arguing in terms of dignity requires some caution.

As a first step, we need to try to get a clear idea of what dignity is, before we can draw any conclusions about how to respect or promote dignity. For a start, we will distinguish between 'being dignified' and 'having or being treated with dignity'. Being dignified involves presenting oneself in a particular way to others. To use some rather outmoded language, it is about being a lady or a gentleman. Dignity in this sense is a social rather than an ethical idea. Having dignity or being treated with dignity, on the other hand, is a matter of possessing a certain attribute or quality (or having it respected), and when this attribute is given ethical value, then dignity becomes an ethical concept.

But what is this attribute which has ethical value? In the past, dignity was seen as an external attribute—something bestowed on a person by virtue of their position in society, or the regard in which they were held by others. Now we tend to see it as an internal feature—a quality which people have inside themselves, by virtue of being human, regardless of their social status. But this still does not tell us what sort of feature or quality dignity is, nor how to respect it.

The attempt to tie down the meaning of dignity usually leads to a connection with autonomy or self-respect. So dignity is seen as residing in a person's quality of being autonomous (or self-governing), or in having self-respect or a sense of their own worth. For the autonomy connection, this would mean that respecting a person's dignity involves allowing them to be self-governing, and treating them accordingly. For the self-respect connection, respecting dignity would mean giving people whatever conditions they need to uphold their self-respect.

This may seem all very unproblematic so far, but there are some complications. Quite apart from the question of why we bother to speak about dignity at all if we really mean autonomy, one complication is this: concerns about respecting or preserving dignity are most often expressed in the context of patients who actually lack the ability to be self-governing. Those with dementia, or severe intellectual disability, the unconscious, even the dead—these are the ones for whom the ethical injunction to respect dignity seems most pertinent. How can we respect the dignity of these people if dignity relies on autonomy, and they are non-autonomous?

This suggests that dignity must rely on something more basic to human beings than autonomy. (The only other possibility is that many patients do not have any dignity, but this is a very unpalatable conclusion.) However, there has been very little time spent in nursing ethics working out what this basic quality might be. Rather, it has simply been assumed that everyone knows what dignity is and how to respect it. This is one of the pitfalls associated with ethical reasoning based on dignity—people may sound as if they agree with each other when really their views are quite different. To illustrate this problem, we now turn specifically to the 'dying with dignity' issue.

Some people, including some nurses, have quite concrete and specific ideas about what it means to die with dignity. These include dying without pain or fear, accepting death rather than fighting it, not being attached to any life support equipment during the dying process, being conscious and in control of what happens and so on. It is also felt that people can 'lose all dignity' in the dying process by, for example, becoming dependent on others for their physical needs (such as eating, dressing or going to the toilet), becoming incontinent, having an offensive odour, or being unable to think straight or speak clearly. There are some definite problems with having such specific views about dignity. These fall into two broad categories: some make dying with dignity a matter of luck rather than ethics, while others risk ignoring the wishes of those who are actually dying.

Firstly, if dying with dignity depends on physical matters such as not being in pain, not being incontinent, not having an offensive odour and so forth, then many terminally ill people will simply be unable to die with dignity. The nature of their illnesses will mean that, no matter what medical or nursing care is given, they will lose control of their bodily functions and become physically dependent. The unpleasant implication of this seems to be that dying with dignity is a matter of luck, which no amount of ethical deliberation or ethical action on the part of nurses can influence. However, the flaw in this line of thinking can be seen by referring to the distinction made earlier between being dignified and having dignity. Patients who are incontinent may well be undignified in the social sense, but this does not equate with having no dignity in the ethical sense. Associating dignity solely with external appearance or social acceptability in this way is one pitfall to avoid.

The second sort of problem is ethical rather than definitional, and in some ways is even more significant. The specific meanings which nurses may attach to 'dying with dignity' can be at odds with what dying patients actually want for themselves. For example, take the very common view that a dignified death is a peaceful death, where the person has come to accept rather than fight what is happening. What does this mean for those patients who have been fighters all their lives and want to fight this last battle to the very end? Would it really be dying with dignity for them to meekly sit back and accept death? Or what about patients who do not mind being physically dependent on others—do they lose dignity when they lose independence? If we accept in these cases that what counts as a dignified death depends on what the dying person wants and cares about, then this sounds a warning about developing too fixed an interpretation of dying with dignity. But it also leads us back to the connection with autonomy, which we noted earlier as quite problematic.

We cannot solve the puzzles about dignity here, but this does not mean that we regard dignity as a useless or meaningless concept. On the contrary, it does seem to be an attempt to recognise some deep and ethically important feature of human beings, which it is important for nurses (and others) to regard with respect. Our point is that this idea of dignity is still a very vague one to the vast majority of people, and so caution must be exercised in using it to draw conclusions about specific questions, such as what forms of care should be provided for individual patients.

Exercise 15.1

The following passages are adapted from newspaper articles, letters to the editor of both newspapers and nursing journals, and conversations with nurses. For each passage, answer the following questions:

a. What is the author's conclusion?
b. What interpretation of the key value term (in bold) is used to reach this conclusion?

c. Could a different conclusion be reached if a different interpretation of this term were used? Explain how.

1. That lovely old lady has lost all **dignity** now—there's tubes sticking out of every orifice, she's so doped up she doesn't know where she is. And look how thin and curled up she is—hardly looks human at all, more like a corpse. I don't know why her husband insists that the doctors keep going. They should just turn everything off now.
2. It's **duty of care** in the end. If that man has a fall, or gets hit by a bus, or God knows what else, it will be our fault. So there's no choice—we have to make sure he doesn't get out of the front door.
3. As nurses, the **well-being** of the client is our goal. Clients are guided and directed in the rehabilitation process by the expert nurse managing their case, so that optimal well-being is achieved. Thus it is inappropriate for clients to plan their own programs.
4. To the editors: In response to your correspondent in the previous issue, I have this to say. The women under our care know their own **best interests** and do not need us to tell them. If your correspondent's clients do not believe that it is in their best interests to space out future pregnancies, then that should be the end of the matter. Your correspondent has no business trying to persuade them otherwise.
5. These people may have advanced dementia, but they should still be treated with **dignity**. So I want to see all of the ladies properly dressed, with hats and gloves, and properly made up, too, before the outing.

Playing God

If you have ever heard or read an argument against euthanasia, experimenting on embryos or genetic technology, you will very probably have encountered the phrase 'playing God'. This is one of the most emotive and least informative expressions in contemporary ethical debate. Usually it is little more than a slogan which conveys intense and instinctive disapproval. However, those who use it presumably intend it to mean something, so it is worthwhile to spend a little time considering what that might be. In the process, we have two questions to ask: what sort of action counts as playing God, and why is playing God wrong?

The definition of 'playing God' seems to vary according to the context. In relation to euthanasia and resource allocation, it seems to mean any decision which results in a person's life being shorter than it might otherwise have been. For example, in resource allocation, a decision to fund coronary care rather than liver transplantation might be labelled 'playing God', because it means that those who need a liver transplant will die, but those needing coronary care will have a chance of survival. (Of course, if the funding decision went the other way, the same objection would apply, so perhaps it is really an objection to making any allocation decisions at all!) The reason why playing God (as it is used in this example) is held to be wrong is somewhat more obscure. An explanation sometimes given (even by those who do not believe in God!) is that it is God who decides when people should die: it is not up to us to make this choice. One obvious problem here (even if we accept that there is a God and this is what he does) is that the objection is never made to decisions that *prolong* life, only to those that shorten life. This seems inconsistent. We could of course just say straight out that it is wrong to shorten lives (or, put differently, that human life must always be prolonged). This would at least specify the reason for the objection, but since this really has nothing to do with God at all, it would also be better to drop the 'playing God' terminology altogether, and state the objection plainly.

In the context of reproductive technology and genetic manipulation a different definition of 'playing God' appears to be operating. Here, it seems to mean any action which creates life or significantly changes the characteristics of a living being. Again, the common explanation for the wrongness of such actions is that it is God's prerogative to do these things, and human beings should not encroach on it. And again, the objection applies inconsistently. Insofar as any human being can create life, this is what couples do whenever sexual intercourse results in conception; but this is never denounced as playing God. To get around this inconsistency, we might say that it is *unnatural* methods of creating life that are wrong, or that it is wrong to interfere with natural genetic processes when doing so might cause unexpected but enormous disasters. As before, if this is what is wrong with playing God, then it would be better to say so straightforwardly, without any reference to God, since God really appears to be irrelevant to the matter.

In summary, then, the term 'playing God' is really better avoided. At best it appears to be a metaphor for some other value-claim, and at worst it really has no meaning at all. If confronted with this term in an argument, the appropriate strategy is to ask what values lie behind the phrase 'playing God': what precisely does the author think is wrong, and why? Be alert to the possibility that the author has no reason to offer for his claim that something is wrong, and the 'playing God' terminology is simply functioning to cover this up. Alternatively, the author may have a meaning which actually has nothing to do with God or religion at all. If tempted to use the phrase yourself, remember that it is really so vague and so laden with emotive connotations that a valid conclusion cannot be drawn from it. Much better to think carefully about what you actually have an objection to, and say that instead.

Exercise 15.2

The following passages, adapted from letters to the editor in various newspapers, all contain the phrase 'playing God'. For each passage, give an explanation of what the author's argument might be (that is, what the author thinks is wrong, and why), without using this term.

1. Recent reports that scientists have found a way to detect so-called abnormalities in IVF embryos are appalling. It's time scientists stopped playing God and left baby-making to nature.

2. There is a moment for death, just as there is a moment for birth. Who knows what peace and joy may come upon a person at the moment of death. It seems to me that doctors are playing God by trying to hasten this moment. It is cheating, a denial of choice and opportunity.
3. My daughter was born eight weeks premature in a regional hospital 400 km from Adelaide. Thanks to a politician's decision that neo-natal intensive care beds are not cost-efficient outside the metropolitan area, she also died there. If politicians are going to play God, they should at least come and see the results for themselves.

Conscientious Objection

Conscientious objection is a refusal to perform or participate in a procedure for reasons of personal moral conscience. For example, a nurse who believes that abortion is wrong might well make a conscientious objection to assisting in an abortion procedure. In doing so, she would essentially be saying that her own moral standards are different from those of the other health professionals involved, or of her profession in general, or of society at large. What is generally regarded as acceptable, she regards as wrong. So conscientious objection is not in itself a specific ethical value, but rather an ethical decision not to do something.

Conscientious objection is often thought to be specifically related to religious beliefs, and it is sometimes treated as a quite mysterious phenomenon. But in fact there is nothing mysterious or particularly religious about conscience. One's conscience is simply one's set of moral values. Acting according to one's conscience is simply a matter of acting upon these values, however they have been acquired. In other words, conscientious objection is just a form of ethical disagreement, although it is often experienced in an intensely emotional way.

The term 'conscientious objection' is particularly applied to situations where ethical disagreement is accepted: where it is believed to be acceptable for a nurse (or other person) to refuse to comply with the instructions of a superior or an employer for ethical reasons, without incurring a penalty like demotion or dismissal. Traditionally this acceptance has been in the areas of abortion, contraception and sterilisation. More recently, organ transplantation and euthanasia have been added to the list. The common feature of all these areas is that they are the subject of moral disagreement within the community at large: it is known that differing views are held, and no way has yet been found to reconcile them. Of course, conscientious objection need not come in the form of a blanket moral objection to all procedures of a certain kind. A dialysis nurse might have a conscientious objection to dialysing a particular patient (perhaps because the patient has indicated that he does not want dialysis, or because the nurse believes that dialysis would actually be harmful to him). She need not believe that dialysis in general is wrong. In this example, it is easy to see that conscientious objection is nothing more than a decision that it is ethically wrong to perform a certain action, and a consequent determination not to do it.

Since the term 'conscientious objection' carries such powerful overtones of *justified* refusal to perform an action, it is vital to be able to distinguish between genuine refusals on ethical grounds, and other sorts of refusals. It is also important to have some way of dealing with the question of whether all genuine ethical refusals should be accepted in an organised working environment, or where patients' well-being is a stake. This last question is specifically addressed in the Code of Ethics for Nurses in Australia, which affirms the right of nurses to conscientious objection, but also recognises limits to this right.

Let us take the example of HIV/AIDS to illustrate the issue of ethical versus non-ethical refusals. Suppose that a nurse were to refuse to be involved in the care of a patient who is homosexual and HIV positive. Would this count as conscientious objection? This is an important question to the nurse concerned, since it means the difference between being quietly transferred to another ward, or being instructed to nurse the patient against her wishes or suffer the consequences. To know whether this refusal is a case of conscientious objection, we need to know the nurse's reasons for refusing to care for the patient. One possible reason is that she is worried about being infected with HIV herself. But this is not an ethical reason, at least as ethical reasons are normally understood. Instead (assuming that the hospital has suitable infection control procedures in place) it seems to be a case of excessive concern for oneself overriding the legitimate moral rights of a person in need. Another possible reason is that she believes that homosexuality is wrong, and so it would be contrary to her values to care for this patient. Again, this is not straightforwardly an ethical reason for refusing care. After all, no one is asking the nurse to engage in homosexual behaviour herself, or even to approve of it—simply to care for someone who happens to be homosexual. It seems more likely that the refusal is based on personal dislike rather than conscience. Finally, a third possible reason for refusing to care for this patient is that the nurse believes that, in the context of a tight health care budget, people who have knowingly engaged in lifestyles which cause ill-health should have lowest priority for health care. Hence, she believes it is wrong for this patient to be given hospital care when others who have not brought their own illness upon themselves are waiting. Now this *is* an ethical reason, rather than one based on feelings of personal dislike or desire for self-preservation. The nurse's argument is based on a particular interpretation of the ethical principle of justice, which here conflicts with the ethical principle of beneficence. So we have a case of ethical disagreement, or in other words, conscientious objection. But should conscientious objection in this form be permitted? It is important to see that this is a legitimate question, but it is not easy to see how to answer it.

The reasons for not forcing a nurse (or any other employee) to do something to which they have a conscientious objection are partly ethical and partly practical. On the ethical side, the main argument is the principle of autonomy, or the right to freedom. These values apply to everyone, not just patients. So just as it can be wrong to force patients to do something which they do not want to do, it can be wrong to force nurses to do so. In particular, it would be a severe infringement of nurses' autonomy to make them do something to which they have a strong objection, based on deeply held moral values. Moreover, if forced to act against their conscience, nurses may lose their integrity, and slide into doing other things which they really think to be wrong. However, against this, it must be remembered that there are limits on the right to freedom, and that autonomy is only one of a number of fundamental ethical principles. Nurses, in choosing to pursue a career in nursing, have already given up their right to do whatever they want, and in addition they have taken on certain special obligations to their patients, their profession and the health care system which employs them.

There are a number of practical reasons for not forcing nurses to be involved in forms of care to which they object. Nurses who are forced to perform tasks will probably not perform them well, and may develop a resentment to the rest of their work, or worse, to their patients. Being forced in this way also tends to work against the development of independent judgement. Further, it is better to have a workforce of nurses who are concerned to do the right thing—this will promote better patient care and help reduce unethical practices within the hospital. However, most of these arguments also apply to refusals for non-ethical reasons—they do not offer special support to conscientious objection. And, in response, it can be argued that the hospital cannot run efficiently and provide high quality care to all its patients if nurses are able to refuse to provide care whenever they have some objection.

The traditional response to these competing arguments is to permit conscientious objection without penalty in areas which are acknowledged to be morally controversial, and where no satisfactory resolution has been achieved. This would include procedures like abortion, organ retrieval and euthanasia, which were mentioned earlier. Conscientious objections to procedures which are in general not morally controversial would not receive the same response. For example, if a nurse had a conscientious objection to being involved in caring for any patient who had undergone surgery, on the grounds that, as a Christian Scientist, she believed surgery to be wrong, it would be unlikely that an employer would feel obliged to find other nursing duties for her. In this instance, her moral beliefs are virtually incompatible with being a nurse. In between these two types of situation lie conscientious objection to the medical management of particular patients. Here, there is really no general agreement, and nurses who speak out in these instances may well find themselves without much support, even though their objection is based on widely accepted ethical principles.

In summary, then, when the idea of conscientious objection is raised in an ethical discussion, there are two questions to ask, rather than simply accepting that if someone claims a conscientious objection, that is the end of the matter. Firstly, ask whether the objection is really based on ethical reasons, and secondly, even if it is based on genuine ethical reasons, ask whether it is really right to reorganise hospital arrangements to accommodate it, especially if this may endanger the well-being of patients.

Accountability

References to accountability are often heard in contemporary nursing circles, although the idea is by no means unique to nursing. Demands for accountability are made in all kinds of contexts—politics, business, health care, fundraising and so on. In nursing, there seems to be very wide acceptance that nurses ought to be accountable, and that accountability is good for nursing. For example, the Code of Ethics for Nurses in Australia puts great emphasis on accountability, devoting one of its six primary value statements to it. Since the requirement for accountability is clearly related in some way to how nurses ought to act, it is in some sense an ethical concept. But there is more, and less, to accountability than merely ethics.

To be accountable is to be held responsible or answerable for one's actions. It means that one can be required to give an account of what one has done, by giving reasons which explain it. It also means that one can be praised or blamed for one's actions, in whatever way is appropriate in the context.

This might make accountability sound like something to be avoided rather than sought, but it is valued in nursing because of its link to professionalism. One of the distinguishing features of professionals, as you may remember from our discussion in Chapter 1, is that they work independently, making their own decisions rather than acting on the instructions of others. It is people who are free to make their own decisions in this way who are accountable for their actions—if one's actions are totally controlled by someone else, one cannot be held accountable for them (except in the very limited sense of being at fault if one fails to obey instructions).

The ethical concept behind accountability is that of moral responsibility. Moral responsibility is not an ethical value in the sense that it gives direction about what it is right or wrong to do. Rather, it is a term which describes a specific feature of people—namely, whether or not they can be held to account for the moral quality of their actions, and thus whether they are open to praise or blame for what they have done. In general, people are held to be morally responsible for most of what they do, but there are some obvious exceptions. For example, we do not hold babies or small children responsible for what they do—it would be nonsensical to blame a baby for wetting a clean nappy! Likewise, we do not hold people responsible for what they do in their sleep, or under anaesthetic, or for things over which they have no control—it would be nonsense to say that it is the patient's own fault if his or her blood pressure drops during surgery!

One important question about moral responsibility for nurses and other health professionals is whether or not they are morally responsible for the adverse events which may happen to patients under their care. For example, suppose a person has an epileptic fit and falls over and fractures his skull, while waiting for an appointment with the Occupational Health and Safety nurse. She has been delayed on the factory floor by a discussion about finger-guards on machinery: is she morally responsible for his injury? We will give a very brief explanation of how this question would be approached in ethics, using the idea of moral responsibility, and then contrast this with accountability as it is currently used in nursing.

The question of moral responsibility is standardly discussed by considering what a person is normally morally responsible for, and then looking at special circumstances which might remove moral responsibility in some instances. So normally, people are held to be morally responsible for all their actions, and their omissions to act (but only those where a reasonable person would be expected to act), and also for the consequences of these actions and omissions (but only those which were reasonably foreseeable—not the ones that no one in their position could have foreseen). This does not apply to situations where they could not have acted differently; for example, where they were threatened or coerced, or had no physical control over what happened, or if acting differently would have required knowledge which they could not reasonably have been expected to have. In those cases they would not be morally responsible for what they did (or failed to do), or for any of the consequences. According to this account of moral responsibility, the OHS nurse is not morally responsible for failing to prevent the man's fractured skull, given that his fracturing his skull was not a reasonably foreseeable consequence of her arriving five minutes late for her appointment. The fractured skull is an accident, not a harm caused by her, and she should not feel guilty.

As you can see from this explanation of moral responsibility, the primary question is 'What am I responsible *for*?' The answer to this question tells me about my moral position. If I know I am responsible for some bad occurrence, I will know that it is appropriate for me to feel guilty, to try to rectify the situation, to make sure I do not act in the same way again and so on, depending on the situation. However, 'accountability', as it is currently used, implies a bit more than this. With accountability, there are actually three pertinent questions to ask:

1. For what am I accountable?
2. To whom am I accountable?
3. In what terms am I accountable?

Note that the last two questions do not really apply to moral responsibility because there is one obvious answer—I am accountable to myself, in moral terms. But a range of answers is possible to these questions when accountability is at issue, so it is vital to know precisely what sort of accountability is being required.

Nurses may be accountable to different people, for different things and in different terms, and these need not be ethical at all. Such a situation can lead to stress and conflict. For example, consider Marcus, a nurse working in a nursing home for the frail elderly. Marcus may be accountable to the administrators of the nursing home for all consumables used during his shift. So he would be required to explain why certain items or certain quantities were used, and to do so in largely financial terms (for example, 'We used two bibs for every resident unable to eat properly, because this is more cost effective than using extra nursing time to assist them.') Marcus may also be accountable to the Director of Nursing for how he spends his time. So he would be required to explain why, for example, he spent forty minutes feeding Mrs Ramirez, when the DON's policy is that a maximum of twenty minutes is to be spent per resident on feeding. His explanation would need to be in terms of procedures: perhaps most residents need only ten minutes' help, so that what he saves on them he can give to Mrs Ramirez without any overall loss of time. And in addition to this, Marcus may feel accountable to Mrs Ramirez' family, who are paying a lot of money for her to live in this nursing home. In this case, he might need to be able to explain why she was being helped with eating for only forty minutes, when it sometimes took her an hour to finish her meal, and in this case he would need to do so in terms of what was the best care for her, or value for money for the family. And amongst all this, Marcus may also feel accountable to himself, for his actions as a nurse: he may feel the need (and it would presumably be generally agreed that he should feel the need) to be able to explain to himself in ethical terms why he is giving Mrs Ramirez this form of care, and whether he would be responsible if her nutritional status deteriorated (or improved). Only this last sense of accountability is moral responsibility as we described it above.

It is easy to see that Marcus may get himself caught in conflicting demands for accountability, since he is accountable to different people, who have quite different standards which they require him to meet. Moreover, the first three types of accountability described above, which are not actually *ethical* accountability (although accountability to the family comes close), may conflict with his personal sense of moral responsibility (ethical accountability to himself). This causes two problems in speaking generally of accountability. Firstly, before reaching any conclusion about accountability, and especially before endorsing, requiring or accepting it in general terms, it is vital to know what sort of accountability is being proposed. Otherwise, you will not really know what you are agreeing to. Secondly, you need to be aware that non-ethical forms of accountability can run contrary to accepted notions of moral responsibility. For example, the employer of the OHS nurse may hold her accountable for the man's fractured skull, despite the fact that she is not morally responsible for it. If she accepts being accountable for all injuries in the workplace, then she is agreeing to being open to some sanction like a reprimand or demotion for events for which she is not morally responsible. Similarly, Marcus may be held accountable for the cost-effective running of his shift even though, as a nurse, he has no training in cost-management, could not reasonably be expected to know about it, and thus cannot be morally responsible for any failures in this area. This is an important caution to sound for the nursing profession, which is on the whole keen to embrace accountability: the sort of accountability which is expected may go well beyond what is required by moral responsibility.

Advocacy

Advocacy is not an ethical term in itself, but it has important connections with ethics, as we shall see. The basic meaning of advocacy is 'speaking on behalf of another'. An advocate is someone who speaks for another person, and represents their interests. Advocates belong most commonly in legal or bureaucratic settings (indeed, in some places a lawyer is actually called an advocate), where ordinary people feel that they lack the knowledge and skills to speak effectively for themselves. The connection between advocacy and nursing may seem obscure at this point but, since the 1980s, advocacy has been adopted by a large number of nursing theorists as a philosophy of nursing. The motivation for using this quasi-legal concept is that patients are seen to be in a situation similar to that of ordinary people in a court of law: because of their illness and lack of knowledge, they are not in a good position to look after their own interests and influence what happens to them, so they need someone to speak on their behalf.

There are a number of different accounts of precisely how advocacy functions as a theory of nursing, each giving its basic aims and methods. Among the most influential nursing theorists in the area of advocacy are Leah Curtin, Sally Gadow and Mary Kohnke. Here we can only give a very brief summary of the important common features of their views, in order to discuss the relationship between advocacy and ethics. But if you are interested in the idea of advocacy, it is much better to read some of their writings (see the list of suggested readings at the end of this part of the book).

In brief, the role of the nurse as advocate is to support patients in exercising their freedom and making their own choices. Among other things, this involves reassuring patients that they have the right to make their own decisions, helping them to clarify their own values (so they will know what choice they really want to make) and providing them with information. Advocacy, according to most theorists, does not mean fighting patients' battles for them, but rather enabling them to fight for themselves. The obligation of nurses to be advocates stems from their special relationship with the patient, as the ones who provide direct care to the patient and know the patient most closely.

Proponents of advocacy as a philosophy of nursing generally regard advocacy as different from, and more important than, ethics. However, as this brief account shows, advocacy is closely related to ethics. Not only is advocacy functioning as an ethical value in the sense that it gives direction as to how nurses ought to act, but more specifically, it only makes sense if certain ethical values are assumed. Advocacy is basically about giving patients a voice, but there is only a reason to do this if it is already accepted that patients have a right to autonomy and nurses have a correlative duty to respect and promote patients' autonomy.

Advocacy, then, while it is not an ethical value as such, is something like a mechanism or procedure for promoting an ethical principle, namely the principle of autonomy. Once seen in this way, it is clear that advocacy cannot be the complete answer to ethical problems in nursing, unless autonomy is taken to be the only ethical value. Regarding autonomy as the only ethical value is implausible, for a number of reasons. Firstly, it allows no room for questions about what is in patients' best interests, which, as we saw in the first part of this chapter, cannot be fully explained in terms of what patients prefer. Secondly, it glosses over the legitimate ethical limits to the exercise of autonomy: limits based on the equal rights of others to exercise their autonomy. And thirdly, it does not give any guidance for dealing with patients who are non-autonomous, a problem which we have pointed out before in relation to the autonomy-based interpretation of dignity.

Taking advocacy to be one part of a wider ethical picture is thus a more reasonable position than regarding it as taking over the whole role of ethics. However, even within the domain of advocacy there are still some questions to be asked before concluding that one should act as an advocate. Is it the case that all patients will want nurses to act as their advocates? If there is a significant difference in cultural, religious or other values between nurse and patient, the patient may not want the nurse's assistance in making his own decisions, nor may the nurse be able to give it, if she strongly objects to the patient's values. For example, if a patient wants to have her newly born son circumcised, and the nurse objects to circumcision, then the nurse may not really be able to help the patient clarify her own values and make her own decision. It is also worth asking whether the nurse ought to do this, when promoting circumcision would compromise her own moral conscience. Another question: is the nurse really best placed to act as the advocate, even for a patient who wants such advocacy? Nurses often know and relate to patients better than anyone else, but this is not always the case. Also, nurses do not always have the information which patients need to make their own decisions, and they may not know how to obtain it. So it is important for nurses to ask themselves, for any particular patient, whether they are the best person for the task of advocacy.

To sum up: advocacy functions as an ethical concept specifically linked to the principle of autonomy, even though it is not originally an ethical term at all. The major pitfall in thinking in terms of advocacy is to assume that it encompasses *all* the ethical obligations of a nurse. A second pitfall is to assume that nurses should act as advocates for *all* patients in all circumstances. Advocacy can be a helpful idea provided that it is not taken as an absolute or even a universal principle.

Caring

Caring, like advocacy, is a concept sometimes used to provide a philosophical foundation for nursing. Unlike advocacy, it is an explicitly ethical concept: indeed, proponents of the caring theory of nursing often speak of an 'ethic of care'. However, it is an ethic which does not sit comfortably with the approach to ethics described in this book, namely a process of reasoning using ethical values. Caring is not an idea that can simply be taken up and slotted into an ethical argument or decision-making process, as if it were parallel to values like autonomy or privacy. Instead, caring represents a totally different way of looking at the world of ethics.

In this section, we will give a brief account of the classic theory of caring in nursing, as put forward by a group of influential nursing theorists, in order to explain the challenges that caring poses to traditional (that is, reason-based) ethics. Then we will consider some objections to the idea of caring, and finally, we will suggest a way of integrating caring and reasoning into a unified approach to ethics.

The idea of caring as a totally different way of thinking about ethical problems began with the publication in 1982 of a book by Carol Gilligan called *In a Different Voice*. In this book, Gilligan challenged the theory of Lawrence Kohlberg[3] that moral development occurred in ranked stages, with reasoning using abstract principles of justice being the highest or 'adult' stage. Kohlberg had done empirical research using moral dilemma scenarios which in his view showed that males reach the adult stage of moral development earlier and more easily than females. Against this, Gilligan argued that the women who thought in terms of personal relationships in order to resolve the dilemmas were not actually inferior in moral development, even though this type of approach only rated at Stage 3 in Kohlberg's six stages. Rather, they were using a completely different, but equally valid, approach to ethics. This idea of a feminine ethics of caring was taken up by Nel Noddings in her highly influential book *Caring: A Feminine Approach to Ethics and Moral Education*, published in 1984. Other important authors in the field of caring are Jean Watson, Madeleine Leininger, Sara Fry and Sally Gadow. You may wish to read some of their work in order to gain a more comprehensive understanding of their theories (although you may find some of the writing rather dense and complex). Here, we will give only the briefest of overviews, sufficient just for the purpose of discussing the relationship between caring and ethical reasoning as described in this book.

Caring is essentially about personal relationships. It emphasises the feeling of connection between the person doing the caring and the person receiving the caring, and the accompanying emotions, such as sympathy and compassion. The response of the carer is not primarily thought of in terms of what the carer *does*, but rather what the carer *feels*, or more precisely, how the carer *is*. So the theorists mentioned above often talk of caring as a way or state of being. This state of being is a natural one: caring is a natural human sentiment which motivates particular caring relationships. The caring relationship is an intimate one, characterised by mutual openness and self-giving. The carer focuses on the one being cared for, and responds to the unique features of that person and that relationship. There are no abstract rules or principles to guide caring: caring is whatever happens in the caring relationship.

As can be seen from this description, caring as conceived by these theorists is not one ethical value among many, but a self-contained and quite different approach to the world of ethics. In fact, the ethic of care involves an explicit rejection of ethical reasoning and so-called 'rational principles'. Caring, according to this view, has nothing to do with critical thinking. For example, Jean Watson maintains that 'If we have to justify our caring, it hardens our compassion.'[4] In other words, the process of justification, or giving reasons to explain actions, which is central to critical thinking and ethical reasoning (and particularly to accountability), does not belong in the world of caring. Nel Noddings is even more specific: immediately following her claim that everything depends on the ideal of caring, she states 'Indeed, I shall reject ethics of principle as ambiguous and unstable.'[5] Thus the idea of caring poses a challenge to the whole idea of ethics as it is traditionally conceived, and as we have explained it in this book. Caring is not an especially tricky part of ethical reasoning, nor a concept that needs further clarification before valid conclusions can be drawn from it. Instead, it constitutes a rejection of the idea that drawing conclusions from premises containing ethical values is an appropriate method for achieving ethical practice in nursing.

In order to suggest a way of understanding the challenge of caring, we will now turn to look at some of the objections which have been made against an ethics of care as a sufficient foundation for nursing ethics. One main objection is that the concept of caring is too vague and ill-defined to be useful. Different theorists give different descriptions of what caring is, and most of them are so general and abstract that it is hard to see how they could differentiate between caring and non-caring. Leininger's account of caring is a good example of this: '[caring is] the creative, intuitive or cognitive helping process for individuals and groups based upon philosophic, phenomenologic and objective and subjective experiential feelings and acts of assisting others'.[6] However, caring theorists could rightly respond that this objection comes from a framework of ethical reasoning, where definitions are important because of their effect on what conclusions can be drawn, whereas they are quite explicitly not talking about reasoning, so precise definitions are not important. This response also points to one major pitfall in thinking in terms of caring, namely confusing the two different approaches of caring and reasoning, and so trying to slot caring into a framework of reasoned argument.

Other objections to caring are not so easily dealt with, since they relate to the actual practice of caring, and not the failure of caring to live up to the standards of reasoning. Amongst these objections is the observation that it is placing an excessive demand on nurses' emotional resources to ask them to enter into such an intimate relationship with each of their patients. Further, not all patients may want such a relationship. And even if both nurses and patients were willing and able, the brief stay in hospital of the vast majority of patients, combined with the current style of staffing arrangements, would probably prevent any significant relationship from forming. In response, the care theorists may say that all this represents a misunderstanding of what the caring relationship is; but in that case, some clarification of the idea of caring really is needed. However, even with clarification, it is hard to see how caring can guide nurses in situations where patients are literally unable to form any relationship at all, because they are in a coma, or have severe dementia, or brain damage and so on. Caring as described by the theorists seems to be reaching its limits here.

Another significant problem for caring is that it appears to be such a personal experience that it cannot be properly articulated or conveyed to others. Perhaps this would not matter if nurses worked alone in a setting where they had complete freedom to care for patients in whatever way they thought best. Unfortunately this is very far from being the case in modern health care. Nurses do need to communicate with others about the management of patients' medical and nursing care, and they do need to be involved in policy discussions in their places of employment. It is one of the real deficiencies of caring that it seems to provide no language for this communication. This is no mere theoretical problem: it can have real and extremely negative effects on patients, and for this reason is justifiably described as ethical deficiency.

A graphic illustration of this deficiency in ethics of care can be found in an article called 'Nurses' stories',[7] which was actually written to affirm the notion of caring in nursing. The author is a nurse and begins by telling the story of Mike, a patient suffering from complications of a leg amputation made necessary by severe diabetes. She was assigned to care for Mike, and one of her tasks was to change the dressing on the wound, which needed to be done frequently. Although Mike was unable to communicate verbally, his screams were enough to show that this process was extremely painful. Over a period of time, Mike's condition deteriorated, and the nurse came to believe that Mike no longer wanted to endure the dressing changes, and was ready to die. This belief arose out of the caring relationship she had established with him, even though all his communication with her was non-verbal. At this point, however, things began to go wrong because the nurse was unable to communicate her views to the medical personnel in charge of Mike's treatment. In her words, 'I tried to explain my rationale but found myself fumbling for the right words. How could I translate my own moral experience into traditional moral language?' (p. 33) As a result of her inability to convey her reasons for her view, she was unable to have done for him what she thought right. Moreover, she was not even able to maintain the caring relationship, because the nurse in charge of the ward dealt with her refusal to participate in any further dressing changes by transferring her to another ward. The end result was that Mike gave up hope, and a week later 'died in pain, frightened and alone' (p. 34).

This is surely an extremely unsatisfactory outcome in traditional ethical terms: Mike suffered harm, and was treated against his wishes (thus contravening the principles of non-maleficence and autonomy). It is also unsatisfactory in terms of ethics of caring, because the caring relationship broke down. The main message of Mike's story seems to be that the ability to engage in ethical reasoning is vital, even if ethical reasoning is not the sole basis on which to make decisions about what is right. If this nurse had been able to use ethical reasoning to persuade the doctors of what it was right to do for Mike, his story would have turned out very differently. By giving up on ethical reasoning, she gave up any chance of achieving this.

With this sort of situation in mind, we propose that there is a place for both reasoning and caring in nursing ethics: they are not mutually exclusive. Nurses do not have to choose one or the other; they can have both, and indeed by doing so their ability to make sensitive ethical decisions will be enhanced. Caring is essentially an emotional response or attitude, which is highly appropriate for nurses to have towards the vulnerable and suffering people under their care. But having such an emotional stance does not prevent anyone from thinking rationally at the same time, unless it is taken to extreme levels. In fact, when one considers all the factors that go into ethical decision making, a nurse who cares in a personal way about her patients is much more likely to be able to make ethically sensitive decisions than one who is totally detached, or committed only to following institutional procedures. The nurse who operates from a perspective of care will know more about each patient, especially about personal matters such as their response to pain, their feelings about their treatment, their hopes and goals for the future and so on. Knowledge of these sorts of things is precisely what enables general principles like autonomy and beneficence to be appropriately applied to real-life situations. Without this personal, particular knowledge, ethical reasoning is indeed in danger of being the abstract, alien, dehumanising process which proponents of caring find so objectionable. For example, without personal understanding of the patient's feelings, reactions and aspirations, a nurse will not really know what will be beneficial to the patient and what won't. Without some insight into his thinking, she will not really know whether he is exercising his autonomy or not. And without a generally positive regard for him, she may not be bothered, or even able, to think creatively about different options for dealing with a situation which raises ethical problems: but such creative thinking is a hallmark of sensitive ethical decision making.

This positive way of looking at the relationship between caring and reasoning in ethics would not satisfy the theorists whom we have discussed above. They reject attempts to fit caring into any other sort of ethical theory, or to reconcile it with the 'ethics of rational principles'. For them, caring is not caring unless it is utterly different from reasoning-based ethics. So it is important to be aware that if you accept our approach, you will not be endorsing caring in the way that its proponents intend. However, we feel that it is a reasonable position which enables nurses to take up the insights of ethics of care without giving away the vital skills of ethical reasoning.

Exercise 15.3 (Revision)

1. What is conscientious objection?
2. What is the difference between conscientious objection and other forms of refusal to carry out instructions? Why does this difference matter?

3. What is accountability?
4. How does moral responsibility differ from accountability?
5. What questions should be asked before accepting that someone is accountable?
6. What is advocacy?
7. What is the relationship between advocacy and ethics?
8. What questions would a nurse need to ask before concluding that she should act as an advocate for a particular patient?
9. Why can't the concept of caring, as used by nursing theorists, be slotted into the framework of standard ethical reasoning?
10. What problems can arise when nurses adopt caring as their only ethic, and do not use standard ethical reasoning?

NOTES

1. Kuhse, Helga & Singer, Peter, 'Euthanasia: a survey of nurses' attitudes and practices', *Australian Nurses Journal*, 12, 8, 1992, pp. 21–22.
2. Kuhse, Helga & Singer, Peter, 'Doctors' practices and attitudes regarding voluntary euthanasia', *Medical Journal of Australia*, 148, 1988, pp. 623–626.
3. Kohlberg, Lawrence, *The Philosophy of Moral Development*, San Francisco, Harper & Row, 1981.
4. Watson, Jean, 'The moral failure of the patriarchy', *Nursing Outlook*, 38, 2, 1990, p. 64.
5. Noddings, Nel, *Caring: A Feminine Approach to Ethics and Moral Education*, Berkeley, University of California Press, 1984, p. 5.
6. Leininger, Madeleine, 'Caring: a central focus of nursing and health care services', *Nursing and Health Care*, 1, 1980, p. 143.
7. Parker, Randy Spreen, 'Nurses' stories: the search for a relational ethic of care', *Advanced Nursing Science*, 13, 1, 1990, pp. 31–40.

Chapter 16
Ethical Decision Making

This chapter sets out a standard decision-making strategy, involving a series of ten steps, and explains how this can be used as a framework for ethical decision-making. Extended examples indicate the sorts of practical considerations that are involved at each step in the strategy.

Ethical decision making is an important part of nursing practice, as we illustrated at the beginning of Chapter 12. The ability to analyse and evaluate ethical argument, which we discussed at length in Chapters 13, 14 and 15, is part of the process of ethical decision making. Having this ability will enable you to understand the arguments which other people put forward—arguments perhaps seeking to persuade you to act in certain ways, or hold certain opinions. The skills of analysis and evaluation will help you to decide whether or not there is good reason to be persuaded by these arguments, and this in turn will affect the way in which you practise as a nurse. The same skills will also help you to formulate and put forward sound and reasonable arguments of your own, if you have a view about what is the right thing to do, and you want or need to persuade others to accept this view.

However, critical analysis of ethical argument is not quite the same as the process of ethical decision making. In many practical nursing situations, your problem may not be to convince others to accept your view about what ought to be done, but rather to make up your own mind and come to a view in the first place. This chapter will suggest a strategy for ethical decision making which uses the concepts of principles, rules, rights and duties, but in a less formal way than that discussed in the preceding chapters. This strategy is intended to be practical, and can be used by people with different ethical viewpoints. It is modelled on a standard strategy for decision making in all contexts, and simply involves working through a number of steps.

A General Decision-making Strategy

Decision making as a general process has been widely investigated, and various strategies for successfully completing the process have been formulated. Here is one very standard strategy for decision making or problem solving, involving a series of steps which may be familiar to you from other contexts. It offers a framework for thinking which will assist you to make a rational or reasonable choice about how to act, in contrast to making a guess or acting on 'gut feeling'. Note that although we refer to this as a strategy for problem solving as well as decision making, we do not mean to imply that you will be able to use it to solve everyone's problems. It is a strategy which guides you in making decisions in problem situations, but it will not make problems disappear.

Step 1: define the problem
Step 2: gather information
Step 3: identify constraints
Step 4: generate possible solutions/courses of action
Step 5: identify criteria for judging best solution
Step 6: evaluate possible solutions/courses of action according to criteria
Step 7: select solution which best fits criteria
Step 8: implement solution
Step 9: check progress of solution
Step 10: modify solution, if necessary

We will now make some comments about how to carry out each of these steps. When you read through them, you may find that they don't carry much meaning for you because they are very general, and do not relate to a specific problem. However, at the end of the general comments you will find an example worked through according to the steps. You may wish to look back at the general comments after reading the example.

The first step, defining the problem, is a vital one which is often neglected. One situation can be seen to involve a number of different problems, depending on the person who is looking at it, what role he or she has in it, and what aims and values he or she has in relation to it. So it is important to clarify which problem you are trying to deal with, since this will determine the sorts of solutions that are possible. Remember that different problems have different sets of possible solutions. It is also important to define the problem in an open rather than a closed way, so that the range of possible solutions is maximised. For example, if you say 'The problem is whether to do A or B', this closes off a whole range of possibilities. It is preferable to say, 'The problem is how to achieve X.'

The second step is to gather information about the situation which is relevant to whatever problem has been identified. This information will be used in the later steps of generating and evaluating possible solutions. At this early stage in the decision-making process, it is often difficult to see what you will need to know later in the process, and so the information gathering may be somewhat unfocused. This is not a great problem, provided that you remember to be ready to seek more information later on, when it becomes clearer what sort of knowledge is needed, or is lacking. A second important part of this information-gathering step is to begin to organise what you find out. Small pieces of information can be grouped into categories, which will not only make them easier to remember, but more importantly will help to build up a coherent understanding of the situation. For example, if your problem concerns the care of a patient, you might group together in one category all information relating to a patient's physical health, and in another information relating to family supports.

The third step is to identify any constraints on possible solutions. A constraint is something which limits your options—something which either forces you to act, or forces you to avoid acting in a particular way. Some constraints are external, others are self-imposed. External constraints include facts about the situation which cannot be changed, or at least cannot be changed within the time and resources available for dealing with the situation. Examples of common external constraints include lack of time, lack of money or other resources, hospital policy, administrative procedure, people's state of mental and physical health and so on. Self-imposed constraints are really decisions by the problem-solver to put limits or requirements on her own options, for her own reasons. They represent an unwillingness to do something, based on serious reasons. Examples of self-imposed constraints include unwillingness to break the law, betray a secret, allow oneself to be used or abused by others and so on.

The purpose of identifying constraints is essentially practical—when there is a real situation to be dealt with, there is no point in thinking up wonderful solutions which are impossible to put into practice. However, take care not to be too pessimistic or narrowminded when looking for constraints, because every constraint cuts off a whole range of possible courses of action.

The fourth step is to generate possible solutions. At this stage in the process, the aim is to think of as many different courses of action as possible. This requires creative thinking, and will be helped by input from other people who may be able to contribute different ideas because of their different background and experience. Virtually all possibilities should be considered at this stage, even if they do not seem very sensible: they can always be ruled out later in the process. One important possibility to keep in mind is non-action: in a practical profession like nursing it is easy to forget that non-intervention may sometimes be the best way to deal with a situation.

The fifth step is to work out how to tell which possible solution or course of action is best: what are the pros and cons? (The pros and cons are the advantages and disadvantages, or positive and negative features, of a possible course of action.) Put more formally, this means identifying the criteria which will be used to evaluate the possible solutions. The appropriate criteria will vary widely, depending on the nature of the situation at hand. It is not really possible to set out any general set of criteria. But what we can say is that the criteria chosen should be related to the goals or aims of the problem-solver. In some situations, this will be an entirely personal matter. Suppose that you are trying to decide which postgraduate nursing course to take. The criteria which you will use to judge the different courses will depend partly on your own personal tastes—whether you prefer to study on-campus or off-campus, full-time or part-time, at a large institution or a small one and so on—and partly on your ambitions—whether you want your career to advance in certain directions or whether you are seeking a promotion, for example. However, if you are trying to decide what type of dressing to put on a wound, the criteria will not depend on your tastes or hopes at all—it won't matter what brand or colour or style of dressing you prefer, because the appropriate criteria will relate to the aim of rapid healing of the wound. Once you have identified your criteria, you will need to decide whether they have any order of importance, or whether they are all equally important. For example, in choosing a course, the most important criterion for you may be how close the campus is to your home, and other criteria about the size of the institution and the range of subjects offered might come much lower in order of priority.

Sometimes this step of identifying the criteria can be a very difficult one, especially if you are not clear about what your aims are in a particular situation. Without criteria for evaluating options, it is impossible to make a decision, so the step cannot be skipped entirely. However, it may be easier to discover what your criteria are by working on concrete ideas, rather than by thinking in the abstract. So you could move on to the next step of actually evaluating possible solutions, and try out one or two in a very general way. List the pros and cons as they seem to you, and then ask yourself why these features seem like advantages or disadvantages. This process will uncover what your criteria are.

The sixth step is to evaluate the options which you generated in step 4. To complete the whole decision-making process successfully, this step needs to done thoroughly. The basic idea is to take each possible solution separately, and list its advantages and disadvantages (in relation to the criteria identified in the previous step). In order to do this, you may need to supplement the information which you gathered in step 2. Note that in order to produce a sensible result, the same set of criteria must be consistently applied to each and every possible solution. The process will produce only a jumble if you use different criteria to evaluate each different option. Two special matters to check on for each proposed solution are effectiveness and practicality: will the solution actually achieve what is wanted, and does it violate any of the constraints identified earlier?

The seventh step is really the culmination of the sixth, namely to choose the best solution from those you have thought of and evaluated. If you earlier identified an order of importance in your criteria (or if you can now see an order), this is where that order comes into effect. The best solution will be the one which best meets the most important criterion. If one or more solutions are equal with respect to the first criterion, then judge them according to the second, and so on down the line until one emerges as the 'winner'. If the criteria do not have any special order of importance, then choosing the best solution is a matter of weighing up the extent to which each solution meets all of the criteria. This is something like producing an overall 'score' of how well each solution has done, by 'adding up' its performances on each of the criteria. For example, let us imagine that you have identified three different but equally important criteria for choosing a postgraduate course (say, location, size of institution and range of subjects). Then Course A, which rates as good on two but poor on one (for example, good on location and range of subjects, but poor on size of institution), will clearly be better than Course B, which rates as good on one but poor on two (for example, good on size of institution but poor on location and range of subjects).

When trying to choose the best solution, keep in mind the possibility that two different solutions could be equally good. It is not necessarily the case that there will be one obvious winner. This is not a difficulty—on the contrary, it means that you have a choice between two equally good or sensible things to do.

Steps 8, 9 and 10 are fairly straightforward. After choosing a solution or option, you need to actually put it into action in an efficient and effective way. Once the solution has been implemented, it needs to be monitored to ensure that it is working out as expected. If it is not, then it needs to be modified. On many occasions, small modifications may be sufficient to correct whatever is going wrong. The key to successful modification is to determine what factors are preventing the chosen solution from working properly. If a large change is necessary, this may pose problems. Changing to a different option is not always easy: it is not always possible to simply go back and select another option from your list of proposed solutions. For example, if you have actually started one postgraduate course, you may not easily be able to swap to a different course whenever you feel like. So what you have now is a different, though related, problem, and you will need to work through this new situation right from the first step.

Example 16.1

Now that we have described the decision-making framework in general terms, it will be helpful to use it to work through a specific example. Imagine that Laura, a student nurse, has been asked to take the temperature of one of the patients in a general medical ward. The patient's name is Mr Brno, and he doesn't speak English.

The first step is to define the problem. Laura might actually see a number of different problems in this situation, depending on her knowledge, outlook and goals. Here are some of the possibilities:

1. The problem is how to communicate with Mr Brno.
2. The problem is how to take a patient's temperature accurately.
3. The problem is how to avoid upsetting Mr Brno.
4. The problem is where to find the thermometer.

For the sake of this example, we will select just one of these problems to work on: the problem of how to communicate with Mr Brno. In reality, Laura may have to deal with all of these problems, and she would have to solve each one separately, because they are all different.

Having identified the problem to be solved, the next step is to gather information which is relevant to the problem. Laura might want to find out all sorts of things: what language Mr Brno does speak, what his general state of mind is, whether he has any family, whether anyone has tried to communicate with him before, what methods there are for communicating with people who do not speak English and so forth. She will find this process easier to manage if she organises the information into categories, such as information about Mr Brno, and information about methods of communication. The information gathered at this stage will give her a starting point for the next steps in the strategy, but it is very unlikely that she will find out everything she needs to know. So she will probably need to seek further information later on.

The third step is to identify constraints which limit the solutions or strategies which Laura can employ. One obvious constraint is lack of time. Laura is not able to spend the whole day on this one task; in fact, she may have only a few minutes. Another is lack of knowledge. Laura does not know how to speak Lithuanian and, given the constraint of time, she cannot go away and learn it, or find someone to teach Mr Brno to speak English. A possible self-imposed constraint might be that Laura believes that it would be uncaring to take Mr Brno's temperature without him knowing what she was doing—so she rules out for herself the option of simply not communicating with him at all.

The fourth step is to generate, or think of, possible solutions. The trick for Laura at this stage is to remember to be creative and wide-ranging in her thinking, and not to worry too much if the ideas she comes up with do not seem very sensible or practical—that can be sorted out later. With this is mind, here are four suggestions, out of the wide range of possibilities:

1. Call an official interpreter.
2. Ask a family member to interpret.
3. Speak loudly and slowly in English
4. Use non-verbal communication, such as hand gestures and drawings.

Once possible solutions have been generated, the next step for Laura is to work out the criteria by which she is going to judge these solutions. This might cause Laura to hesitate—she may not be very sure what sort of features a good solution would have. At this point, she needs to think about what her aims are in this situation. A good solution is one which will achieve these aims. Perhaps Laura has as her two main aims to communicate accurately with Mr Brno, and to avoid upsetting him. Her third aim, perhaps somewhat less important, is to appear to be a good student in front of her clinical tutor. In this case, her criteria for a good solution would be the following:

1. To promote accurate communication of her message.
2. To not upset Mr Brno.
3. To win the approval of the clinical supervisor (for example, by demonstrating time-efficiency or good nursing practice)

Now that Laura has identified at least some of her criteria for a good solution, she can take the next step of evaluating each of her proposed solutions. One fairly easy way for her to do this is to try to list (in her mind) the pros and cons of each solution, and then compare them with her list of criteria for a good solution. In doing so, she may find herself lacking some of the information which she needs, so this is an appropriate point at which to gather more information, now that she has a better idea of what she needs to know. At the end of the evaluation process, Laura might come up with something like the following:

Solution 1: Call an interpreter

Pros	Cons
ensures accurate communication	takes time—delays procedure
in line with hospital policy	brings in a stranger—perhaps upsetting
can do something else while waiting (?)	too trivial for interpreter

Solution 2: A family member interprets

Pros	Cons
familiar to patient	translation not accurate?
could be quicker	perhaps demeaning
less formal—not threatening	no family member present

Solution 3: Speak loudly and slowly in English

Pros	Cons
easy and quick to do	Mr Brno won't understand
no other person involved	may cause fear, anxiety
	may make Mr Brno feel stupid

Solution 4: Use non-verbal communication

Pros	Cons
maintains privacy—no third person involved	perhaps time-consuming
recognises Mr Brno as an individual	not so accurate?
good chance of being understood—idea is simple	may cause confusion
probably not upsetting	

The next step, Step 7, is to select the solution which best fits the criteria. With all the criteria identified and each possible solution evaluated, it might seem perfectly straightforward to select the best solution. But, as you can see, this is not necessarily so. In fact, it is often the most difficult step; certainly, it is the step for which it is hardest to give simple rules. One of the problems for Laura here is that she has to make an educated guess about the effect on Mr Brno of her various plans of action—she cannot know for sure what will happen. Another problem is that each solution may partly fulfil one or more of her criteria, so she must somehow weigh up all these partial fulfilments against each other, to find the one which does best overall.

Laura's thinking at this step may be along the following lines: 'No solution seems to be obviously better than all the others—but the "speaking loudly" one does seem to be the worst, since it doesn't fit any of my criteria. So I will rule that one out. Of the remaining three, calling an interpreter is best at accurately conveying my message to Mr Brno, but it is more likely than the others to upset him, because it brings in a complete stranger. It is also quite likely not to win favour with my clinical tutor, because it would take time to organise and may not be appropriate procedure. The other two solutions are more "middle of the road". Using hand gestures scores moderately well on communicating my message accurately, and fairly high on not upsetting Mr Brno (assuming that I'm skilful at non-verbal communication). Getting a family member to interpret also scores relatively well on communicating (but it does depend on the family member, of course). It's a bit harder to tell how well it meets the criterion of not upsetting Mr Brno—it depends on his feelings towards his family. So the hand gesture solution looks a little bit better. And in addition, I think my clinical tutor would approve of the hand gesture solution more than the family member solution, because it is more sensitive and shows more initiative. So it comes down to choice between getting an interpreter, which is very good on one criterion but fairly poor on the other two, and using hand gestures, which seems moderately good on all of them. Overall, I think the hand gestures solution is best.'

As you can see, choosing the best solution is not a precise mathematical process. On the contrary, it is fairly rough and subjective. The best way to look at it is as a skill which you will be able to develop with practice.

Implementing the solution is fairly straightforward, although Laura may need some assistance or extra information here. Once her chosen solution has been implemented, she will need to monitor its progress. If, for example, she has chosen to use hand gestures to convey her meaning to Mr Brno, she will need to pay attention to whether or not this appears to be achieving the goals which it was intended to achieve. It was supposed to be effective in communicating, without upsetting Mr Brno. But if, after ten minutes of hand gesturing, Mr Brno is simply looking bewildered and agitated, Laura will have reason to believe that the solution is not working as expected. She will need to modify what she is doing, or even switch to a different plan of action. This is where so-called 'contingency plans' are useful. A contingency plan is a plan about what to do in case the chosen solution does not work. Laura's contingency plan might be to seek the assistance of a family member if she makes no progress in communicating after five minutes. She would have decided on this before implementing her chosen solution, rather than leaving it until the heat of the moment, when the first plan was failing. With practice, a contingency plan can be built into a solution, so that the step of choosing the best solution includes the process of deciding what to do if the first plan does not work.

This example should have made clearer what is actually involved in going through the steps in the decision-making framework. Before we move on to use the framework in relation to ethical problems, there are two final points to note about putting the framework into practice. The first is about the order of the steps. Although the steps are presented in numerical order, as if they should be followed from start to finish in one smooth progression, things will not always work out this way in practice. Sometimes you may want to go back and modify your thoughts on a previous step. For example, as you go through the step of evaluating the solutions, you may suddenly think of a new possibility, or you may realise that something you had previously identified as a constraint really is not a constraint at all. This is not a failure or a mistake; on the contrary, it is quite natural and can be expected to happen. Just return to the appropriate step, or incorporate the change as you go. Provided that you are aware of what you are doing, this will not cause any difficulties.

The second point concerns the settings in which this strategy for decision making is useful. The strategy can be used in a semi-formal way, where written notes are taken at each stage, or quite informally, as a series of quick internal thought processes, probably without a word being spoken. Occasions for both types of use will occur in nursing. The quick informal process is likely to be the most common, since nurses make many decisions every day about how to handle the situations that they face, and mostly they do so within seconds or minutes. The more formal written procedure is useful in dealing with an ongoing and difficult problem, where there is more time available before something must be done. It is also helpful in guiding a group discussion. For example, a team meeting about how to manage the care of a patient who is aggressive towards staff might be a suitable setting in which to use the written procedure. It will help rational reflection on the situation, and provide a means of bringing together the knowledge and ideas of all the different team members in a structured way.

Ethical Decision Making

This same decision-making strategy can be applied to ethical problems. The advantage of dealing with practical ethical problems using this sort of process is that it is broad-ranging and flexible, whereas formal ethical argument is more narrow and rigid. In particular, using a decision-making process rather than formal argument allows you to consider a range of ethical values and positions at the one time, whereas formal argument requires you to follow through one ethical position to its logical conclusion, before looking to see what other ethical positions might be relevant to the issue.

Using the decision-making process for ethical problems is very similar to using it for other sorts of problems: the content and the order of steps is the same. One starts by identifying the problem, then looking for possible solutions, having clarified what constraints there might be, and what criteria will be used to evaluate the solutions. Again, creativity and broad thinking are important in coming up with a wide range of solutions. Then one chooses the solution which best fits the criteria for a good solution, implements it, checks its progress and modifies it if necessary. The main difference is that some special considerations of an ethical nature come in at some steps, especially in identifying constraints and the criteria for a good solution.

One particular feature of ethical problem solving or decision making is that it tends to be even more complex than ordinary problem solving, and often does not produce clearcut or generally agreed outcomes. In ethical problem solving, it is important to develop a tolerance for reasonable disagreement amongst rational people. As we take a closer look at the special features of ethical problem solving, you will be able to see more clearly where and how these disagreements can arise. In order to make the following discussion clearer, we will refer on occasion to the following example.

Example 16.2

> Mr Jones is a 79-year-old man who has never married, and has no living relatives. He has multiple medical problems, including diabetes and cancer of the prostate. His life expectancy is about three months. He was admitted to a nursing home six months ago. About two months ago, he had a fall which resulted in a fractured arm. The fracture is healing poorly, partly because Mr Jones refuses to keep it in a sling. For the past two weeks he has been refusing to eat or drink, and has become aggressive or distressed when attempts are made to assist him at meal times. On several occasions he has made comments about being tired of living, and seeing no point in continuing. He is now 5 kg below an appropriate weight, and his health is deteriorating rapidly.

As with ordinary problem solving, the step of identifying the problem is a vital and often overlooked one. A common mistake is to think loosely of a problem as an ethical one, but then try to solve it as if it were a legal or bureaucratic one. For example, when Mr Jones refuses food, the nurse assigned to care for him may ask herself, 'Should I try to force or persuade this patient to eat?' This sounds like an ethical problem. But if the nurse then goes on to solve the problem by considering only what legal rules might apply, or what hospital policy requires her to do, she is actually solving a different problem, namely a legal or bureaucratic one. So it is important in ethical problem solving to formulate the problem so that it is clearly an ethical one, and then try to solve it according to ethical considerations. Matters of law or hospital policy may come into the process, but they will not be overriding. In fact, an ethical problem may well be of the form, 'Should I do X, even though it is contrary to hospital policy or the law?'

Solving a problem according to ethical considerations requires special attention to three steps in the decision-making process. The first of these is identifying constraints. For ethical problems there may be some constraints of an ethical nature, which rule out certain solutions before they are even considered, or mean that certain things must never be done, no matter what. For example, it is felt by many people that the wrongness of killing is an ethical constraint. This would mean that a solution to an ethical problem could never involve deliberately killing a human being. So if it were proposed that the best solution in the case of Mr Jones would be to give him a lethal injection to bring about the death which he obviously wants, this would be rejected without any further consideration because it violates the constraint. However, as we saw in Chapter 13, the idea of an *absolute* rule against killing is not universally accepted. So not everyone would agree that the wrongness of killing constitutes an ethical constraint. Different views about constraints are one of the sources of disagreement in ethical decision making.

The next step which calls for special attention in ethical decision making is step 4, where the criteria for a good solution must be identified. This is where the ethical nature of the problem really becomes evident. In ordinary problem solving or decision making, the criteria for evaluating the possible solutions can be largely personal and subjective. They will naturally vary from person to person, and will depend on personal goals, outlook and attitudes. However, the criteria for deciding what counts as an ethically good solution are somewhat more fixed than this. In fact, they are just the sorts of ethical rules and principles, rights and duties which we discussed in Chapters 13, 14, and 15, although they might be expressed in rather less formal ways when ethical decision making occurs in a practical context. As we saw in Chapter 12, these ethical values, however expressed, are more than simply personal taste or opinion: they can usually be measured against some sort of external standards. In terms of ethical decision making, this means that the criteria for evaluating solutions cannot be whatever the decision-maker wants them to be. If the decision is to be an ethically sensitive and reasonable one, the criteria used to produce it must represent a set of generally accepted ethical values.

What are the ethical values which form this set of criteria for ethical decision making? This is one place in which codes of ethics can offer assistance. The Code of Ethics for Nurses in Australia sets out six value statements, together with explanatory notes, which give an indication of an appropriate set of values for nurses to use in their decision making. These value statements refer to respect for individuals, regardless of their background, the right of patients to make their own choices, the obligation of nurses to provide quality nursing care and to maintain confidentiality, and the promotion of well-being. As is pointed out in the introduction to the code, these value statements may not cover every ethical consideration which nurses should take into account, but they do provide a good starting point.

The precise form of expression of particular values is not significant in terms of the whole decision-making process, because there is no single line of logical argument which must be followed. In the Code of Ethics you will find rights-claims, principles and rules expressed in a variety of ways. For the purposes of ethical decision making, this variety of value expressions could be summarised as a series of principles; for example, non-discrimination, privacy, dignity, confidentiality, informed choice, quality care and promotion of well-being. Or it could be summarised as a series of rights: the right to non-discriminatory treatment, the right to privacy and so forth. In ethical-decision making, it is the basic idea that counts, not the precise form of words.

In choosing a set of ethical criteria, there are some significant considerations to take into account. For a professional making decisions in a professional setting, conformity with the expectations and standards of the profession is important. An individual nurse has good reason to be guided by the ethical values contained in a nursing code of ethics or similar document. However, nurses must also be able to maintain their own integrity, which means making decisions on the basis of values which they truly endorse, rather than on the basis of values which they are told to adopt by someone else. Hence, the importance of conscientious objection, which was discussed in the previous chapter. Choosing and endorsing a set of values is an ongoing process, rather than a once-in-a-lifetime event, so professional nurses need to reflect on their own values and be prepared to change them in response to their own experience. However, at any one point in time, consistency is vital in ethical decision making. Each ethical problem should be dealt with according to the same set of criteria, and all the criteria relevant to the situation must be considered. One cannot pick and choose criteria to suit the situation as this would be quite arbitrary, and thus open to the charge of being unethical in itself.

This account of identifying the criteria which will be used to evaluate solutions as ethically good or poor shows up another possible source of disagreement over ethical matters. Different people may have different ethical values, and thus may identify different criteria for evaluating solutions. Inevitably, therefore, they will sometimes end up with different preferred solutions.

The next step at which there are special considerations in ethical decision making is the step of evaluating possible solutions. At this step, the very general ethical values which have been identified as criteria must be applied to a particular situation. Each possible solution to an ethical problem must be evaluated in terms of the extent to which it respects or promotes that general value. This is not always straightforward, because the precise meaning and application of a principle is not always evident. Let us take the principle of beneficence (producing benefit) as an example. It would be reasonable to identify this as one of the criteria in making an ethical decision about Mr Jones, the patient in Example 16.2, even though it is not explicitly referred to in the Code of Ethics for Nurses in Australia.

This is because beneficence is clearly one of the principles lying behind concerns for provision of quality care, and promotion of an environment conducive to well-being which the Code does name. But having identified beneficence as one of our general ethical criteria, we must apply it to the specific situation of Mr Jones. One possible course of action here is simply to go along with his refusal to eat, and allow him to die. Another possible course of action is to insert a naso-gastric tube to provide for his nutritional requirements. How do these courses of action rate in terms of beneficence? This depends on what is meant by beneficence. If we are talking about purely physical benefit, then we have to compare the amount of benefit produced by using an uncomfortable and distressing form of treatment to prolong life, with the benefit produced by allowing a slow decline and death. Even here there will be disagreement. Some, for example, will say that continued life must always count as more beneficial than death—death is a state of nothingness, and cannot be of any benefit. Others will say that death can sometimes be a benefit, when compared with the life that is being endured. Difficult though this matter is to resolve, it is only one facet of the interpretation problem. Another question is whether beneficence refers only to physical benefit, or also to other dimensions, such as psychological, emotional, social and even spiritual benefit. If these other dimensions are to be included, then we also need to ask whether a slow decline and death might be psychologically or spiritually beneficial to the patient, even if physically non-beneficial.

So, at the stage of evaluating possible solutions, there are at least two sources of uncertainty for one person or disagreement between two people, even if a set of ethical criteria has been clearly identified and agreed upon. Firstly, it can be unclear what a particular ethical value actually means (for example, what kinds of benefit are meant by the principle of beneficence?). Secondly, it can be unclear whether a particular state of affairs really promotes or exemplifies the value (for example, is death an example of a benefit or not?). These sources of uncertainty potentially exist no matter what value we are trying to apply. For instance, in Mr Jones' case there is also a problem about the principle of informed choice. Does this principle mean *any* choice based on adequate information, or must it be a choice made in a rational frame of mind? The meaning of informed choice needs to be clarified. And even if it is clarified, there is still a question as to whether Mr Jones' refusal to eat really constitutes an informed choice. Does he really have enough information on which to base a choice? Is he really making a serious choice, or is he just expressing his unhappiness in a rather forceful way? Reasonable people could well have different views on these matters.

The step of choosing the best solution also brings with it some difficulties in ethical decision making. Here, there are two main problems—do the criteria have any order of priority, and if not, how do we weigh them against each other? For example, suppose that we have evaluated the possible courses of action in the case of Mr Jones, using criteria based on the Code of Ethics for Nurses in Australia. One of these possible courses of action, namely accepting his refusal and allowing him to die, we might rate highly on the criterion of informed choice, on the grounds that it respects his wishes and his right to control his own life. But we might rate it as low on the criterion of beneficence, since it will result in an unpleasant death. Another course of action, inserting a naso-gastric tube, could be seen as high on beneficence, since it prolongs his life, but low on informed choice, since it would appear to be directly contrary to his wishes. Which course of action is the best one according to the criteria we have identified? It is not easy to say.

At this point, there are two main ways of thinking this through. One is to say that there is an order of priority in our criteria. For example, we might say that informed choice has the highest ranking, so the course of action which best promotes it is the best solution, even if other solutions do better on other values. (So allowing Mr Jones to die would be the ethically best course of action, even if it did not produce as much benefit for him as inserting a naso-gastric tube.) Of course, this is an obvious source of disagreement or uncertainty in ethical decision making, because it is by no means self-evident that autonomy really is the most important ethical value. Others might reasonably think differently, and the Code of Ethics gives no direction on this issue. For example, they might hold the view that promoting benefit is the most important value, or that there is no single value which is more important than any other.

This last view represents the alternative approach to thinking in terms of an order of priority; that is, the approach of regarding all criteria as equal and looking for the solution which provides the greatest overall fulfilment of all criteria. As we described this process earlier in the chapter, it involves something like producing an overall 'score' of how well each solution has done, by 'adding up' its performances on each of the criteria. A solution which does fairly well on four different criteria will be better than one which does very well on one criterion, and very poorly on the other three. However, as we also saw earlier, this process of producing an overall score is not precise, and is very much open to individual interpretation. How do we tell just how much benefit Mr Jones will gain from having a naso-gastric tube inserted? How do we subtract from this the amount of informed choice that he will lose, to produce the overall score? This process of producing an overall score is clearly another source of disagreement or uncertainty in ethical decision making.

This discussion may have made ethical decision making seem very complex and difficult indeed. Whilst it is important not to minimise or ignore the complexity, it is also important not to give up in despair. Professional nurses must become competent ethical decision-makers. But just like skill in ordinary decision making, or in any other area of nursing, skill in ethical decision making will increase with practise. You cannot expect to be expert right from the start. Finally, bear in mind that competence in ethical decision making does not mean always producing the one and only right answer to the problem. Rather, it means arriving at a reasonable decision which is sensitive to the relevant features of the situation: a decision which has been made thoughtfully and which you can explain to others, giving reasons for adopting this solution rather than the others which were open to you.

Exercise 16.1

Use the decision-making strategy to plan a course of action in the following scenarios. For each scenario, identify one problem only and work on that. Indicate explicitly whether the problem is ethical or not. Propose and evaluate at least three different possible solutions, and choose the best one according to the criteria which you have identified. Use steps 1 to 7 of the strategy, but note that you will not really be able to gather much further information: you will need to rely on what is given in the scenario and the general knowledge which you already have. (It may help to make some assumptions about the facts of each situation—simply state what assumptions you have made.)

1. Conrad is a student nurse on clinical placement in a nursing home. While he is walking along the corridor, he happens to look into Mrs Forster's room, because the door is open wide. Inside, he sees Mrs Forster lying on the bed, with a man lying next to her. Conrad thinks the man is Mr Faldoni, an Italian widower who has only recently moved into the nursing home. Both are fully clothed, they are not talking or making any noise, and they seem unaware that anyone can see them.
2. John has gone out to dinner with the other students in his clinical placement group to a Chinese restaurant. The other students go out together every Friday night, but John is rather shy, and this is the first time he has had the courage to go along, although they have frequently asked him to, and they seem genuinely friendly. Half way through the meal, John realises that he has left his wallet somewhere, perhaps at the hospital or in the train they caught, and he has no money with him at all.
3. Cora is a third-year nursing student on a clinical placement in a small private hospital. Over a period of about a week, she comes to know one of the patients, Mrs Vanston, quite well. Mrs Vanston is in her fifties, and has emphysema. Sometimes she has difficulty speaking, but she seems to enjoy talking to Cora. In fact, the nurses on the ward have told Cora that Mrs Vanston is always wanting to know when Cora will be on duty again, and prefers to have Cora rather than anyone else wash her and help her to the toilet. Cora is pleased and quite proud that she has managed to win the trust of a patient so firmly. One day, during one of her 'chats', Mrs Vanston reveals to Cora that she is still smoking, although she told her doctors that she gave up a year ago. She wanted to share her little secret with someone, she says, and knows that she can trust Cora not to tell anyone that she is being 'naughty'.

4. Mei Lai is a trained nurse originally from Hong Kong, who has just started a new job in the maternity ward of a large public hospital. This is the first job she has had in Australia since completing her conversion course. On her second day, she is asked to help the new mothers to bath their babies. But one of them violently refuses, snatching up her baby boy and shouting that she is not going to let any 'dirty Chink' near him.
5. Patrick is a nurse working at a rehabilitation centre where a number of the long-term patients are young people with head injuries. One of these patients is Jim, who for some reason has recently started to refuse to have a shower. Jim is in a wheelchair and not able to speak, but is quite mentally alert, and can make his meaning clear on simple matters by various forms of non-verbal communication. The nursing unit manager is getting fed up with Jim's refusals, which are time-consuming and disruptive, and one morning tells Patrick (who is tall and strong-looking) to go and get Jim in the shower, no matter what.

Chapter 17
Critical Thinking in the Working Context

This chapter outlines some of the difficulties encountered by nurses in their attempt to be critical thinkers. It suggests how to recognise the extent of these difficulties and gives possible strategies for change.

Previous chapters have described the basic methods of critical thinking as well as highlighting some of the more difficult areas associated with ethical decision making. As stated in Chapter 1, in the world of clinical practice there will be occasions when a degree of risk taking is involved in attempting to apply this knowledge, and this will be most evident when other people simply do not want to listen to your opinion or do not invite your contribution. As discussed in earlier chapters, the right attitude is pivotal to developing and accepting a reasoning process based on sound judgement and deliberation. Many situations in the professional arena militate against the use of critical thinking and may either block one's ability to think critically in the first place or impinge on desired outcomes. Some of these situations will be outlined in this chapter and possible strategies for overcoming the difficulties will be suggested towards the end.

Difficulties Encountered in the Nursing Context

The demands of shiftwork and poor rostering systems for nurses within many institutions can lead to sleep deprivation and fatigue, and these can be major factors in an inability to think clearly and deliver appropriate care. Some of you may be aware that changing your sleep-wake pattern results in conflicting environmental time cues (alteration in circadian rhythm by being awake at night and asleep during the day), and intensifies the adverse effects of sleep deficit on your performance ability and sense of well-being. Many of you will find it far more difficult to make complex drug calculations or think through the solution to a problem between 3 and 5am on your second night of night duty than to approach the same tasks during the day after a regular sleep-wake pattern. Similar although less severe fatigue-associated difficulties can also occur towards the end of a busy shift, making critical thinking more arduous.

Demands of the day-to-day workload can be excessive to the point of preventing critical thinking. Lack of time may be so pressing that you think completing the vital tasks may be your only survival strategy. Trying to equate quality care with the demands of case-mix may result in a situation which seems so overwhelming or impossible that ticking off chores and completing the necessary paper work on a busy unit is all you feel can be achieved during that shift. A small amount of stress tends to improve performance, but the perceived level of distress associated with lack of time, heavy workloads and unrealistic demands can lead to poor judgement and decisions made on less than optimal information.

Distractions can divert your thinking away from the job at hand and can easily disrupt your careful planning or time management strategies. Examples of these types of situations include intrusive demands from other health professionals, sudden requests for assistance from another colleague, an emergency situation, an unexpected admission or transfer, or a glitch in the computer system during data entry. During a busy shift, distractions may be numerous and the resulting loss of concentration, especially with complex tasks, can lead to frustration, irritability and a level of distress which interferes with your ability to reason.

Peer pressure to conform to a certain pattern of behaviour which discourages critical thinking on a ward level or within an institution can be a very difficult obstacle to overcome. You may experience this situation as an undergraduate or postgraduate student when, due to fear and ignorance, your peers view pursuit of study, privileges of study leave or upgrading of qualifications as a personal threat. This is an especially onerous problem for novice practitioners who have a strong need to feel accepted by their colleagues and, despite previous learning, discover the quickest route to this goal is to follow the leader and not upset the status quo. This socialisation process can also apply to experienced nurses who transfer to new areas where they are no longer regarded as 'the experts'. Loss of prestige can foster a strong need to regain stature within the new group. Pressure to conform can also occur when successful application to a higher position or progression is dependent on personal attributes that complement, rather than challenge, the beliefs and values of the hierarchy.

Regardless of age and stage of professional development, self-doubt (your negative attitude about yourself) will always act as a barrier to critical thinking. Self-doubt may be due to lack of experience in a particular situation or lack of suitable colleagues to use as a sounding board. On the one hand, feeling inferior to other more senior staff may prevent you from discussing a logical approach to a problem. On the other hand, if you are in charge of a shift and your team consists mainly of junior or agency staff, you may decide not to act on a reasonable solution (and thus prolong a problem) until you have shared your thoughts with other more senior colleagues. Some thoughts associated with self-doubt include an inability to believe any praise you receive; imagining all the things that can go wrong in a shift; convincing yourself that if you are not an over-achiever, you are a failure; never admitting that you do not know how to do something or not verbalising that you need help, and worrying about the performance of people to whom you have delegated tasks. The end result

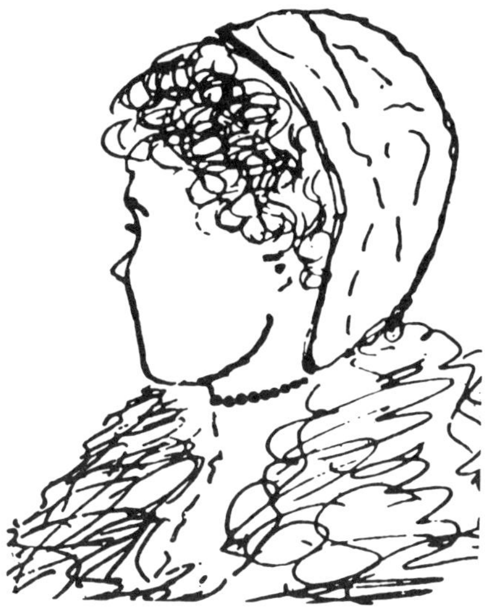

Figure 17.1

of this belief is that you generate or increase your level of distress and may show poor judgement in attempting to solve a problem.

As outlined in preceding chapters, conflict is a felt struggle between two or more individuals over perceived incompatible differences in beliefs, values and goals, or over differences in desires for control, status and affection. If conflict is viewed as a necessary evil or something to be avoided at all costs instead of a healthy approach to change, then the uncomfortable and threatening feelings associated with personal opposition can obstruct critical thinking. The potential causes of conflict within the nursing profession are numerous and are related to issues of power, influence, time, money, esteem, control, affiliation, jealousy and fear, to name a few. Lack of assertive behaviour can make handling of conflict situations extremely difficult, and responsible assertion is a skill that can only be learned over time through practice and a sound knowledge base of critical thinking skills.

Exercise 17.1

Make a list of the most difficult people, obstructions, feelings as well as clinical, educational and personal situations that you think are major barriers to critical thinking.

Exercise 17.2

In order to gain more insight into the extent of the above difficulties impinging on your ability to think critically:

a. Review reflective communication in Chapter 2.
b. Keep a reflective journal for two to three weeks and honestly describe every situation where you are aware of uncomfortable feelings or thoughts in relation to implementing the knowledge from this book.

(A second part to this exercise occurs toward the end of the chapter).

A Different View

Think about your perception of the environment in which you work, that is, how you actually *see* and interpret a clinical situation. Perceptual messages may differ significantly from one colleague to another, with the result that interventions may not always be based on sound judgement. We assume that the way we see things is the way they really are, or the way they should be, yet the brain's interpretation of what is perceived can differ significantly from person to person (think about the mechanics of vision and our dependence on the strength of a light source). The old saying 'seeing is believing' is not always true and it is extremely hard to grasp the fact that what we see is not necessarily what is so in our complex clinical world. As previously pointed out, if you are so personally involved in your own approach to a particular situation and what you think you see, then you will have difficulty considering alternatives.

Exercise 17.3

In order to successfully complete this exercise you will need a partner.

a. Firstly, *you* are to look closely at the picture in Figure 17.1 for about twenty seconds.
b. Now look at the picture in Figure 17.2 and describe in writing what you see in Figure 17.2.
c. After you have completed this task get your partner to look closely at the picture in Figure 17.3 for about twenty seconds.
d. Now your partner is to look at the picture in Figure 17.2 and describe in writing what they see in Figure 17.2.
e. Compare notes and discuss what you both saw in Figure 17.2.
f. How do you explain your interpretations of what you both saw in Figure 17.2?
g. What impact do you think this type of situation could have on judgements made in the clinical area?

Exercise 17.4

Look back at your reflective journal and identify areas where your thinking was impaired by what you thought you were seeing.

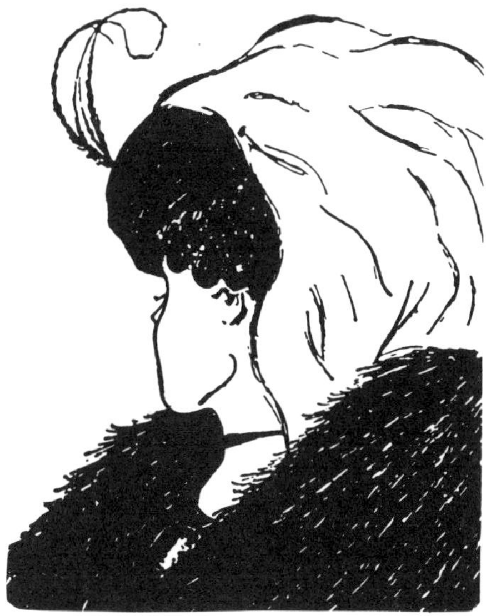

Figure 17.2

Some Strategies for Change

There are no 'quick fix' solutions or advice. Like all things worthwhile it takes time and persistence to make changes, and the first change needs to be within yourself (remember how attitude affects critical thinking). Think of the number of hours you have spent perfecting complex clinical skills or becoming computer literate. The information literate person is a lifelong learner and the basic methods described in this book are building blocks which need to be practised and revised on a day-to-day basis. Expect to make some mistakes along the way but review the situation, gather more complete and accurate information, learn from it, integrate this new information into your existing body of knowledge, then re-evaluate the situation and use your extended knowledge base for the next situation. Health professionals have been educated to identify and solve problems as quickly and cost effectively as possible. Unfortunately, some of the difficulties outlined above that impact on nurses are chronic in nature. But the more people attempt 'quick fixes' and focus only on the acute problems, the more the underlying chronic problem will grow.

Exercise 17.5

Look back at the reflective journal you wrote in Exercise 17.2 and complete the following:

a. Identify your existing knowledge and highlight your problem areas.

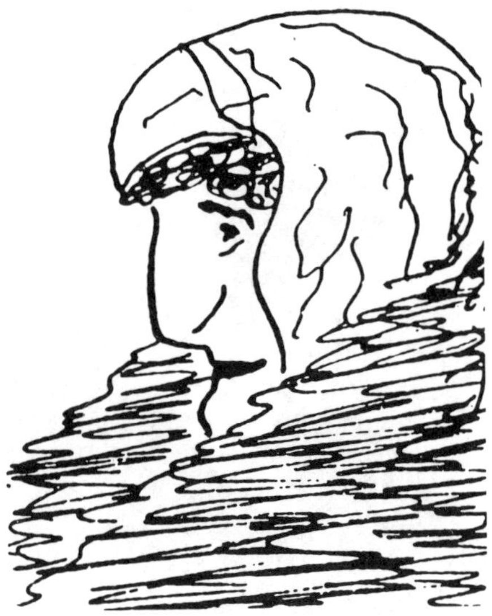

Figure 17.3

b. Are there any patterns to your behaviour that emerge over that time?
c. Prioritise your personal deficits from most to least significant.
d. How can these be overcome? What is lacking? What alternatives could you use to improve the situation?
e. Integrate your new-found knowledge with your existing knowledge and predict the likely consequences of your future actions.

As a result of the above exercise, some of you may have identified that you need to:

- pursue other skills (which are beyond the scope of this book) such as assertiveness training, stress management, conflict resolution or time management
- review certain management aspects of clinical care in more detail and develop a more conceptual understanding of illness or dedicate more practice time to perfecting complex skills
- rethink how adversely you are affected by shiftwork and make changes for yourself, or consult the extensive occupational health and safety literature on this issue in order to mount a sound argument for change for everyone in your work area
- review the organisation of work in your area and critically analyse which aspects take priority and which are just part of a traditional routine that could be improved
- stop and take the time to think before acting.

The next step is to develop and to judge your new perspective further by applying your new knowledge and skill in similar situations. Keep utilising a reflective journal approach to your day-to-day living in order to recognise strengths and weaknesses in your critical thinking and where you need to make changes.

Today's reality is that the health care industry is in a state of restructuring driven by economic constraints. With this major emphasis on cost saving, reflected by shortened lengths of time in hospital for patients and a staff mix with varying levels of skill, the challenge to provide quality care requires the ability to think critically about all aspects of nursing. One of the major reasons for writing this book is our belief that critical thinking is pivotal to the profession of nursing and that few existing texts provide basic methods and skills applicable within the nursing context. We hope students and clinicians alike will recognise that the heavy responsibility of patient care, and the quality of that care, depends on how health professionals think, and the subsequent decisions that come from that thinking.

Suggested Further Reading for Part Three

Australian Nursing Council Inc., *Code of Ethics for Nurses in Australia*, 1993.
Copies of the code, which is printed in pamphlet form, should be available from the Australian Nursing Council, GPO Box 1907, Canberra ACT 2601; or from the Royal College of Nursing or the Australian Nursing Federation.

Beauchamp, Tom L. & Childress, James F, *Principles of Biomedical Ethics* (4th edition), New York, Oxford University Press, 1994.
The standard work on the principles-based approach to bioethics. Contains detailed chapters on autonomy, beneficence, non-maleficence and justice. The introductory chapters discuss the nature of rules, principles and rights. Includes over 30 case studies.

Benjamin, Martin & Curtis, Joy, *Ethics in Nursing* (3rd edition), New York, Oxford University Press, 1992.
Includes two chapters on rights, as well as discussions of particular ethical issues in nursing.

Chadwick, Ruth & Tadd, Win, *Ethics and Nursing Practice: A Case Study Approach*, London, The Macmillan Press, 1992.
A short book which discusses the nurse's professional relationships as well as different approaches to the life cycle. The case study approach provides useful material for discussion.

Charlesworth, Max, *Life, Death, Genes and Ethics*, Sydney, ABC Books, 1989.
A very readable overview of the ethical issues involved in reproductive technologies, euthanasia and gene technology. (Australian.)

Curtin, Leah L., 'The nurse as advocate: a philosophical foundation for nursing', in Chinn, P.L. (ed.), *Ethical Issues in Nursing*, Rockville, Maryland, Aspen Systems, 1986.
An important article on advocacy in nursing.

Davis, Anne J. &Aroska, Mila A., *Ethical Dilemmas and Nursing Practice* (3rd edition), Norwalk, Connecticut, Appleton & Lange, 1991.
This book, which is fast becoming a standard, includes discussion of ethical principles, rights and obligations, as well as substantive ethical issues.

Gadow, Sally, 'Existential advocacy: philosophical foundation of nursing', in Murphy, C.P. & Hunter, H. (eds), *Ethical Problems in the Nurse-Patient Relationship*, Boston, Allyn and Bacon, 1983.
An influential early article on advocacy in nursing.

Johnstone, Megan-Jane, *Bioethics: A Nursing Perspective* (2nd edition), Sydney, Harcourt Brace Jovanovich, 1994.
The best Australian reference on ethical issues in nursing. Especially useful on rights, advocacy, caring, conscientious objection and dignity. Addresses some substantive ethical issues, including not-for-resuscitation orders, euthanasia, organ transplantation and abortion.

Kohnke, Mary F., *Advocacy: Risk and Reality*, St. Louis, C.V. Mosby, 1982.
One of the most influential early works on advocacy in nursing.

Leininger, Madeleine, *Care: The Essence of Nursing and Health*, Thorofare, New Jersey, Slack, 1981.
One of the classic works on caring as an ethical basis for nursing.

Mitchell, Kenneth R. & Lovat, Terence J., *Bioethics for Medical and Health Professionals*, Wentworth Falls, Social Science Press, 1991.
A simplified exposition of the standard ethical principles, with some introductory discussion of ethical concepts and a large number of case studies. (Australian)

Noddings, Nel, *Caring: A Feminine Approach to Ethics and Moral Education*, Berkeley, University of California Press, 1984.
One of the classic works on the ethics of caring.

Reich, W.T. (ed.), *Encyclopaedia of Bioethics*, New York, The Free Press, 1978.
A very useful starting point for further discussion of any of the concepts or issues raised in this part of the book.

Schon, D., *The Reflective Practitioner* (2nd edition), San Francisco, Jossey & Bass, 1991.
This book provides a background knowledge for reflective practice and shows how to learn about your strengths and weaknesses in clinical practice, through reflection.

Singer, Peter (ed.), *A Companion to Ethics*, Oxford, Basil Blackwell, 1991.
A collection of introductory articles on moral philosophy and ethics, written by internationally known philosophers. Relevant topics include rights, relativism, virtue ethics, Kantian ethics, duties, feminist ethics, abortion and euthanasia.

Smedes, Lewis B., *Choices: Making Right Decisions in a Complex World*, San Francisco, Harper, 1986.
Presents an interesting and personal approach to making complex ethical decisions without feelings of guilt.

Sterba, James (ed.), *Morality in Practice*, Belmont, California, Wadsworth, 1991.
An edited collection of relatively short readings on a variety of ethical issues, including abortion, euthanasia, gender equality, AIDS and privacy, gay and lesbian rights and animal liberation.

Thomas, S., Wearing, A. & Bennett, M., *Clinical Decision Making for Nurses and Health Professionals*, Sydney, Harcourt Brace Jovanovich, 1991.
Provides theories and principles for decision making as it relates to nursing, and elaborates on specific clinical problems referred to in this book.

Watson, Jean, *Nursing: Human Science and Human Care: A Theory of Nursing*, Norwalk, Connecticut, Appleton Century Crofts, 1985.
A standard work on ethics of care in nursing.

GLOSSARY OF TERMS

The following are descriptions of the way key terms are used in this book. They are not definitions of the terms which accord with general usage, nor are they descriptions of how these terms might be used in other contexts. Parentheses indicate the chapters in which the terms are defined and explained. Words in bold are terms that have their own entries in the glossary.

$\Rightarrow$ Symbol meaning 'therefore' or 'if . . . then'. (Chapter 6)

Absolute Refers to a property of a **principle** or **rule** which means that it always applies, must always be obeyed, and is never overrideable. (Chapter 13)

Accountability The state of being held answerable or responsible for what one does; of being required to given an explanation to justify one's actions. (Chapter 15)

Ad hominem arguments **Arguments** which (mostly unfairly) attack the **author**. Usually a fallacy. (Chapters 4, 5)

Advocacy In general, speaking on behalf of another, or representing their interests. Sometimes used to describe the nurse's task. (Chapter 15)

Aesthetic value Attitude or evaluation based on an appreciation of beauty. (Chapter 12)

Affirming the antecedent Valid form of the **syllogism** in which the first occurring term in an 'if . . . then' statement is said to obtain, or in which x, in the formula x $\Rightarrow$y, is said to have an instance. (Chapter 6)

Affirming the consequent Invalid form of the **syllogism** in which the second occurring term in an 'if . . . then' statement is said to obtain, or in which y, in the formula x $\Rightarrow$y, is said to have an instance. (Chapter 6)

Ambiguous terms The fallacy arising from using unclear language. (Chapter 5)

Ambiguous variables A **fallacy** in **induction** or statistical reasoning in which what is being counted or studied is not clearly defined or where items being compared are not defined in the same way. (Chapters 7, 11)

Appeal to pity The fallacy of using inappropriate **emotive** language or appealing to the sympathy or other emotions of the **audience**. (Chapter 5)

Argument Structured reasoning in which **premises** lead to a **conclusion**. (Chapter 3)

Argument by analogy An argument which appeals to a similarity between what is being talked about and something else. If the similarity is not **warranted**, then the argument is a **fallacy**. (Chapter 7)

Argument by coercion A **fallacy** in which the **author** uses threats to persuade the **audience**. (Chapter 5)

Argument from authority A **fallacy** in which the expertise or reputation of the **author** or persons associated with the author are used to persuade the **audience**. The authority is 'connected' when the expertise or reputation is relevant to the matter of the argument and 'disconnected' when it is not. (Chapter 5)

Argument from ignorance A **fallacy** in which the **conclusion** is supported only by the claim that there is no known argument or evidence against it. (Chapter 5)

Argumentum ad hominem *see* **ad hominem arguments**

Assertion Label used in a **logical outline** for an **informative premise** which is offered without adequate support or evidence. (Chapter 3)

Assumption A **premise** in an argument which is not stated. A 'hidden' premise. (Chapter 3)

Audience The person or persons to whom an **author** is addressing a **communication**. (Chapter 2)

Author The speaker or writer of a **communication**. (Chapter 2)

Autonomy The ability of a person to be self-governing, or to make their own decisions about how to run their life. As an ethical **principle**, it means respecting and promoting this ability. (Chapter 13, 16)

Average A statistic in which a snapshot is given of a group by indicating a value that applies to the whole group. A 'mean' average is calculated by adding the values that apply to each individual and dividing by the number of individuals in the group. A 'median' average is calculated by ordering the group according to the individual values and finding the value of the individual that falls in the middle of the list. (Chapter 7)

Background condition A **condition** which is **necessary** for an **effect** to occur and which is usually taken for granted. (Chapter 10)

Begging the question The fallacy of using the **point of contention** as a premise, whether explicitly, or as an **assumption**. (Chapter 5)

Beneficence As an ethical **principle**, the producing or promoting of benefit. (Chapters 13, 16)

Caring A philosophy or ethics of nursing which is based on committed and concerned interpersonal relationships. (Chapter 15)

Causal model of explanation Explaining an event by identifying what caused it. (Chapter 9)

Causality The power to produce an **effect**. Sometimes defined as a **necessary and sufficient condition**. (Chapter 10)

Chain of justification A series of increasingly general explanations or justifications of an ethical **rule** or **principle**. (Chapter 13)

Changing the question The fallacy of arguing for a **conclusion** which differs from the **point of contention**, or of distracting the audience with irrelevant points. (Chapter 5)

Classification model of explanation Explaining something by saying what kind of thing it is, or what class it belongs to. (Chapter 9)

Communication An instance of an **author** conveying information (or narratives, values, exhortations and so forth) to an **audience**. (Chapter 2)

Composition (fallacy of) The fallacy of attributing to a group or class properties which belong to an individual member of that group or class, when there is no further reason for that attribution. (Chapter 5)

Conclusion The **proposition** to which an argument leads. (Chapter 3)

Condition A state of affairs (event or entity) which may be identified as a cause (*see* **causality**). *See also* **variable**. (Chapter 10)

Confusing cause and effect The fallacy of attributing **causality** to an **effect** rather than to a **condition**. (Chapter 11)

Conscientious objection A refusal to perform or be involved in a procedure, based on a conviction that it would be ethically wrong to do so. (Chapter 15)

Constant correlation The phenomenon of finding **conditions** occurring together all or most of the time. (Chapter 10)

Constraint Something which limits one's options. (Chapter 16)

Context The background knowledge or attitudes of **author** and **audience** in a **communication**, along with the purposes and social situation of that communication. (Chapter 2)

Contingent Opposite of **necessary** and meaning 'could have been otherwise'. A property of informative propositions and of conclusions of arguments which are not proofs. (Chapter 7)

Controlled experiment A testing procedure for a causal **hypothesis** in which all relevant **variables** and **conditions** are kept constant except those mentioned in the hypothesis. (Chapter 10)

Controversial premise A **premise** with which an **audience** is apt to disagree or about which there is no social consensus. (Chapter 4)

Correlation The phenomenon of **variables** or **conditions** occurring together. It may be a 'statistical' correlation discovered by induction, constant (*see* **constant correlation**), or 'coincidental' which is when no cause can be found to explain the correlation. (Chapter 10)

Correlative duty A **duty** arising out of a **right**; the duty of others to do or give what the right requires. (Chapter 14)

Covering law model of explanation Explaining something by saying that it enjoys constant correlation with another, better understood, **condition**. (Chapter 9)

Criteria Features on which an evaluation or assessment is based during decision making. (Chapter 16)

Crucial premise A premise without which the **conclusion** would only be **warranted** weakly or not at all. (Chapter 4)

Debate A **communication** between different **authors** in which **arguments** are offered for conflicting or differing **points of contention**. The **authors** challenge the **conclusions** reached by the other authors and compromises may be sought. (Chapter 4)

Deduction A form of **argument** in which the **conclusion** spells out what is already implicit in one or more of the **premises**. (Chapter 6)

Denying the antecedent Invalid form of the **syllogism** in which the first occurring term in an 'if . . . then' statement is said not to obtain, or in which x, in the formula x ⇒y, is said not to be instantiated by the entity in question. (Chapter 6)

Denying the consequent Valid form of the **syllogism** in which the second occurring term in an 'if . . . then' statement is said not to obtain, or in which y, in the formula x ⇒y, is said not to be instantiated by the entity in question. (Chapter 6)

Division The fallacy of attributing to an individual member of a group or class properties which commonly belong to that group or class, when there is no further reason for that attribution. (Chapter 5)

Duty An ethical obligation to do something, whether one wants to or not. (Chapter 14)

Duty of care As a legal term, the obligation to exercise a reasonable standard of care and expertise in relation to others. As an ethical term, the obligation to produce benefit for others and refrain from harming them. (Chapter 15)

Effect The **condition or variable** which is said to be caused (*see* causality) by another condition or variable. (Chapter 10)

Emotive communication Communication in which rhetoric is used to move the audience emotionally. (Chapter 2)

Emotive language The fallacy of using **emotive communication** to persuade an audience, rather than **argument**. (Chapter 5)

Ethical premise Premise of an argument which contains or refers to an ethical value, labeled in a **logical outline** as a value or an exhortation. (Chapter 12)

Ethics The systematic study of morality. *See also* **moral philosophy**. (Chapter 12)

Evaluating arguments The set of activities involved when an **audience** asks whether the **premises** in an **argument** are true or reasonable and whether the reasoning is sound. May also involve the offering of alternatives. (Chapters 4, 12)

Evaluative communication **Communication** which conveys the author's attitudes and values about the matter at hand. (Chapter 2)

Exhortation Label used in a **logical outline** for **premises** which urge an audience to act in certain ways. An instance of **hortatory communication**. (Chapter 3)

Explanation A **communication** which solves a puzzle such as 'how did that happen?' or 'what is that?' and so forth. (Chapter 9)

Expressive communication A communication which articulates what the **author** is feeling. (Chapter 2)

Extrapolating beyond an appropriate range of cases The fallacy of extending **explanations** to cases to which they do not apply. (Chapter 11)

Fact Label used in a **logical outline** for an **informative premise** with which the **audience** agrees. (Chapter 3)

Fallacy An error in reasoning. Includes 'informal fallacies' such as dirty tricks and mistakes in the use of argument, 'formal fallacies' which are errors in the form of a deductive argument such as **denying the antecedent** and **affirming the consequent**, errors in attributing **causality**, and errors relating to ethical arguments. (Chapters 4, 5, 6, 11, Part Three)

False dilemma The fallacy of arguing for a **point of contention** by alleging that the only alternative would be disastrous. The alternative given is usually exaggerated or **implausible**. *See also* **straw man argument**. (Chapter 5)

Formal logic The study of the forms of **argument** (as opposed to the content of arguments). (Chapters 4, 6)

Frequencies Statistical data showing how many instances of a **variable** occur, or how often a variable occurs, in a given population, as compared to a different population. (Chapter 7)

Hasty generalisation The fallacy of drawing an inductive inference (*see* **induction**) from too small a **sample** or with inadequate evidence. (Chapter 7)

Hidden premise *see* **assumption**

Hortatory communication A **communication** which urges an audience to act in ways intended by the **author**. (Chapter 2)

Hypothesis A suggestion as to what might be causing a puzzling phenomenon. When a hypothesis survives rigorous testing or is widely accepted by the scientific community, it becomes known as a theory. (Chapter 8)

Hypothetical communication A **proposition** which says what would happen if something else happened. An 'if . . . then' statement. (Chapter 2)

Hypothetico-deductive method The most frequently occurring method in scientific research in which **hypotheses** generate **predictions** by **deduction** which are then tested, and in which numerous tests give inductive **warrant** to the **conclusion**. (Chapter 8)

Ignoring a common cause The fallacy of attributing **causality** to a **condition** because it is correlated with the condition to be explained, when in fact there is a third condition causing both. (Chapter 11)

Imperative communication A communication in which the author gives an order to do something or an instruction to an audience. *Also known as* 'directive communication'. (Chapter 2)

Implausible Unlikely to be the case; refers to a property of a **proposition** which elicits immediate disagreement on the part of the **audience**. (Chapter 7)

Implication Any **proposition** which may be deduced from another or from the meaning of a word. *See also* **inference**. (Chapter 4) Also, a **condition** which may be deduced from a **hypothesis**. (Chapter 8)

Improper analogy The fallacy of drawing a conclusion about something on the basis of its similarity with something else where the similarity is weak or inappropriate. *See also* **argument by analogy**. (Chapter 5)

Inappropriate purposive explanation The fallacy of explaining a phenomenon by saying what purpose it served or goal it pursued when the entity in question is not one which can act purposefully or entertain goals. Unjustified use of **purposive model of explanation**. (Chapter 11)

Incidental effect An effect which is not part of the causal **explanation** being sought. (Chapter 10)

Induction A form of reasoning in which a general conclusion is drawn from a number of instances or from a representative **sample**. (Chapter 7)

Inference The process of drawing a **conclusion** from **premises**. Or a way of referring to the conclusion that is drawn. (Chapter 3)

Informal logic The study of informal fallacies (*see* **fallacy**) and of ways of persuading others that do not rely on **deduction**. (Chapters 4, 5)

Informative communication Descriptions of states of affairs in the world or features of people, places and things which may or may not be true. The truth of informative communications is established by observations, evidence or testimony. (Chapter 2)

Interpretation model of explanation Explaining something by saying what it means. (Chapter 9)

Interrogative communication Asking questions. (Chapter 2)

Invalid Opposite of **valid**. Negative appraisal of an **argument** (as opposed to **conclusion**) on the grounds that the form of the argument is wrong (for example, **denying the antecedent**), or that key words in it have been wrongly understood, or that methodological rules (for example those relating to **samples** in the rules for **induction**) have been flouted. (Chapter 6)

Issue *see* **point of contention**

Jargon The fallacy of using technical terms in a way that causes confusion or in order to impress others. (Chapter 5)

Joint method A method for finding causes which combines the **method of** agreement and the **method of difference** so as to identify **necessary and sufficient conditions**. (Chapter 10)

Justice As an ethical **principle**, this means fairness. It is usually meant in the distributive sense, referring to a fair or just distribution of resources. (Chapter 13)

Logic The study of reasoning.

Logical outline A description in point form of a **text** which identifies the **point of contention** and demonstrates the form of the **arguments** in it. (Chapter 3)

Major premise The general **proposition** in a **syllogism** of which the **minor premise** is an application and from which the **conclusion** is drawn. (Chapter 6)

Metaphor A means of describing or emphasising the properties of something by calling it something else to which it is similar. Use of metaphors is a fallacy when the similarity is not appropriate or when the metaphor is used to distract scrutiny away from the matter at hand. *See also* **improper analogy**. (Chapters 5, 15)

Method of agreement A method for finding causes which looks for a **condition** which a range of cases has in common. Used to identify **sufficient conditions** for the **effect** to occur. (Chapter 10)

Method of concomitant variation A method for finding causes when variables cannot be completely isolated. Changes in **conditions** and **effects** which correlate with each other are noted. Used to identify **necessary and sufficient conditions**. (Chapter 10)

Method of difference A method for finding causes which looks for a condition without which the **effect** would not occur. Used to identify **necessary conditions**. (Chapter 10)

Method of remainders A form of deduction in which alternatives are eliminated leaving only the conclusion. *See also* **straw man argument**. (Chapter 6)

Method of residues A method for finding causes when the effect is out of proportion to the known causes. It involves looking for a missing **condition**. (Chapter 10)

Middle term The feature by virtue of which two things are similar in an **argument by analogy** or in the use of a **metaphor**. (Chapter 7)

Minor premise The particular **proposition** in a **syllogism** which applies the **major premise** to the particular case about which the **conclusion** is drawn. (Chapter 6)

Misuse of language The class of fallacies that involves unclear words, misleading terms and other rhetorical tricks and incompetencies. (Chapter 5)

Moral philosophy The branch of philosophy which involves the study of morality, including the meaning of moral terms, the foundations of moral values and rights, the reasonableness of principles and rules and so on. It is often referred to as **ethics**. (Chapter 12)

Moral responsibility Being held responsible for what happens, and so open to praise for doing or bringing about something morally good, or blame for something morally bad. (Chapter 15)

Narrative communication A description of a series of events in temporal sequence together with the links between those events. The telling of a story. In the context of art, can be linked to poetic communication. (Chapter 2)

Necessary Refers to the property of a relationship between **premises** and **conclusions** such that one cannot disagree with the conclusion if one agrees with the premises. A feature of **proofs**. (Chapter 6)

Necessary and sufficient condition A **condition** without which the **effect** would not occur, and with which it always does. (Chapter 10)

Necessary condition A **condition** without which the **effect** would not occur. (Chapter 10)

Negative right A **right** to be free from interference or hindrance, to be left alone to do what one wants. It imposes a negative **correlative duty** on others to refrain from doing anything which would interfere. (Chapter 14)

Nested conclusion A label used in a **logical outline** to identify a **conclusion** which then becomes a **premise** from which a further **conclusion** is drawn. (Chapter 3)

Non-maleficence As an ethical **principle**, this means not causing harm or protecting from harm. (Chapter 13)

Objection A proposition which opposes the **point of contention**. (Chapter 4)

Objective Based on standards which are independent of the desires, attitudes, or opinions of individuals. Opposite of **subjective**. (Chapter 12)

Overlooking complexity The fallacy of attributing **causality** to a **condition** which itself is an **effect** of more significant causal conditions. (Chapter 11)

Patients' rights Specific **rights** which patients have, based on general human rights. (Chapter 15)

Performative communication A statement which produces an effect by virtue of the saying of the words. (Chapter 2)

Persuasive communication A set of statements intended to change the attitude, knowledge, plans or point of view of the **audience**. (Chapter 2)

Plausible Refers to a property of a **proposition** which elicits immediate agreement on the part of the **audience**. (Chapter 7)

POC *see* **point of contention**

Point of contention (POC) The proposition that an author wants to persuade the audience of. The issue or question that is being discussed or debated. Identifying the point of contention is the first step in writing **a logical outline**. (Chapter 3)

Positive right A **right** to have or be provided with something. It imposes a positive **correlative duty** on others to do or provide something specific. (Chapter 14)

Post hoc fallacy The fallacy of attributing **causality** to a **condition** on the grounds that the **effect** (regularly) occurs after it. *See also* **hasty generalisation**. (Chapter 11)

Postulating an undiscoverable cause The fallacy of attributing **causality** to a **condition** which cannot be identified apart from the **effect**. (Chapter 11)

Practical syllogism An argument in the form of a **syllogism** in which the **conclusion** or **point of contention** concerns what should be done or some other practical matter. (Chapter 6)

Prediction A proposition which states what will happen in the future on the basis of drawing an **implication** from a **hypothesis**, a theory or an item of general knowledge. (Chapter 8)

Premise A **proposition** that leads to a **conclusion**. (Chapter 3)

Prima facie Refers to a property of a **principle** or **rule** which means that it applies, all other things being equal. A prima facie rule or principle can be overridden if there is a compelling reason. It is not **absolute**. (Chapter 13)

Principle (moral) A fundamental ethical value. (Chapter 13)

Principle of falsifiability A methodological rule in science which states that all hypotheses should be able to be tested. Researchers must be able to say what test result or observation would show the hypothesis to be false. A hypothesis that would survive *any* contrary evidence (or where contrary evidence could be explained away), would be a case of pseudo-science. (Chapter 11)

Proof An argument in which the **conclusion** cannot rationally be disagreed with if the premises are agreed with. *See also* **necessary**. (Chapter 6)

Proposition A statement with content that can be supported with reasons of any kind. Includes **facts**, **assertions**, **exhortations**, **value claims, ethical statements** and so on. (Chapter 3)

Proximate cause A **condition** to which **causality** is attributed and which occurs immediately before the **effect**. (Chapter 11)

Prudential value Attitude or evaluation based on what is sensible or in one's own best interests. (Chapter 12)

Purposive model of explanation Explaining a phenomenon by saying what purpose it served or goal it pursued when the entity in question is one which can act purposefully or entertain goals. *Also known as* 'teleological model of explanation'. (Chapter 9)

Quarrel A series of statements in which opposing **propositions** are put forward without reasoned **argument**. (Chapter 3)

Ratios A way of reporting statistical proportions which indicates the number of one class of objects as compared to another. Expressed as a fraction. (Chapter 7)

Reductio ad absurdum A form of argument against a **proposition** in which the implications of that proposition are shown to be unwelcome or absurd, or implausible. *See also* **straw man argument**. (Chapters 4, 5)

Reflective communication A communication in which **authors** articulate their own knowledge, points of view and attitudes, primarily with themselves in mind as the intended **audience**. (Chapter 2)

Relative Refers to a property of a **principle** or **rule** which means that it is relevant only in certain circumstances, such as particular historical periods, societies or cultures; it is not **universal**. (Chapter 13)

Remote cause A **condition** to which **causality** is attributed and which has effects which are themselves causes of the **effect** which is under investigation. (Chapter 11)

Representative sample A **sample** which contains individuals with the same type and mix of features which are present in the whole population being studied. (Chapter 7)

Right An ethical entitlement to do or have something if one wants to. (Chapter 14)

Rule (ethical) A way of expressing a fundamental ethical value. The terms **rule** and **principle** are often used interchangeably. (Chapter 13)

Sample A number of individuals in a population being studied, from which an inductive inference can be drawn about the whole population. (Chapter 7)

Side comment A label used in a **logical outline** to identify propositions which are not relevant to the **conclusion**. (Chapter 3)

Signposts Indicator words which show the nature and status (including logical status) of propositions within **texts** and **arguments**. (Chapter 2)

Slogans Pithy propositions, frequently **hortatory** in nature, with which most people are inclined to agree, but which are vague in meaning. They can be fallaciously used in argument to persuade. *See also* **misuse of language**. (Chapter 5)

Social identification The fallacy of seeking to persuade others by appealing to their wish to be seen as not different from others or as having socially desirable qualities. (Chapter 5)

Statement *see* **proposition**

Statistical model of explanation Explaining something by saying that it has a statistical **correlation** with another **condition**. It is usually expressed as a probability. (Chapter 9)

Statistics A means of presenting, classifying and interpreting information and data, using numbers and mathematical formulae. (Chapter 7)

Straw man argument A version of **false dilemma** using **reductio ad absurdum**, in which a proposition is argued for by positing and then attacking an **implausible** alternative. (Chapter 5)

Subjective Based on an individual's own particular perspective, attitude, or opinion. Opposite of **objective**. (Chapter 12)

Sufficient condition A **condition** which is always followed by a given **effect**. A condition which is sufficient to make the effect occur. (Chapter 10)

Syllogism An argument form in which there is a **major premise**, a **minor premise**, and a **conclusion** drawn by **deduction**. (Chapter 6)

Teleological model of explanation *see* **purposive model of explanation**

Text Any **proposition**, or set of propositions, written or spoken by an author for an **audience**. (Chapter 2)

Topical outline A description in point form of a **text** which summarises the content of the **propositions** in it. (Chapter 3)

Totals Statistical data showing the number of members of a group or class. (Chapter 7)

Trend Statistical data showing changes in totals or other statistical data over time. (Chapter 7)

Universal Refers to a property of a **principle** or **rule** which means that it is relevant in all circumstances, regardless of historical time or place. (Chapter 13)

Unwarranted Opposite of **warranted**. *see* **warrant**. (Chapters 7, 8, 12)

Using an inappropriate explanatory model The error of offering an explanation using a model that does not fit the phenomenon in question. (Chapter 11)

Vague terms Fallacy arising from use of unclear language. *See also* **ambiguous terms** and **misuse of language**. (Chapter 5)

Valid Refers to the property of an **argument** (as opposed to a **conclusion**) when it is correct by virtue of its form, its methodological rules or the meanings of its key terms. An argument is either valid or not (*compare with* **warrant**). *See* **invalid**. (Chapter 6)

Value A proposition expressing an attitude or evaluation on the part of the **author**. (Chapter 3)

Variable A **condition** which, when it varies, will produce corresponding variations in the **effect**. (Chapters 7, 10)

Veracity The ethical **principle** of truthfulness. (Chapter 13)

Warrant A property of a **conclusion** (as opposed to an **argument**) when the argument for it is **valid** and the evidence for it is strong. In an induction the sample needs to be large and representative. In an ethical argument the terms have to be correctly used and their implications correctly drawn. Conclusions can be strongly or weakly warranted. *Also called* 'warranted assertability'. (Chapters 7, 8, 12)

INDEX

G

H

I

J

K

L

M

N

O

P

Q

R